Atlas of INFECTIOUS DISEASES

FUNGAL INFECTIONS

Atlas of INFECTIOUS DISEASES

FUNGAL INFECTIONS

Editor-in-Chief

Gerald L. Mandell, MD

Chief, Division of Infectious Diseases
University of Virginia Health Sciences Center
Charlottesville, Virginia

Editor

Richard D. Diamond, MD

Department of Infectious Diseases
Boston Medical Center
Boston, Massachusetts

With 26 contributors

DEVELOPED BY CURRENT MEDICINE, INC.
PHILADELPHIA

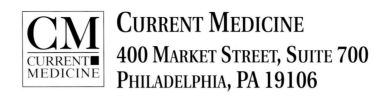
Current Medicine
400 Market Street, Suite 700
Philadelphia, PA 19106

© Copyright 2000 by Current Medicine, Inc. All rights reserved. No part of this publication may be reproduced, stored in a retrieval system, or transmitted in any form by any means electronic, mechanical, photocopying, recording, or otherwise, without prior consent of the publisher.

Library of Congress Cataloging-in-Publication Data

Atlas of fungal infections / Richard D. Diamond, editor.
    p. ; cm.
    Includes bibliographical references and index.
    ISBN 1-57340-136-6 (alk. paper)
    1. Mycoses--Altases. I. Title: Fungal infections. II. Diamond, Richard D., 1942-
    [DNLM: 1. Mycoses--Atlases. WC 17 A8805 2000]
  RC117 .A86 2000
  616.9'69--dc21
                                                                                                          99-056628

For more information please call 1-800-427-1796 or email us at inquiry@phl.cursci.com
www.current-science-group.com

Development Editor:	Marian A. Bellus
Editorial Assistant:	Annmarie D'Ortona
Design and Layout:	Christine Keller-Quirk
Illustration Director:	Ann Saydlowski
Illustrators:	Marie Dean, Andra Ross, Ann Saydlowski, Larry Ward
Managing Editor:	Charles Field
Books Supervisor:	Fran Klass
Commissioning Supervisor/Books and Journals:	Nicole Garron
Production Director:	Lori Holland
Assistant Production Manager:	Simon Dickey
Indexer:	Alexandra Nickerson

Although every effort has been made to ensure that drug doses and other information are presented accurately in this publication, the ultimate responsibility rests with the prescribing physician. Neither the publishers nor the author can be held responsible for errors or for any consequences arising from the use of the information contained therein. Any product mentioned in this publication should be used in accordance with the prescribing information prepared by the manufacturers. No claims or endorsements are made for any drug or compound at present under clinical investigation.

Printed in Hong Kong by Paramount Printing Group Limited
10 9 8 7 6 5 4 3 2 1

PREFACE

The diagnosis and management of patients with infectious diseases are based in large part on visual clues. Skin and mucous membrane lesions, eye findings, imaging studies, Gram stains, culture plates, insect vectors, preparations of blood, urine, pus cerebrospinal fluid, and biopsy specimens are studied to establish the proper diagnosis and to choose the most effective therapy. The *Atlas of Infectious Diseases* will be a modern, complete collection of these images. Current Medicine, with its capability of superb color reproduction and its state-of-the-art computer imaging facilities, is the ideal publisher for the Atlas. Infectious diseases physicians, scientists, microbiologists, and pathologists frequently teach other healthcare professionals, and this comprehensive atlas is an effective teaching tool.

Dr. Richard Diamond is an internationally recognized expert in laboratory and clinical aspects of fungal diseases. He has assembled a roster of expert authors who have prepared superbly informative chapters. The coverage is comprehensive and the illustrations are very useful as aids for clinical diagnosis and therapy. This *Fungal Infections* volume will be a valuable resource for clinicians caring for patients and teachers in fields related to clinical mycology. Specialists in infectious diseases HIV/AIDS, pulmonary medicine, dermatology, oncology, clinical pathology, and neurology will find this volume of special interest.

Gerald L. Mandell, MD

Contributors

Neil M. Ampel, MD
Professor
Department of Medicine
University of Arizona;
Staff Physician
Southern Arizona Veterans Affairs Health Care System
Tucson, Arizona

Arnaldo Lopes Colombo, MD, PhD
Associate Professor
Department of Medicine
Escola Paulista Medicina-UNIFESP
Sao Paulo, Brazil

Laurie Anne Chu, MD
Fellow, Infectious Diseases
Department of Medicine
Harbor-UCLA Medical Center
Torrance, California

Hans E. Einstein, MD
Professor Emeritus
Department of Medicine
University of Southern California
Los Angeles, California;
Attending Physician
Kern Medical Center
Bakersfield, California

Scott G. Filler, MD
Associate Professor
Department of Medicine
UCLA School of Medicine
Los Angeles, California;
Physician Specialist, Infectious Disease
Harbor-UCLA Medical Center
Torrance, California

John N. Galgiani, MD
Director
Valley Fever Center for Excellence;
Professor of Medicine
University of Arizona;
Program Director for Infectious Diseases
Southern Arizona Veterans Affairs Health Care System
Tucson, Arizona

John R. Graybill, MD
Professor
Department of Medicine/Infectious Diseases
University of Texas Health Science Center of San Antonio
San Antonio, Texas

Andreas H. Groll, MD
Senior Clinical Fellow
Immunocompromised Host Section
Pediatric Oncology Branch
National Cancer Institute
Bethesda, Maryland

Roderick J. Hay, DM, FRCP, FRCPath
Mary Dunhill Professor of Cutaneous Medicine
St. John's Institute of Dermatology
London, England

Carol A. Kauffman, MD
Professor
Department of Internal Medicine
University of Michigan;
Chief, Infectious Diseases
Ann Arbor Veterans Affairs Healthcare System
Ann Arbor, Michigan

El Sheikh Mahgoub, MD, PhD, FRCPath
Professor
Department of Pathology
Faculty of Medicine
Jordan University of Sciences and Technology
Irbid, Jordan

Patricia P.C. Pacheco, MD
Fellow in Infectious Diseases
Infectious Diseases Service
Department of Medicine
Santa Maria Hospital
Lisbon, Portugal

Demosthenes Pappagianis, MD, PhD
Professor
Department of Medical Microbiology and Immunology
University of California, Davis, School of Medicine
Davis, California

Peter G. Pappas, MD
Associate Professor
Department of Medicine/ Infectious Diseases
University of Alabama, Birmingham
Birmingham, Alabama

John R. Perfect, MD
Professor
Department of Medicine
Duke University School of Medicine
Durham, North Carolina

Flavio Queiroz Telles, MD, PhD
Associate Professor
Department of Infectious Diseases
Federal University of Parana
Curitiba, PR, Brazil

Michael G. Rinaldi, PhD
Professor of Pathology, Medicine, Microbiology, and Clinical Laboratory Sciences
Fungal Testing Laboratory
Department of Pathology
University of Texas Health Sciences Center at San Antonio
San Antonio, Texas

Thira Sirisanthana, MD
Professor
Department of Medicine
Chiang Mai University
Chiang Mai, Thailand

Jack D. Sobel, MD
Professor
Department of Internal Medicine
Wayne State University;
Chief, Division of Infectious Diseases
Detroit Medical Center
Detroit, Michigan

Alan M. Sugar, MD
Professor
Department of Medicine
Boston University School of Medicine
Boston, Massachusetts;
Director, HIV/AIDS Program
Cape Cod Hospital
Hyannis, Massachusetts

Khuanchai Supparatpinyo, MD
Associate Professor
Department of Medicine
Chiang Mai University
Chiang Mai, Thailand

Deanna A. Sutton, MS, MT, SM (ASCP), RM, SM (NRM)
Assistant Professor
Department of Pathology
University of Texas Health Sciences Center
San Antonio, Texas

Peter D. Walzer, MD
Professor
Department of Medicine
University of Cincinnati;
Associate Chief of Staff for Research
Veterans Affairs Medical Center
Cincinnati, Ohio

Thomas J. Walsh, MD
Senior Investigator and Chief
Immunocompromised Host Section
Pediatric Oncology Branch
National Cancer Institute
Bethesda, Maryland

Joseph Wheat, MD
Professor of Medicine
Department of Medicine
Indiana University
Indianapolis, Indiana

Marion A. Wieden, PhD
Adjunct Professor (Retired)
Department of Medical Technology
University of Arizona;
Consultant
Valley Fever Center for Excellence
Tucson, Arizona

Contents

Chapter 1
Histoplasmosis
Joseph Wheat

EPIDEMIOLOGY AND PATHOGENESIS	2
CLINICAL MANIFESTATIONS	5
LABORATORY EVALUATION FOR DIAGNOSIS	16
INDICATIONS FOR TREATMENT	19

Chapter 2
Coccidioidomycosis
Neil M. Ampel, Hans E. Einstein, John N. Galgiani, Demosthenes Pappagianis, and Marion A. Wieden

EPIDEMIOLOGY	24
DISEASE MANIFESTATIONS	27
Pulmonary Manifestations	28
Cutaneous Manifestations	29
Extrathoracic Coccidioidomycosis Due to Dissemination	30
DIAGNOSIS	33
TREATMENT	36

Chapter 3
Blastomycosis
Peter G. Pappas

PULMONARY BLASTOMYCOSIS	42
CUTANEOUS BLASTOMYCOSIS	44
OSTEOARTICULAR BLASTOMYCOSIS	47
OTHER FORMS OF BLASTOMYCOSIS	48

Chapter 4
Paracoccidioidomycosis
Arnaldo Lopes Colombo, Flavio Queiroz-Telles, and John R. Graybill

GEOGRAPHIC DISTRIBUTION	54
LIFE CYCLE AND ECOEPIDEMIOLOGY	55
PATHOPHYSIOLOGY	56
CLINICAL MANIFESTATIONS	56
LABORATORY DIAGNOSIS	62

Chapter 5
Sporotrichosis
Carol A. Kauffman

CAUSATIVE ORGANISM AND EPIDEMIOLOGY	66
MANIFESTATIONS	68
LYMPHOCUTANEOUS SPOROTRICHOSIS	68
PULMONARY SPOROTRICHOSIS	72
OSTEOARTICULAR SPOROTRICHOSIS	73
SPOROTRICHOSIS IN HIV INFECTION	74
DIAGNOSIS	76
TREATMENT	76

Chapter 6
Cryptococcosis
John R. Perfect

LIFE CYCLE AND DISTRIBUTION	81
YEAST CHARACTERISTICS	82
CLINICAL EPIDEMIOLOGY	83
INITIATION AND DISSEMINATION	84
TREATMENT	85
CULTURE AND HISTOPATHOLOGY	87
CLINICAL MANIFESTATIONS	90

Chapter 7
Systemic Candidiasis
Laurie Anne Chu and Scott G. Filler

EPIDEMIOLOGY	97
MICROBIOLOGY	98
PATHOLOGY	100
HEPATOSPLENIC CANDIDIASIS	101
HEMATOGENOUS *CANDIDA* ENDOPHTHALMITIS	102
CUTANEOUS LESIONS	105
CANDIDA ENDOCARDITIS	106
CANDIDA MYOCARDITIS	107
GENITOURINARY CANDIDIASIS	108
CENTRAL NERVOUS SYSTEM CANDIDIASIS	110
CANDIDA OSTEOMYELITIS	111
CANDIDA PNEUMONIA	113
MANAGEMENT	114

Chapter 8
Mucocutaneous Candidiasis
Jack D. Sobel

VULVOVAGINAL CANDIDIASIS	118
Epidemiology	119
Etiology	120
Pathogenesis	120
Clinical Manifestations	122
Differential Diagnosis	123
Diagnostic Procedures	123
Treatment	125
OROPHARYNGEAL CANDIDIASIS	126
ESOPHAGEAL CANDIDIASIS	128
Differential Diagnosis	129
Treatment	129
CUTANEOUS CANDIDIASIS	130
CANDIDA ONYCHOMYCOSIS	131
HEMATOGENOUS CANDIDIASIS	132
DRUG-RESISTANT CANDIDIASIS	132

Chapter 9
Aspergillosis
Andreas H. Groll and Thomas J. Walsh

DESCRIPTION OF THE ORGANISM AND SPECTRUM OF DISEASES	137
NONINVASIVE DISEASE MANIFESTATIONS OF ASPERGILLOSIS	140
INVASIVE ASPERGILLOSIS	142
Classification and Epidemiology	142
Experimental Pathogenesis and Clinical Risk Factors	143
Invasive Pulmonary Aspergillosis	147
Extrapulmonary Manifestations of Invasive Aspergillosis	153
Treatment	156

Chapter 10
Mucormycosis and Entomophthoromycosis
Alan M. Sugar

RHINOCEREBRAL MUCORMYCOSIS	165
PULMONARY MUCORMYCOSIS	166
INVOLVEMENT OF THE STOMACH IN DISSEMINATED MUCORMYCOSIS	167
TREATMENT OF MUCORMYCOSIS	167
CUTANEOUS MUCORMYCOSIS	168
CONIDIOBOLUS INFECTION	169

Chapter 11
Penicillium marneffei Infections
Khuanchai Supparatpinyo and Thira Sirisanthana

INCIDENCE AND DISTRIBUTION	172
CLINICAL APPEARANCE	173
MICROSCOPIC APPEARANCE	175
CULTURE	177
ROUTE OF INFECTION	179
TREATMENT	180

Chapter 12
Mycetoma
El Sheikh Mahgoub

DEFINITION AND CLINICAL APPEARANCE	183
RADIOGRAPHIC APPEARANCE	186
BIOPSY SPECIMEN	187
HISTOPATHOLOGY	188
DIAGNOSTIC TESTS AND TREATMENT	189

Chapter 13
Dermatophytoses and Other Superficial Mycoses
Roderick J. Hay

DERMATOPHYTE INFECTIONS	193
SCYTALIDIUM INFECTIONS	200
MALASSEZIA YEAST INFECTIONS	202
RARER SUPERFICIAL INFECTIONS	202

Chapter 14
Pneumocystis carinii Infection
Peter D. Walzer

APPEARANCE AND LIFE CYCLE	206
CLINICAL PRESENTATION	210
DIAGNOSIS	212
TREATMENT AND PREVENTION	215

Chapter 15
Phaeohyphomycosis and Hyalohyphomycosis
Patricia P.C. Pacheco, Deanna A. Sutton, and Michael G. Rinaldi

GENERAL CHARACTERISTICS	219
MAJOR RISK FACTORS	219
CLINICAL MANIFESTATIONS	220
DIAGNOSTIC PROCEDURES	221
SPECIES	228

Index   231

Chapter 1

Histoplasmosis

Joseph Wheat

Histoplasmosis is worldwide in distribution but is more prevalent in certain parts of North and Latin America. *Histoplasma capsulatum* var. *capsulatum* grows best in soil contaminated with bat or bird droppings. Patients often report exposure to microfoci-contaminated materials. Spores or mycelial fragments are inhaled and cause localized or patchy pneumonitis. Hematogenous dissemination to other tissues commonly follows during the first 2 weeks of infection before specific immunity has developed.

Fewer than 5% of exposed individuals develop symptomatic disease after low-level exposure to *H. capsulatum*, whereas most become ill following heavy exposure. Flulike pulmonary illnesses, pericarditis, and arthritis or arthralgia with erythema nodosum are the most common manifestations in the normal host, and those with underlying lung disease develop chronic pulmonary infection. Progressive disseminated infection is common in patients with immune deficiencies. An acute, rapidly fatal course with diffuse reticuloendothelial involvement characterizes the infection in infants and others who are severely immunosuppressed, whereas a chronic course with more focal organ distribution is more typical in nonimmunocompromised children and adults. Cultures, fungal stains, antigen detection, and serologic tests for antibodies are useful diagnosic tools for histoplasmosis. All are reasonably specific and can serve as the basis for diagnosis in patients with compatible clinical findings. Each test has certain limitations that must be recognized if they are to be used correctly. The most sensitive approach to diagnosis uses a combination of these tests.

Antifungal therapy is unnecessary in most patients with acute pulmonary histoplasmosis or rheumatologic syndromes or pericarditis. Some patients, however, may remain symptomatic longer, particularly following more extensive exposure, and they may benefit from treatment. Treatment is indicated in all patients with chronic pulmonary histoplasmosis to prevent progression. The mortality in patients with disseminated histoplasmosis without treatment is 80% but can be reduced to less than 25% with antifungal therapy. Although treatment induces a remission of illness in patients with AIDS, relapse follows if treatment is stopped, thus supporting the need for chronic maintenance therapy.

EPIDEMIOLOGY AND PATHOGENESIS

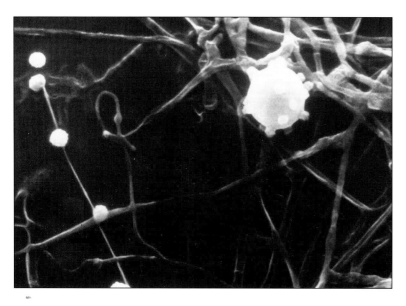

FIGURE 1-1 Scanning electron microgram of the mold phase of *Histoplasma capsulatum*. *H. capsulatum* var. *capsulatum* grows as a mold in the soil and is found primarily in microfoci containing large amounts of bat or bird guano. The mold is characterized by tuberculate macroconidia measuring 8 to 14 µm in diameter. Macroconidia are too large to reach terminal airways and are not involved in the pathogenesis of the disease. Smaller microconidia measuring 2 to 5 µm are the infectious form of the organism.

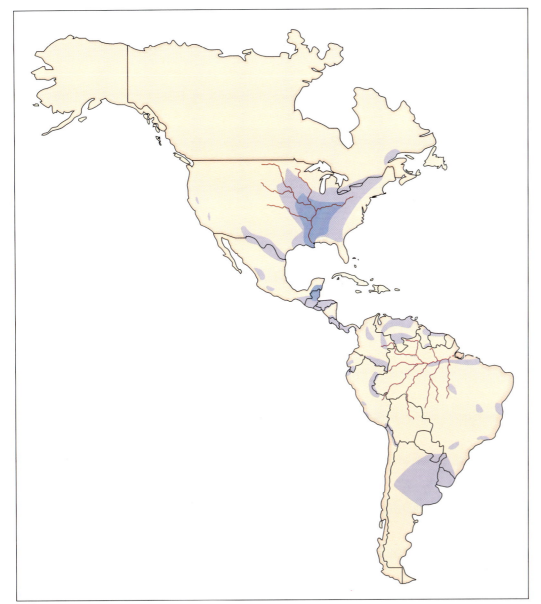

FIGURE 1-2 Endemic distribution of histoplasmosis in the Americas. Histoplasmosis is endemic in the Americas, occurring in regions noted for high humidity and moderate temperatures. In the United States, most cases have been identified within the Ohio and Mississippi valleys. Histoplasmosis also is endemic in parts of Central and South America. (*Adapted from* Rippon [1].)

Sources for Exposure to *Histoplama capsulatum*

Microfocus	Activities
Caves	Spelunking
Chicken coops	Cleaning, demolition, use of bird droppings in garden
Bird roosts	Excavation, camping
Bamboo canebreaks	Cutting cane, recreation
School yards	Cleaning
Prison grounds	Routine activities
Decayed wood piles	Transporting or burning wood
Dead trees	Recreation, cutting wood
Contaminated chimneys	Cleaning, demolition
Old buildings	Demolition, remodeling, cleaning
Laboratories	Research projects

FIGURE 1-3 Sources of exposure to *Histoplasma capsulatum*. Patients with histoplasmosis may recall exposure to environmental sites contaminated by bat or bird droppings or may have been involved in activities known to place them at risk for exposure to *H. capsulatum*.

Fungal Infections

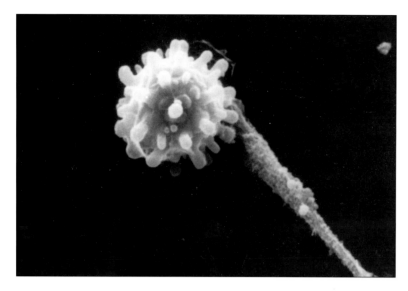

Figure 1-4 Scanning electron microgram of phagocytosis of *Histoplasma capsulatum* yeast. Inhaled microconidia rapidly convert to the yeast phase of the organism within the airways and alveoli. They initially induce a neutrophilic inflammatory response, followed promptly by influx of lymphocytes and macrophages. Pseudopods extend from macrophages to phagocytose the organism. Organisms proliferate within the macrophage during the first few weeks of infection, prior to the development of a specific cell-mediated immune response. With development of specific immunity in the normal host, organisms are cleared from the tissues during the first 2 months of infection. In the immunosuppressed host, however, *H. capsulatum* continues to proliferate in the tissues, causing a progressive and often fatal illness.

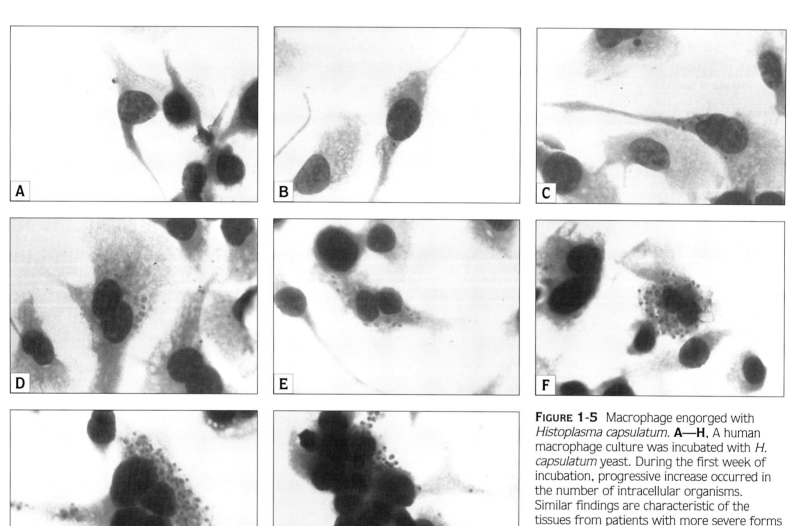

Figure 1-5 Macrophage engorged with *Histoplasma capsulatum*. **A—H,** A human macrophage culture was incubated with *H. capsulatum* yeast. During the first week of incubation, progressive increase occurred in the number of intracellular organisms. Similar findings are characteristic of the tissues from patients with more severe forms of progressive disseminated histoplasmosis.

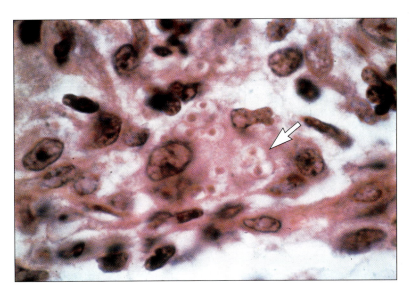

FIGURE 1-6 Hematoxylin-eosin stain of liver biopsy specimen from a patient with progressive disseminated histoplasmosis. The stain shows heavy parasitization with the yeast phase of the organism. The organisms demonstrate an eosinophilic staining central nucleus surrounded by a clear halo (*arrow*), which represents cytoplasmic shrinkage rather than a capsule.

CLINICAL MANIFESTATIONS

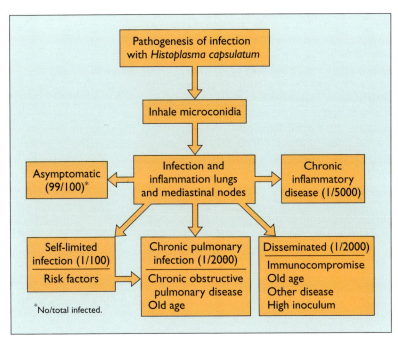

FIGURE 1-7 Course of infection after exposure to *Histoplasma capsulatum*. Inhalation of microconidia causes localized or diffuse pulmonary infection, depending on the magnitude of the inoculum, which is followed by spread to the mediastinal lymph nodes. With low-level exposure in immunocompetent individuals, the infection is asymptomatic in 99% of patients [2]. With heavy exposure, however, most individuals will experience illnesses caused by histoplasmosis. Of symptomatic patients, most manifest self-limited forms of the infection (acute pulmonary and rheumatologic syndromes, pericarditis), whereas those with underlying illnesses may experience chronic manifestations of the disease. Patients with underlying chronic obstructive pulmonary disease often develop chronic pulmonary histoplasmosis characterized by progressive lung damage. Those patients who have underlying conditions with compromised immunity may develop progressive disseminated infection. Some may develop chronic inflammatory manifestations, including granulomatous mediastinitis, fibrosing mediastinitis, and possibly a sarcoidosis-like illness.

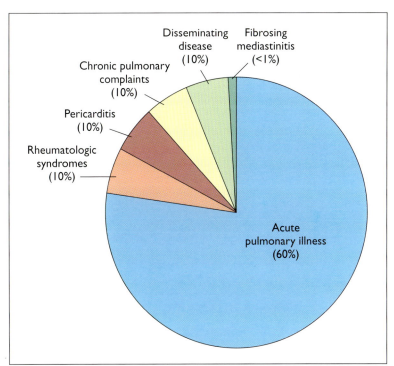

FIGURE 1-8 Clinical manifestations of acute histoplasmosis. Of symptomatic patients with acute histoplasmosis, self-limited illnesses occur in 80% of patients [2]. Most of these individuals exhibit acute pulmonary illnesses characterized by flulike symptoms associated with pulmonary complaints. Less commonly, patients (5% to 10%) may experience rheumatologic syndromes with arthritis or arthralgia associated with erythema nodosum or erythema multiforme or acute pericarditis. Asymptomatic infections usually are identified because of chest radiograph abnormalities found during evaluation of other conditions.

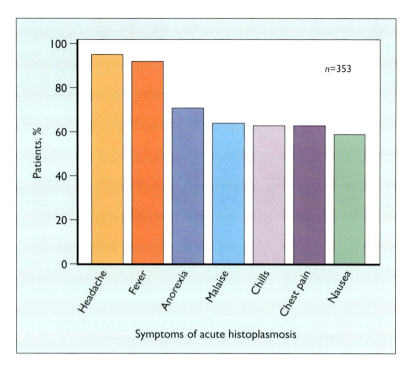

Figure 1-9 Symptoms of acute histoplasmosis. Acute symptomatic histoplasmosis presents as a respiratory disease in the majority of patients. These patients exhibit flulike symptoms highlighted by fever and headache [3]. Pulmonary complaints include chest pain and cough. With heavy exposure causing diffuse infiltrates, patients also may experience dyspnea. The absence of symptoms of upper respiratory infection, including sore throat and coryza, is noteworthy. (*Adapted from* Brodsky *et al.* [3].)

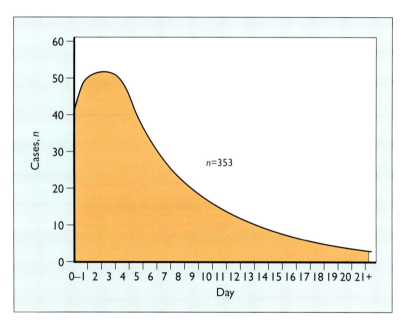

Figure 1-10 Course of resolution of acute symptomatic histoplasmosis. The illness is self-limited in healthy individuals following low-level exposure. In a large point-source outbreak of histoplasmosis in 1970 in Delaware, Ohio, involving 353 individuals who were exposed during clean-up activities celebrating Earth Day, illnesses resolved within 3 weeks in nearly all patients [3]. Symptoms may be more protracted in individuals who have experienced a more significant exposure. These patients may remain symptomatic for months. (*Adapted from* Brodsky *et al.* [3].)

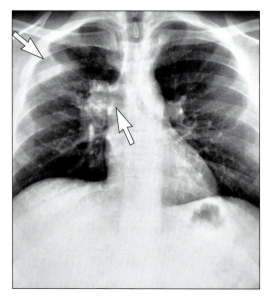

Figure 1-11 Chest radiograph of low-intensity acute pulmonary histoplasmosis. Radiographic findings in acute pulmonary histoplasmosis include mediastinal lymphadenopathy and patchy pulmonary infiltrates. This radiograph shows enlargement of the right hilar lymph nodes (*bottom arrow*) associated with a faint right upper lobe infiltrate (*top arrow*). The patient complained of substernal chest pain and cough. He recovered over a few weeks without treatment.

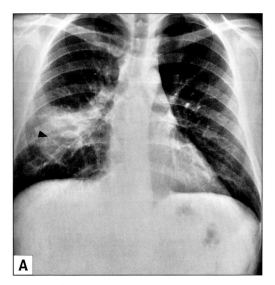
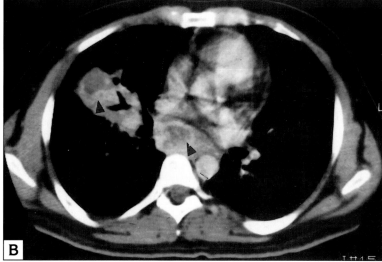

Figure 1-12 **A**, Chest radiograph of acute pulmonary histoplasmosis in a patient who required treatment because of persistent symptoms. This patient complained of pleuritic chest pain, night sweats, productive cough, and a 25-lb weight loss over a 5-month period, during which he received repeated courses of antibiotics for suspected pneumonia. The radiograph shows right hilar lymphadenopathy with a right midlung infiltrate (*arrowhead*). The patient underwent bronchoscopy, which was nondiagnostic on two occasions except for caseating granulomas. Special stains for fungus and mycobacteria were negative, as were cultures. Serologic testing for histoplasmosis was negative initially but positive on follow-up, showing H and M bands by immunodiffusion and complement fixation titers of 1:64 to the yeast and 1:8 to the mycelia antigen. Itraconazole 200 mg twice daily for 6 months led to resolution of the clinical symptoms and improvement in the chest radiograph. **B**, Chest CT scan shows a subcarinal lymph node and right midlung infiltrate with central lucency (*arrowheads*). The central lucency is believed to represent caseous necrosis, although a biopsy was not performed. Prolonged illnesses related to persistent mediastinal adenitis occur in a small percentage of patients with acute histoplasmosis (less than 10%).

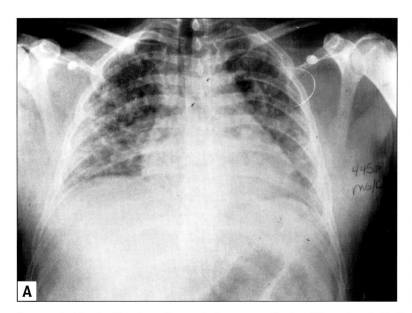
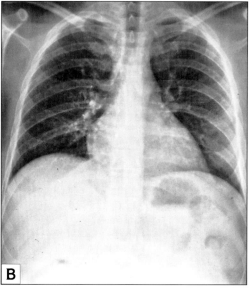

Figure 1-13 **A**, Chest radiograph from a patient with diffuse pulmonary histoplasmosis following heavy exposure to pigeon guano. The patient worked for several hours removing pigeon guano from a bell tower. He presented 5 days later with high fever and dyspnea. The chest radiograph shows diffuse reticulonodular infiltrates. The patient was hypoxic with a pO_2 of 58 torr. Histoplasmosis was suspected based on the clinical history. A bronchial alveolar lavage showed no pathogens. The lavage fluid, serum, and urine were positive for *Histoplasma* antigen, prompting initiation of treatment with amphotericin B and prednisone. He showed marked improvement over the next 4 days. Amphotericin B was stopped, and itraconazole was administered for another 3 months. Serologic tests initially were negative but subsequently were positive showing an M band by immunodiffusion and complement fixation titers of 1:32 to the yeast but nonreactive to the mycelial antigen 4 weeks later. **B**, Follow-up chest radiograph 3 weeks later showed considerable clearing of the pulmonary infiltrates.

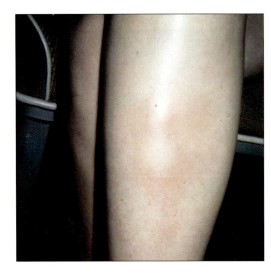

FIGURE 1-14 Erythema nodosum in a patient with rheumatologic manifestations of histoplasmosis. The patient presented with pain in the knees and hips associated with mild swelling of the right knee. Although the patient denied pulmonary symptoms, her chest radiograph showed right paratracheal lymphadenopathy. Examination also showed erythema nodosum. A synovial fluid analysis was unremarkable. Although initially believed to have sarcoidosis, a diagnosis of histoplasmosis was considered because she presented during an outbreak, and serologic tests were positive for histoplasmosis with an M band by immunodiffusion and a complement fixation titer of 1:16 to the yeast and 1:8 to the mycelial antigen. Synovial fluid cultures were negative for fungus. She received 6 months of anti-inflammatory therapy with complete resolution of the arthritis and erythema nodosum. This manifestation of histoplasmosis represents a systemic immunologic reaction to acute pulmonary infection and not dissemination to the joints or skin [4–6]. Rarely, patients have exhibited bone or joint lesions as a manifestation of disseminated histoplasmosis.

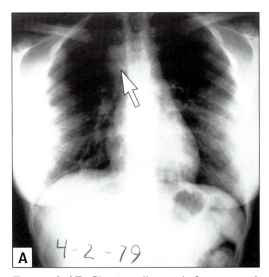
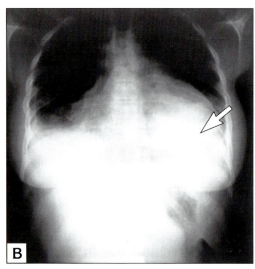

FIGURE 1-15 Chest radiograph from a patient with pericarditis caused by histoplasmosis. The patient presented with cough and substernal chest pain. **A,** The initial chest radiograph showed right paratracheal lymphadenopathy (*arrow*). **B,** Two weeks later the patient complained of shortness of breath, and the chest radiograph now showed marked enlargement of the cardiac silhouette (*arrow*). Pulsus paradoxes was present, as was a pericardial friction rub. The patient underwent placement of a pericardial window. Histopathologic findings showed acute and chronic inflammatory changes but no granulomas, and organisms were not identified by fungal stain or culture. This manifestation represents an inflammatory reaction to histoplasmosis in the adjacent mediastinal lymph nodes rather than dissemination involving the pericardial tissue or fluid [7]. The patient responded to anti-inflammatory therapy with nonsteroidal anti-inflammatory agents and occasionally short courses of corticosteroids. Constrictive pericarditis rarely may be caused by histoplasmosis [7].

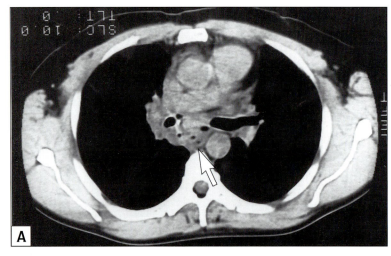
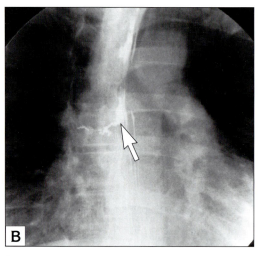

FIGURE 1-16 A, Chest CT scan from a patient with granulomatous mediastinitis showing air bubbles in the subcarinal lymph node. The patient complained of hemoptysis, dysphagia, and pleuritic chest pain. Chest radiograph showed enlargement of the right hilar, and CT showed a subcarinal mass containing air collections (*arrow*). Esophagoscopy demonstrated an extrinsic mass indenting the subcarinal portion of the esophagus with erosion of the esophageal mucosa. A CT-guided needle biopsy of the subcarinal mass showed granulomatous inflammatory changes. Gomori methenamine silver stain revealed organisms consistent with *Histoplasma capsulatum*, and the complement fixation titer was 1:64 to the yeast and 1:128 to the mycelial antigen. The patient received a 35-mg/kg course of amphotericin B, which reduced the size of the mediastinal lymph nodes and decreased the extrinsic compression of the esophagus as determined by esophagraphy. (*continued*)

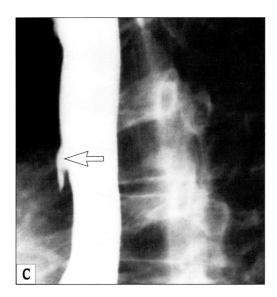

FIGURE 1-16 (*continued*) **B,** Esophagram demonstrated a fistula track between the subcarinal lymph node and the esophagus (*arrow*), explaining the presence of air bubbles in the subcarinal lymph node. Esophagoscopy demonstrated a fistula opening at about 28 cm. Yellow-green material was draining through the opening. Fungal cultures were negative. **C,** Esophagram 4 months after completion of amphotericin B treatment shows a traction diverticulum (*arrow*), confirming the role of mediastinal histoplasmosis in formation of traction diverticuli [8].

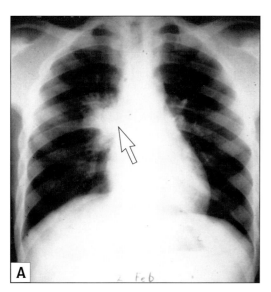
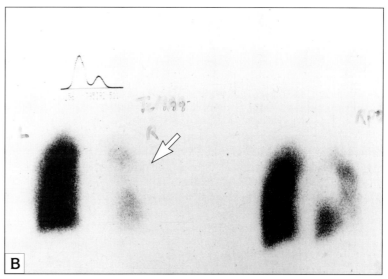

FIGURE 1-17 **A,** Chest radiograph showing right hilar lymphadenopathy in a patient with granulomatous mediastinitis causing pulmonary artery obstruction. The patient presented with complaints of pleurisy. Chest radiograph revealed enlargement of the right hilar lymph nodes (*arrow*), and serologic tests were positive for histoplasmosis. **B,** A lung scan performed to evaluate complaints of pleurisy showed reduced perfusion to the right lung with normal ventilation consistent with pulmonary artery obstruction caused by the hilar lymph node. The clinical course of granulomatous mediastinitis has not been fully characterized. Patients experience moderate morbidity and may benefit from antifungal therapy, perhaps combined with a brief course (2 weeks) of corticosteroids.

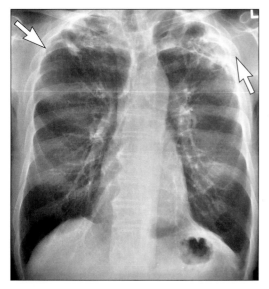

FIGURE 1-18 Chest radiograph from a patient with bilateral apical pulmonary infiltrates (*arrows*) caused by chronic pulmonary histoplasmosis. The patient presented with 20-lb weight loss, night sweats, and cough productive of green to yellow sputum. Work-up included negative tuberculin skin test and negative cultures for mycobacteria. This chest radiograph shows bilateral fibrotic upper lobe infiltrates without mediastinal lymphadenopathy. Work-up included serologic tests for histoplasmosis, which were positive, revealing an M band by immunodiffusion and complement fixation titers of 1:32 to the yeast and 1:128 to the mycelial antigen. Sputum cultures grew *Histoplasma capsulatum*. The patient was treated with amphotericin B administered over a 3-month period. He noted improvement in his cough and resolution of the fevers and night sweats. Chest radiograph showed improvement in the infiltrates but persistent stranding in the upper lobes. Chronic pulmonary histoplasmosis primarily occurs in individuals with underlying chronic obstructive pulmonary disease [9]. Although patients with acute pulmonary histoplasmosis usually recover within a few weeks, those with underlying chronic obstructive pulmonary disease often exhibit chronic progressive pulmonary infection. The clinical syndrome resembles reactivation tuberculosis.

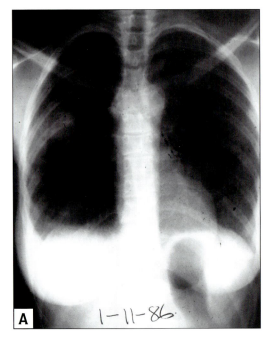 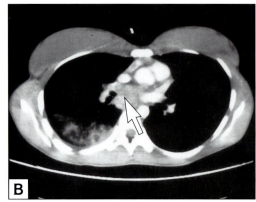 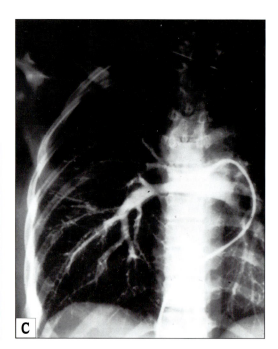

FIGURE 1-19 **A,** Chest radiograph from a patient with fibrosing mediastinitis. The patient complained of shortness of breath and chest pain. Chest radiograph showed a right lower lobe infiltrate and mediastinal widening in the area of the azygos vein. Histoplasmosis was diagnosed serologically, with a complement fixation titer of 1:64 to the yeast and less than 1:8 to the mycelial antigen. **B,** Chest CT scan shows enlarged azygos lymph node with calcification and obstruction of the pulmonary artery (*arrow*). **C,** Pulmonary arteriogram shows absent blood flow to the right upper lung field. The patient was hospitalized 10 years later and continued to have problems with chest pain. Work-up showed continued obstruction of the right pulmonary artery associated with 70% occlusion of the right main stem bronchus. She was experiencing hemoptysis and required embolization of the right bronchial artery. Fibrosing mediastinitis is a rare manifestation of histoplasmosis, which is believed to represent a fibrotic reaction to seepage of antigen from caseous mediastinal lymph nodes [2,10,11]. Fibrosis may obstruct any of the major mediastinal structures, including pulmonary arteries and veins, vena cava, airways, esophagus, and pericardium. The course often is progressive and may be fatal. Antifungal therapy is not believed to be helpful, and surgery is hazardous.

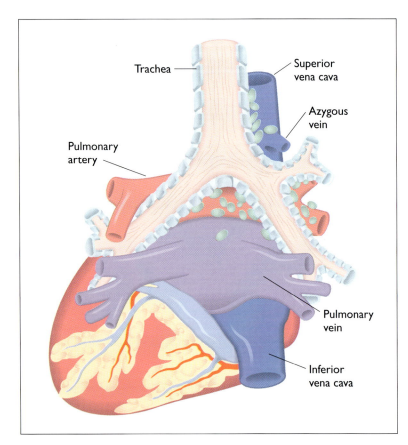

FIGURE 1-20 Relationship of mediastinal lymph nodes to contiguous structures. Fibrosis of the subcarinal nodes involves the major bronchi and pulmonary veins, whereas fibrosis related to the hilar nodes involves bronchi and pulmonary arteries. Fibrosis of the paratracheal nodes may cause occlusion of the superior vena cava, azygos vein, and right upper lobe bronchus [11]. Differentiation between fibrosing mediastinitis and granulomatous mediastinitis may be difficult. Granulomatous mediastinitis usually occurs earlier in the course of infection, whereas fibrosing mediastinitis is a later complication. Masses are more common with granulomatous mediastinitis and calcification with fibrosing mediastinitis. Granulomatous mediastinitis is less likely to obstruct major mediastinal structures and is more likely to respond to antifungal therapy.

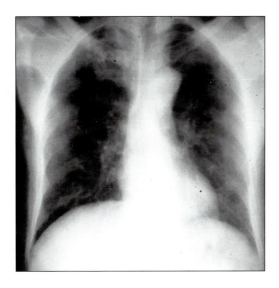

FIGURE 1-21 Chest radiograph from a patient with chronic pulmonary histoplasmosis complicated by adrenal insufficiency. The patient presented with cough and weight loss. Chest radiograph showed a right upper lobe infiltrate. During hospitalization, the patient experienced episodes of hypotension and hyperkalemia, prompting concern about the possibility of adrenal insufficiency.

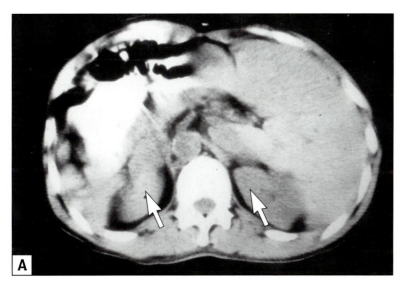
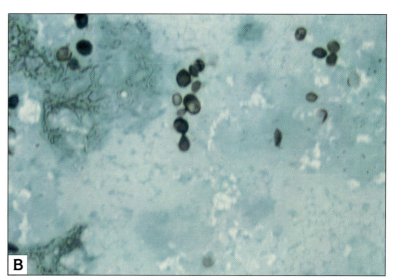

FIGURE 1-22 A, Abdominal CT scan showing bilateral adrenal masses (*arrows*). A fine-needle aspiration biopsy revealed organisms consistent with *Histoplasma capsulatum* yeast on Gomori methenamine silver stain. A diagnosis of disseminated histoplasmosis with adrenal involvement was established. Adrenal involvement is common in patients with progressive disseminated histoplasmosis, although adrenal insufficiency is seen only in those with extensive disease [12]. Histoplasmosis should be considered in the differential diagnosis of bilateral or unilateral adrenal masses. **B,** Gomori methenamine silver stain of fine-needle aspirate shows typical yeast forms of *Histoplasma capsulatum* measuring 2 to 5 μm in diameter with narrow based buds. *H. capsulatum* var. *capsulatum* is ovoid and shows budding at its smaller end.

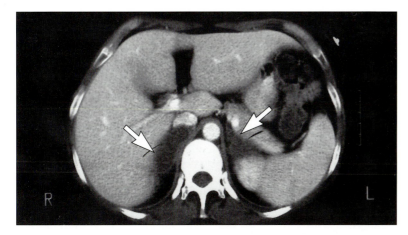

FIGURE 1-23 Abdominal CT scan showing cystic-appearing bilateral adrenal glands in a patient with Addison's disease. The patient presented with typical features of Addison's disease, including dizziness caused by orthostatic hypotension. She had no evidence of histoplasmosis in the lungs or other organs. Abdominal CT scan showed bilateral enlargement of the adrenal glands, which appeared cystic (*arrows*). Fine-needle aspiration showed inflammatory changes, but fungal stains and cultures were negative. Histoplasmosis was diagnosed based on detection of *Histoplasma* antigen in the urine. The patient improved in response to treatment with hydrocortisone, fludrocortisone acetate, and itraconazole. After 1 year of treatment, a slight reduction (about 1 cm) occurred in the size of the adrenal glands. This case illustrates the importance of consideration of histoplasmosis in the etiology of Addison's disease.

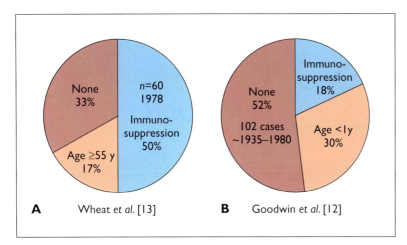

FIGURE 1-24 Risk factors for disseminated histoplasmosis. **A,** During a large outbreak of histoplasmosis in Indianapolis in 1978, immunosuppression and age of 55 years or greater were identified as risk factors for disseminated disease [13]. Of disseminated patients diagnosed during the outbreak, 74% had evidence for immunosuppression. Among nonimmunosuppressed patients, disseminated disease occurred four times more frequently in individuals more than 55 years of age (18%) than in those less than 54 years (4.8%). **B,** In another study, immunosuppression was seen in 18% of cases, and age less than 1 year in 30% [12]. In that study, more than half the patients had no identifiable risk factor. AIDS now is a major risk factor for disseminated histoplasmosis. (Panel A *adapted from* Wheat *et al.* [13]; panel B *adapted from* Goodwin *et al.* [12].)

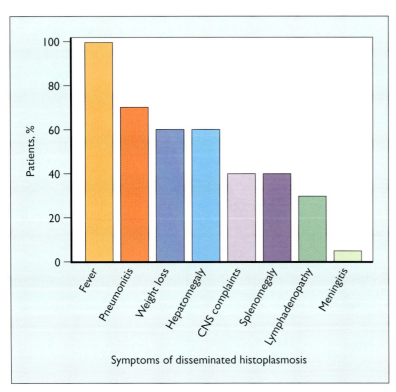

FIGURE 1-25 Clinical findings in disseminated histoplasmosis. Fever was present in all patients identified during the large outbreak in Indianapolis [14]. However, fever is less common in patients with localized manifestations of disseminated disease [12]. Central nervous system (CNS) complaints, including headache and depressed mentation, were relatively common, but evidence for CNS involvement, including meningitis, was seen in only 6% of patients. Other well-recognized manifestations of disseminated histoplasmosis, such as Addison's disease, skin lesions, and mouth or intestinal lesions, were uncommon, occurring in less than 5% of patients in this review. (*Adapted from* Sathapatayavongs *et al.* [14].)

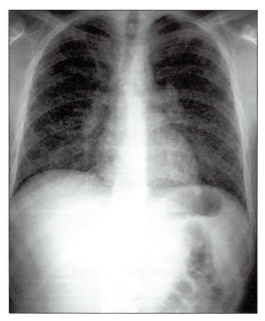

FIGURE 1-26 Chest radiograph showing miliary infiltrate in a patient with disseminated histoplasmosis. The patient presented with fever and weight loss. Anemia, leukopenia, and thrombocytopenia prompted a bone marrow examination, which showed granulomatous changes and contained organisms resembling *Histoplasma capsulatum*. Although diffuse infiltrates may be seen in patients with acute pulmonary histoplasmosis following a heavy inoculum challenge, they suggest disseminated disease in the absence of extensive exposure.

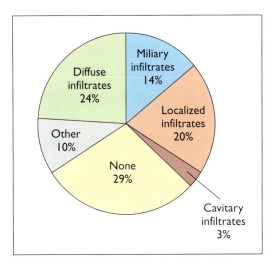

FIGURE 1-27 Summary of chest radiographic findings in disseminated histoplasmosis. Chest radiographs showed diffuse infiltrates or miliary infiltrates in about 40% of cases. Localized infiltrates with or without mediastinal lymphadenopathy also were common. Cavitary infiltrates were seen in only 3% of patients. Radiographs were normal in 29% of patients [14]. (*Adapted from* Sathapatayavongs *et al.* [14].)

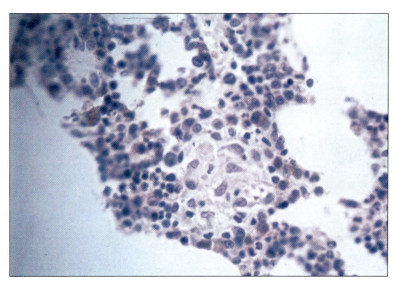

FIGURE 1-28 Bone marrow aspirate from the patient with disseminated histoplasmosis described in Figure 1-5. Hematoxylin-eosin stain shows noncaseating granulomas in this case, whereas silver stains were negative. The *Histoplasma* antigen test was positive, and the bone marrow subsequently grew *Histoplasma capsulatum*. This case illustrates the risk of misdiagnosis of sarcoidosis in patients with disseminated histoplasmosis. Care must be taken to exclude histoplasmosis before initiation of corticosteroid treatment for presumed sarcoidosis in patients with noncaseating granulomas in tissues.

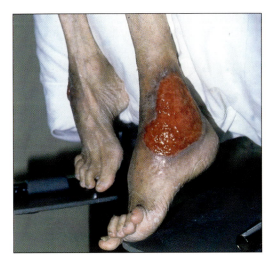

FIGURE 1-29 Skin ulcer in a patient with disseminated histoplasmosis. The patient had a chronic ulcer on her left foot. She was hospitalized for skin graft placement, and evaluation revealed that she had lost weight and exhibited massive hepatosplenomegaly. Bone marrow examination showed yeasts consistent with *Histoplasma capsulatum*, which subsequently were isolated in culture. The skin lesion also grew *H. capsulatum*. The ulcer healed, and the patient regained the lost weight in response to amphotericin B treatment.

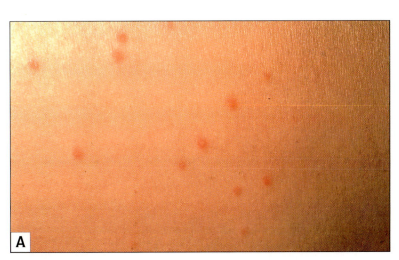
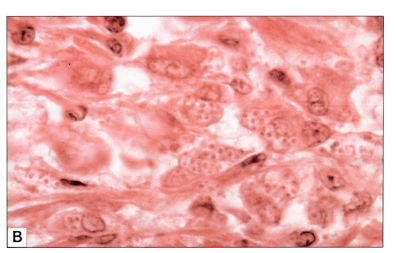

FIGURE 1-30 A, Maculopapular skin lesions in a patient with disseminated histoplasmosis. Numerous small maculopapular lesions were identified on the skin of this patient with AIDS. Biopsy showed intracellular organisms consistent with *Histoplasma capsulatum*. **B,** Hematoxylin-eosin stain of biopsy specimen shows intracellular and extracellular yeast consistent with *Histoplasma capsulatum*. (*Courtesy of* Dr. Tony Hood.)

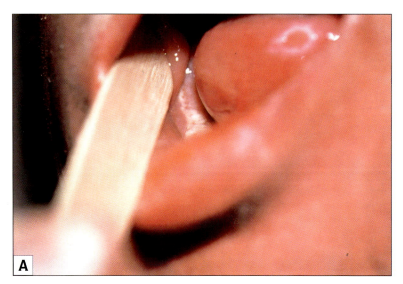 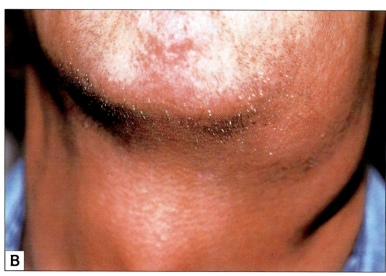

FIGURE 1-31 **A,** Oral ulcers in a patient with AIDS and disseminated histoplasmosis. Examination showed an ulcer on the tip of the tongue and on the lower gums. Biopsy showed organisms consistent with *Histoplasma capsulatum*. The patient also demonstrated marked enlargement of the cervical lymph nodes (**B**). He was treated initially with amphotericin B, followed by itraconazole, and demonstrated complete resolution of these lesions.

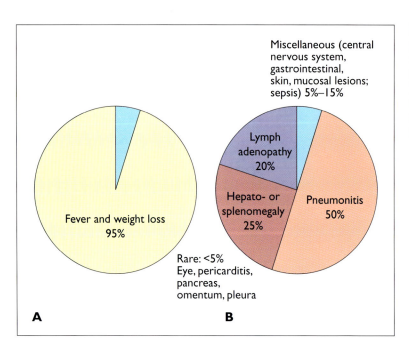

FIGURE 1-32 Clinical findings in disseminated histoplasmosis in patients with AIDS. **A,** Fever and weight loss are the most common manifestation [15]. **B,** Pulmonary involvement occurred in about half of the cases. Hepatosplenomegaly and lymphadenopathy also were common. Miscellaneous manifestations occurred in 15% of patients, including meningitis or focal brain lesions, gastrointestinal or skin lesions, and a syndrome resembling septic shock [15].

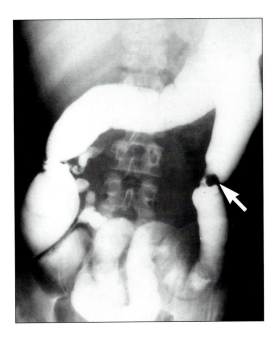

Figure 1-33 Colonic mass in a patient with AIDS and disseminated histoplasmosis. The patient presented with fever and weight loss. He also demonstrated a mass lesion on barium enema (*arrow*), which was found to be caused by histoplasmosis. *Histoplasma capsulatum* causes ulcers, masses, inflammatory changes resembling Crohn's disease, peritonitis, and mesenteric lymphadenitis. (*Courtesty of* Dr. George Sarosi.)

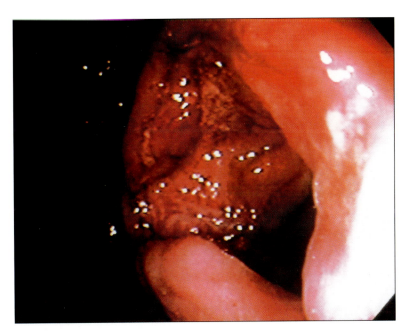

Figure 1-34 Colonic ulcer in a patient with AIDS and disseminated histoplasmosis. The patient experienced rectal bleeding. Colonoscopy demonstrated a large rectal ulcer, which contained organisms consistent with *Histoplasma capsulatum* by fungal stain. (*Courtesy of* Dr. Douglas Dieterich.)

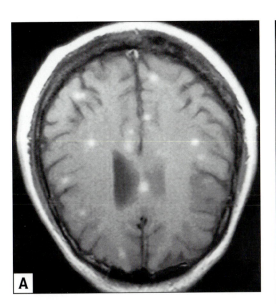
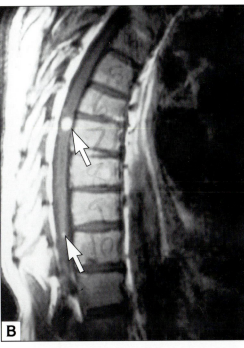

Figure 1-35 A, Head magnetic resonance imaging (MRI) scan showing enhancing lesions. The patient was found to have disseminated histoplasmosis based on positive fungal stains of a skin lesion. He also exhibited mental status changes, cerebellar abnormalities, and loss of sensation in his left leg. Head MRI showed more than 100 lesions involving the brain and cerebellum. **B**, Spine MRI showed lesions at T7 and T10, which accounted for the patient's sensory loss (*arrows*). He was treated with amphotericin B for 3 months and exhibited complete resolution of his neurologic findings as well as clearance of the lesions in the brain and spine after only 3 weeks. He also received dexamethasone during the first 2 weeks of therapy. He exhibited no findings suggestive of meningitis, and his cerebrospinal fluid was normal.

Laboratory Evaluation for Diagnosis

Summary of Diagnostic Test Results in Histoplasmosis

Diagnostic Test	Patients Positive for Acute Pulmonary Disease, %	Patients Positive for Cavitary Disease, %	Patients Positive for Disseminated Disease, %
Antibody			
Immunodiffusion	75	100	63
Complement fixation	89	93	63
Either immunodiffusion or complement fixation	99	100	71
Antigen detection	40–75*	21	92
Culture	15	85	85

*75% with diffuse pulmonary infiltrates.

FIGURE 1-36 Laboratory evaluation for diagnosis of histoplasmosis. The sensitivity of tests for diagnosis of histoplasmosis was determined in an evaluation of cases diagnosed in Indianapolis [16]. Rapid diagnosis can be established by antigen detection in patients with disseminated disease and in those with more severe manifestations of pulmonary histoplasmosis. Cultural methods are most useful in disseminated and chronic pulmonary histoplasmosis, but may provide results too slowly for patients with severe manifestations. Although fungal stain is useful, sensitivity is relatively low. Serologic tests for antibodies are positive in most patients with chronic pulmonary or self-limited forms of the infection but may be falsely negative in immunocompromised patients with disseminated histoplasmosis. The highest yield can be achieved by using a combination of tests, avoiding invasive procedures when possible. (*Adapted from* Williams *et al.* [16].)

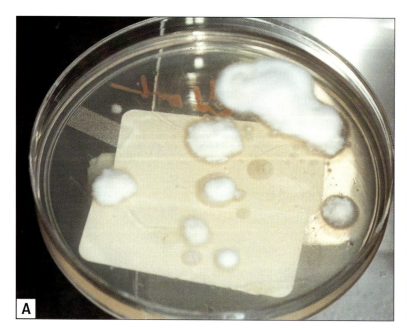 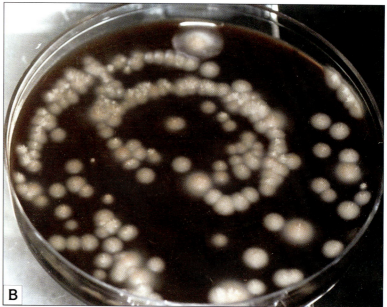

FIGURE 1-37 Mold and yeast culture of *Histoplasma capsulatum*. Fungal cultures are incubated at 25°C in the clinical laboratory, and *H. capsulatum* grows as a mold at this temperature. *H. capsulatum* may grow as early as 1 week but often requires up to 4 weeks to be detected. **A**, Colonies of the mold phase are white or buff in color. Characteristic tuberculate macroconidia are identified by fungal stain (*see* Fig. 1-38). Macroconidia measure 8 to 14 μm in diameter and may resemble those seen with other nonpathogenic molds. **B**, Identification as *H. capsulatum* requires additional testing, including demonstration of conversion of the mold to the yeast on incubation at 37°C and demonstration of *H. capsulatum* exoantigens by immunodiffusion or DNA probe.

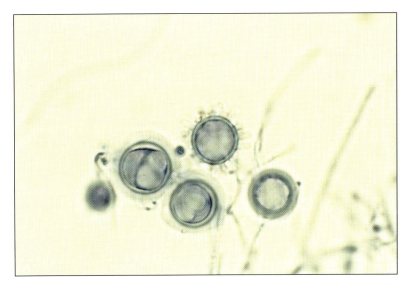

Figure 1-38 Lactol phenol cotton blue stain of the mold phase of *Histoplasma capsulatum* showing tuberculate macroconidia.

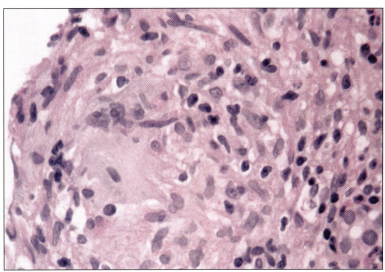

Figure 1-39 Liver biopsy specimen showing granuloma in a patient with disseminated histoplasmosis. Granuloma inflammation is characteristic of histoplasmosis. Both caseating and noncaseating granulomas may be seen. Sarcoidosis may be mistakenly diagnosed based on demonstration of noncaseating granulomas in the liver or other tissues.

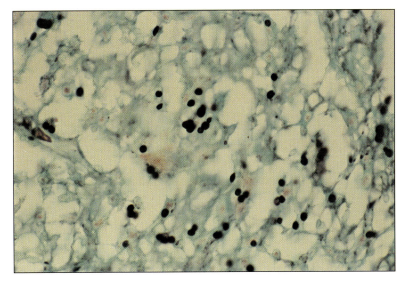

Figure 1-40 Gomori methenamine silver stain of bone marrow in a patient with disseminated histoplasmosis. Organisms may be seen more readily by methenamine silver stain than by hematoxylin-eosin stain (*see* Fig. 1-6). However, other organisms and artifacts may be mistaken for *Histoplasma capsulatum*. Organisms that have been misidentified as *H. capsulatum* include *Pneumocystis carinii*, *Blastomyces dermatitidis*, *Candida glabrata*, *Penicillium marneffei*, *Toxoplasma gondii*, and *Leishmania donovani*. More commonly, however, staining artifact mistakenly is identified as yeasts.

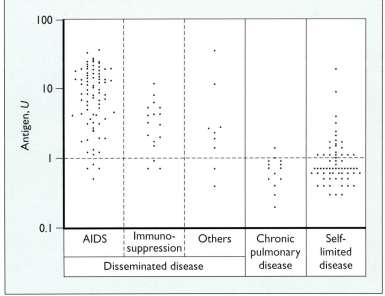

Figure 1-41 Antigen detection for diagnosis of histoplasmosis. Diagnosis based on detection of antigen in urine and blood has become a useful method for diagnosis of the more severe forms of histoplasmosis [16,17]. Antigen can be identified in the urine or blood in more than 90% of patients with disseminated histoplasmosis, especially in those who are immunosuppressed. Antigen also can be found in 40% of patients with acute pulmonary infection. The spectrum of disease in patients with acute pulmonary histoplasmosis ranges from asymptomatic infection to severe disease causing respiratory failure. Sensitivity for diagnosis of acute pulmonary histoplasmosis with diffuse infiltrates is 75%, making it a useful test for rapid diagnosis in patients who require prompt identification and treatment. Antigen detection is insensitive in patients with chronic pulmonary histoplasmosis or fibrosing mediastinitis. Antigen testing is available at the Histoplasmosis Reference Laboratory (1-800-HISTODGN or www.iupui.edu/it/histodgn).

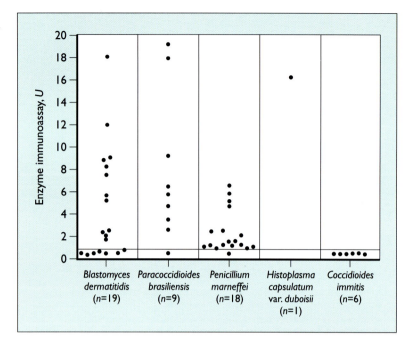

FIGURE 1-42 Cross reactions in the *Histoplasma* antigen assay. Positive results may also occur in patients with blastomycosis, paracoccidioidomycosis, *Penicillium marneffei* infection, and *Histoplasma capsulatum* var. *duboisii* infection, but not in patients with coccidioidomycosis, *Cryptococcus* infection, candidiasis, aspergillosis, or infection with other molds.

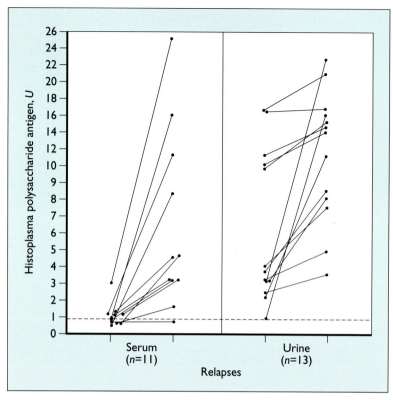

FIGURE 1-43 Antigen detection for diagnosis of relapse. Antigen levels in urine and serum fall in response to effective antifungal therapy and increase at least 2 U in patients with disseminated infection who relapse. Among patients with AIDS who experienced a relapse of disseminated histoplasmosis, an increase in antigen was detected in 90% [18]. Periodic measurement (3 to 6 months) of antigen in urine and serum is necessary to use this test to monitor therapy and assess for relapse.

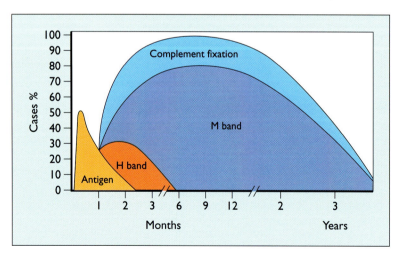

FIGURE 1-44 Diagnosis of milder forms of self-limited histoplasmosis. Tests for antigen usually are negative in patients with mild symptoms and limited pulmonary disease caused by acute histoplasmosis. The diagnosis is established based on measurement of the serologic response using the immunodiffusion and complement fixation test. Elevated concentrations of antibodies usually occur between 4 and 8 weeks following exposure. H bands by immunodiffusion occur in less than one third of patients and disappear over the next 6 months, whereas M bands appear more frequently and persist for several years. The complement fixation tests measuring antibodies to the yeast and mycelial phase of the organism provide the most sensitive serologic assay and are positive in more than 80% of cases [9,14–16,19]. The greatest sensitivity is achieved by measuring the response both by immunodiffusion and complement fixation. Although complement fixation titers of 1:32 provide the strongest basis for diagnosis, titers of 1:8 to 1:16 are found in up to one fourth of patients with active histoplasmosis and thus should not be disregarded.

INDICATIONS FOR TREATMENT

Indications for Antifungal Treatment in Histoplasmosis

Treatment Indicated	Treatment Not Indicated
Acute pulmonary disease with hypoxemia	Acute self-limited syndromes
Acute pulmonary disease >1 mo	Acute pulmonary disease, mildly ill
Chronic pulmonary disease	Rheumatologic disease
Esophageal compression or ulceration	Pericarditis
Granulomatous mediastinitis with obstruction or invasion of tissue	Histoplasmoma
	Broncholithiasis
Disseminated disease	Fibrosing mediastinitis
	Presumed ocular syndrome

FIGURE 1-45 Indications for antifungal treatment in histoplasmosis. In most patients, the manifestations of histoplasmosis are self-limited and treatment is not required. Treatment is mandatory in patients with disseminated or chronic pulmonary infection as well as in those with respiratory compromise caused by acute pulmonary histoplasmosis. Treatment also appears to be helpful in patients with granulomatous mediastinitis but unfortunately not in those with fibrosing mediastinitis.

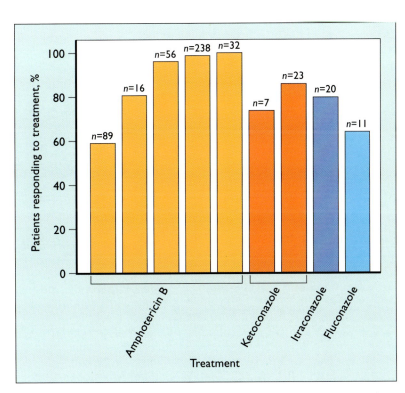

FIGURE 1-46 Response to treatment for disseminated histoplasmosis. Amphotericin B and itraconazole have been shown to be highly effective for treatment of disseminated histoplasmosis. Response rates greater than 80% have been reported in several studies. However, relapse predictably has occurred in patients with AIDS and often in those with other severe and persistent immunosuppressive disorders. Chronic maintenance therapy is recommended in patients with AIDS and should be considered in those who have relapsed despite appropriate treatment. Fluconazole has been less effective for treatment of histoplasmosis because of its reduced in vitro activity and potential for induction of resistance.

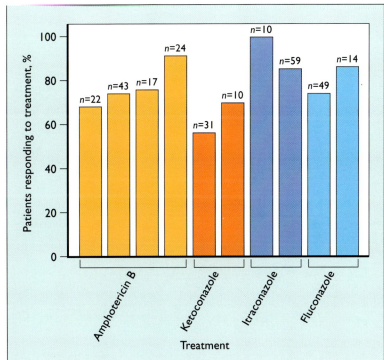

FIGURE 1-47 Response to treatment for chronic pulmonary histoplasmosis. Amphotericin B and itraconazole are highly effective for treatment of chronic pulmonary histoplasmosis, which occurs in 5% to 10% of cases. Thus, prolonged courses of at least 18 months of itraconazole therapy are recommended, and patients should be monitored for relapse.

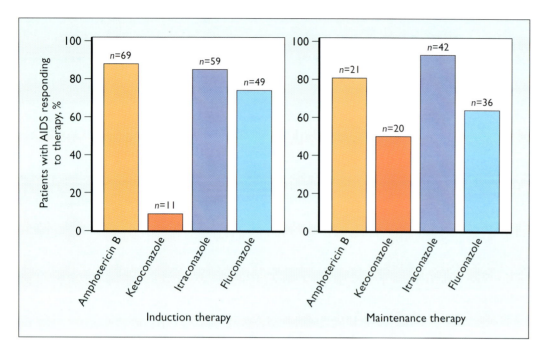

FIGURE 1-48 Treatment of histoplasmosis in patients with AIDS. Amphotericin B and itraconazole have proven to be highly effective for treatment of histoplasmosis in patients with AIDS [15,20,21]. Ketoconazole has not been well studied but appears to be less effective [15]. Chronic maintenance therapy is essential to prevent relapse [15]. Itraconazole has emerged as the most effective maintenance treatment [22,23]. Relapses have occurred in patients receiving fluconazole; these have demonstrated to be caused by resistant organisms that emerged during the course of treatment [21].

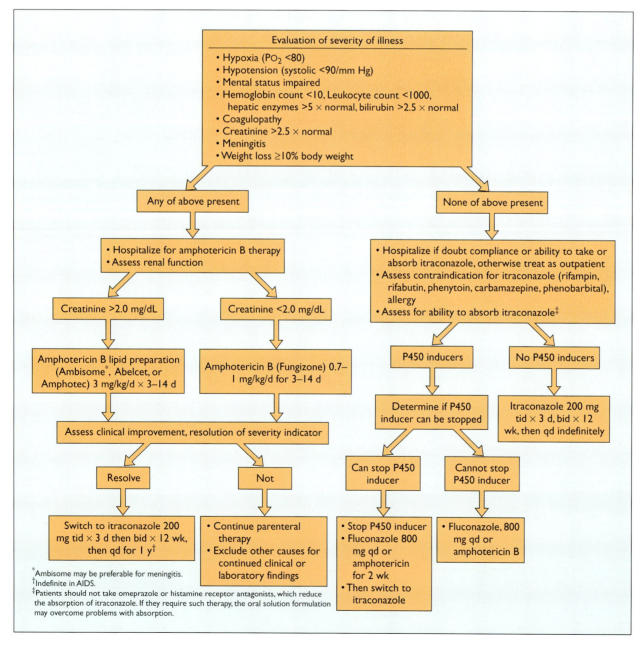

FIGURE 1-49 Guidelines for selection of antifungal treatment for disseminated histoplasmosis. Amphotericin B or one of the lipid preparations should be chosen for initial treatment in patients with severe manifestations of histoplasmosis. Itraconazole is appropriate for patients with mild manifestations or following improvement in response to amphotericin B treatment. Itraconazole usually should be given for at least 1 year in patients with disseminated disease and longer in those with chronic pulmonary disease to reduce the likelihood of relapse. bid—twice a day; qd—every day; tid—three times a day.

References

1. Rippon JW: Histoplasmosis (*Histoplasmosis capsulati*). In *Medical Mycology: The Pathogenic Fungi and the Pathogenic Actinomycetes*. Edited by Wonsiewicz M. Philadelphia: WB Saunders; 1988:381–423.

2. Wheat J: Histoplasmosis: experience during outbreaks in Indianapolis and review of the literature. *Medicine* 1997, 76:339–354.

3. Brodsky AL, Gregg MB, Kaufman L, Mallison GF: Outbreak of histoplasmosis associated with the 1970 Earth Day activities. *Am J Med* 1973, 54:333–342.

4. Ozols II, Wheat LJ: Erythema nodosum in an epidemic of histoplasmosis in Indianapolis. *Arch Dermatol* 1981, 117:709–712.

5. Thornberry DK, Wheat LJ, Brandt KD, Rosenthal J: Histoplasmosis presenting with joint pain and hilar adenopathy: pseudosarcoidosis. *Arthritis Rheum* 1982, 25:1396–1402.

6. Rosenthal J, Brandt KD, Wheat LJ, Slama TG: Rheumatologic manifestations of histoplasmosis in the recent Indianapolis epidemic. *Arthritis Rheum* 1983, 26:1065–1070.

7. Wheat LJ, Stein L, Corya BC, et al.: Pericarditis as a manifestation of histoplasmosis during two large urban outbreaks. *Medicine* 1983, 62:110–119.

8. Coss KC, Wheat LJ, Conces DJ Jr, et al.: Esophageal fistula complicating mediastinal histoplasmosis: response to amphotericin B. *Am J Med* 1987, 83:343–346.

9. Wheat LJ, Wass J, Norton J, et al.: Cavitary histoplasmosis occurring during two large urban outbreaks: analysis of clinical, epidemiologic, roentgenographic, and laboratory features. *Medicine* 1984, 63:201–209.

10. Loyd JE, Tillman BF, Atkinson JB, des Prez RM: Mediastinal fibrosis complicating histoplasmosis. *Medicine* 1988, 67:295–310.

11. Goodwin RA, Nickell JA, des Prez RM: Mediastinal fibrosis complicating healed primary histoplasmosis and tuberculosis. *Medicine* 1972, 51:227–246.

12. Goodwin RA Jr, Shapiro JL, Thurman GH, et al.: Disseminated histoplasmosis: clinical and pathologic correlations. *Medicine* 1980, 59:1–33.

13. Wheat LJ, Slama TG, Norton JA, et al.: Risk factors for disseminated or fatal histoplasmosis. *Ann Intern Med* 1982, 96:159–163.

14. Sathapatayavongs B, Batteiger BE, Wheat LJ, et al.: Clinical and laboratory features of disseminated histoplasmosis during two large urban outbreaks. *Medicine* 1983, 62:263–270.

15. Wheat LJ, Connolly-Stringfield PA, Baker RL, et al.: Disseminated histoplasmosis in the acquired immune deficiency syndrome: clinical findings, diagnosis and treatment, and review of the literature. *Medicine* 1990, 69:361–374.

16. Williams B, Fojtasek M, Connolly-Stringfield P, Wheat J: Diagnosis of histoplasmosis by antigen detection during an outbreak in Indianapolis, Ind. *Arch Pathol Lab Med* 1994, 118:1205–1208.

17. Wheat LJ, Kohler RB, Tewari RP: Diagnosis of disseminated histoplasmosis by detection of *Histoplasma capsulatum* antigen in serum and urine specimens. *N Engl J Med* 1986, 314:83–88.

18. Wheat LJ, Connolly-Stringfield P, Blair R, et al.: Histoplasmosis relapse in patients with AIDS: detection using *Histoplasma capsulatum* variety *capsulatum* antigen levels. *Ann Intern Med* 1991, 115:936–941.

19. Wheat LJ, French MLV, Kohler RB, et al.: The diagnostic laboratory tests for histoplasmosis: analysis of experience in a large urban outbreak. *Ann Intern Med* 1982, 97:680–685.

20. Wheat J, Hafner R, Korzun AH, et al.: Itraconazole treatment of disseminated histoplasmosis in patients with the acquired immunodeficiency syndrome. *Am J Med* 1995, 98:336–342.

21. Wheat J, MaWhinney S, Hafner R, et al.: Treatment of histoplasmosis with fluconazole in patients with acquired immunodeficiency syndrome. *Am J Med* 1997, 103:223–232.

22. Hecht FM, Wheat J, Korzun AH, et al.: Itraconazole maintenance treatment for histoplasmosis in AIDS: a prospective, multicenter trial. *J Acquir Immune Defic Syndr Hum Retrovirol* 1997, 16:100–107.

23. Wheat J, Hafner R, Wulfson M, et al.: Prevention of relapse of histoplasmosis with itraconazole in patients with the acquired immunodeficiency syndrome. *Ann Intern Med* 1993, 118:610–616.

Chapter 2

Coccidioidomycosis

Neil M. Ampel
Hans E. Einstein
John N. Galgiani
Demosthenes Pappagianis
Marion A. Wieden

Coccidioidomycosis represents a spectrum of clinical diseases due to infection with the dimorphic, soil-dwelling fungus *Coccidioides immitis*. The fungus is found in limited regions of the Western hemisphere, with highly endemic areas in the United States located in the San Joaquin Valley of California and the south-central region of Arizona, including the metropolitan regions of Phoenix and Tucson.

Although the vast majority of individuals who become infected with *C. immitis* either are asymptomatic or have self-limited illness, chronic pulmonary infection or persistent infection disseminated beyond the thoracic cavity occurs in approximately 5% of all individuals infected. These latter syndromes cause significant morbidity and occasional mortality and usually require prolonged antifungal therapy.

The development of oral triazole antifungal therapies has widened the therapeutic options for the treatment of many forms of coccidioidomycosis. The emergence of new diagnostic techniques, from magnetic resonance imaging (MRI) to confirmation of diagnosis through the use of genetic analysis, has revolutionized the management of this infection.

Epidemiology

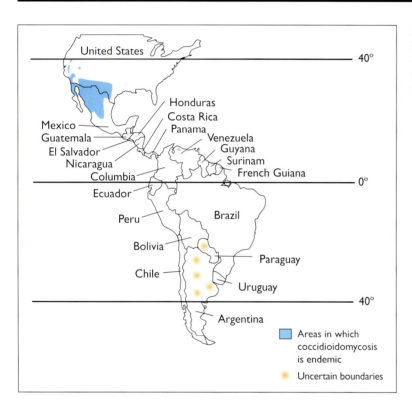

Figure 2-1. Western hemisphere endemic area. Coccidioidomycosis occurs only in the western hemisphere from approximately 40°N 120°W in California to 40°S 65°W in Argentina. The figure depicts the known endemic regions. Not shown is a newly identified area in central Brazil. (*Adapted from* Pappagianis [1].)

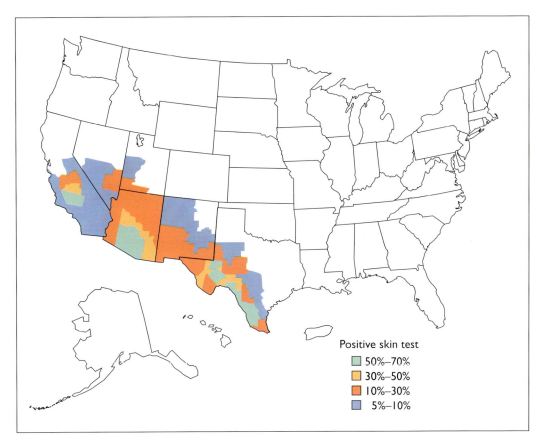

Figure 2-2. Areas of skin-test positivity. In the United States, coccidioidomycosis occurs principally in the San Joaquin Valley and other nearby areas of California and the south-central region of Arizona, including the major cities of Tucson and Phoenix. It also occurs in southern Nevada and Utah as well as in areas of southern New Mexico and western Texas. The figure shows the prevalence of coccidioidal skin-test reactivity in the western United States. *Green areas* depict regions of highest prevalence. These data originally were published in 1957; therefore, prevalence of skin-test positivity may be different today. (*Adapted from* Edwards and Palmer [2].)

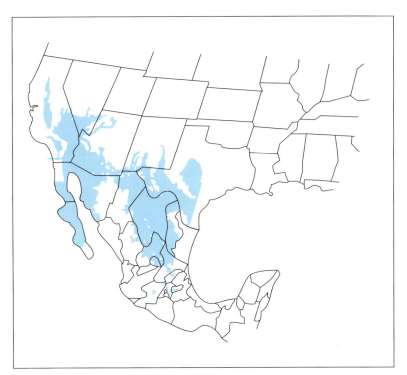

Figure 2-3. The Lower Sonoran Life Zone. Coccidioidomycosis is intimately associated with the Lower Sonoran Life Zone, which is a geoclimatic region of aridity associated with hot summers, mild winters, and alkaline soil. The figure depicts the region of the Lower Sonoran Life Zone that roughly parallels the area of endemicity for coccidioidomycosis. (*Adapted from* Ochoa [3].)

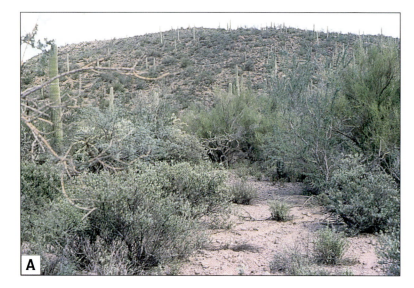
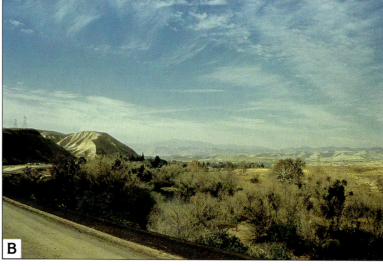
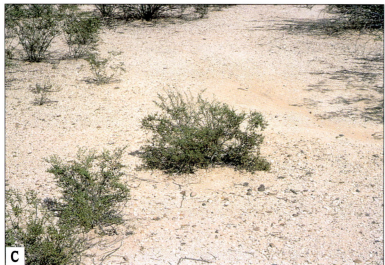

Figure 2-4. Endemic areas for coccidioidomycosis. **A,** The Sonoran Desert in southern Arizona and northern Mexico is located within the Lower Sonoran Life Zone and is highly endemic for coccidioidomycosis. The figure, which is a photograph taken just outside of Tucson, Arizona, displays saguaro cacti, mesquite, and jojoba, which are typical native flora. **B,** The southern portion of the San Joaquin Valley is also a highly endemic region. This area of Kern County, located in the southernmost region of the San Joaquin Valley, is highly endemic for coccidioidomycosis. **C,** Areas where the creosote bush grows have been strongly associated with coccidioidomycosis.

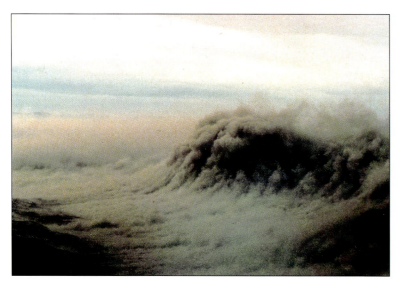

Figure 2-5. Dust storm. Most cases of coccidioidomycosis are acquired through inhalation of airborne soil containing the fungus. As a result, dust storms have been associated with outbreaks of coccidioidomycosis. This photograph was taken 5000 ft above Kern County, California, in December 1977, during a massive dust storm that was associated with a large outbreak of coccidioidomycosis.

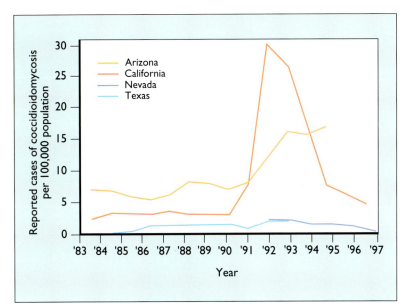

Figure 2-6. Incidence of coccidioidomycosis over the past decade. The greatest impact of coccidioidomycosis during the past decade has been in California and Arizona. During the early 1990s, a marked increase occurred in the number of cases in California, especially in the San Joaquin Valley. This increase has since abated and probably was a result of a prolonged drought followed by rains and a large influx of new residents from nonendemic regions. In Arizona, the number of reported cases has increased steadily. The reasons for this continued increase are not clear, but the largest impact of cases is occurring in the region encompassing the two largest cities in Arizona, Phoenix and Tucson. (Courtesy of Dr. Tom Larwood.)

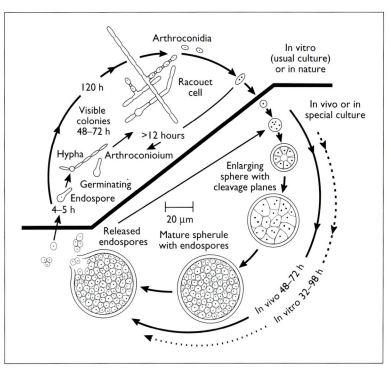

Figure 2-7. Life cycle of *Coccidioides immitis*. The life cycle of the fungus occurs in two phases. In the soil, *C. immitis* exists as a mold in which alternating cells degenerate, leaving barrel-shaped arthroconidia that can become airborne. When inhaled into the lung, arthroconidia undergo profound morphologic changes. The entire structure rounds, the outer wall thickens, and internal septations form. This stage is called the spherule. As the spherule matures, it enlarges and the septations develop into packets of endospores. Endospores may continue to propagate infection within the host by developing into spherules. (Adapted from Pappagianis and Zimmer [4].)

DISEASE MANIFESTATIONS

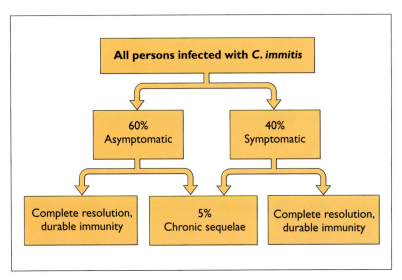

Figure 2-8. Outcomes after infection with *Coccidioides immitis*. At the time of infection with *C. immitis*, about 60% of persons are asymptomatic. In these individuals, the only evidence of infection is a delayed-type hypersensitivity reaction to coccidioidal antigen after skin testing. Approximately 30% of those persons infected have a self-limited pulmonary illness. Chronic pulmonary illness occurs in 5% to 10% of persons infected, and disseminated disease also occurs in 5%. This illness may consist of chronic pulmonary disease or infection disseminated beyond the thoracic cavity. Dissemination may occur in those persons who were initially asymptomatic or symptomatic at the time of infection.

Pulmonary Manifestations

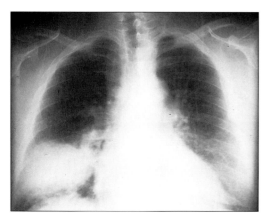

FIGURE 2-9. Radiograph showing primary focal coccidioidal pneumonia. Primary pneumonia due to *Coccidioides immitis*, when symptomatic, usually presents with fever, pleuritic chest pain, and cough. Cough is usually minimally productive. Radiographically, the pneumonia is usually not distinguishable from that caused by a bacterial infection. This patient suffered from alcoholism and initially was believed to have pneumonia owing to *Klebsiella* species. The diagnosis of coccidioidomycosis was subsequently made when spherules were seen on a potassium hydroxide preparation of a sputum sample. Unfortunately, the patient died shortly thereafter.

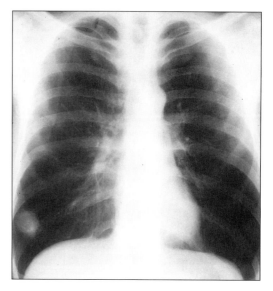

FIGURE 2-10. Radiograph showing coccidioidal nodule. Development of a nodule after coccidioidal pneumonia occurs in fewer than 10% of all patients. The nodule is usually solitary and less than 6 cm in diameter. In a patient not previously known to have had coccidioidomycosis, the major concern of a solitary nodule is whether it represents a malignancy or coccidioidomycosis. Noninvasive tests, including skin testing, coccidioidal serologic tests, and imaging techniques, are usually inconclusive. Similarly, bronchoscopy with analysis of respiratory secretions is almost always unrevealing. Biopsy usually is required to make the distinction. The results of percutaneous needle biopsy may establish the diagnosis in approximately 50% of cases. Histologic examination is more sensitive than culture.

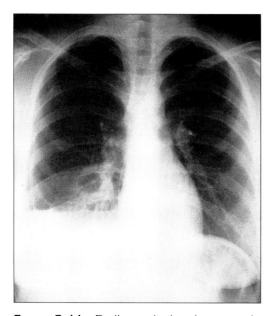

FIGURE 2-11. Radiograph showing an early coccidioidal cavity with surrounding pneumonitis and a pleural effusion. Pulmonary cavities represent nodules that have excavated their inner contents. These cavities are often benign but can be associated with a variety of complications, including hemoptysis and secondary infection. In some instances, surgical extirpation is required. In most cases, however, the cavities close over time without complication.

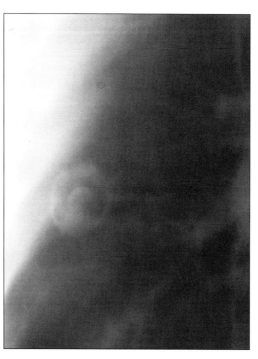

FIGURE 2-12. Radiograph showing coccidioidal mycetoma. Cavities may become secondarily infected with bacteria and fungi, such as *Aspergillus* species. They also may become secondarily infected with *Coccidioides immitis*. Both the cavity and the mycetoma shown in this figure were due to *C. immitis*.

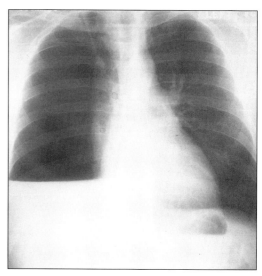

FIGURE 2-13. Radiograph showing pyopneumothorax. Pyopneumothorax is an uncommon complication owing to a rupture of a subpleural coccidioidal cavity into the pleural space. Although surgical therapy usually is required, antifungal therapy generally is not. Pyopneumothorax is not considered a sign of dissemination. (*From* Snyder and Galgiani [5]; with permission.)

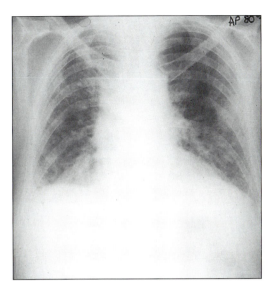

Figure 2-14. Radiograph showing diffuse pneumonia in a patient with HIV infection. Although bilateral pneumonia is sometimes the result of inhalation of a large inoculum of *Coccidioides immitis*, more often it is a reflection of fungemia and overwhelming dissemination. In that form, diffuse coccidioidal pneumonia usually occurs in hosts with underlying cell-mediated immune deficiency, such as in patients with HIV infection, patients who have undergone allogeneic organ transplantations, or patients receiving chronic corticosteroid therapy. Sometimes called reticulonodular pneumonia, the pattern is similar to that seen in miliary tuberculosis. (*Adapted from* Galgiani [6].)

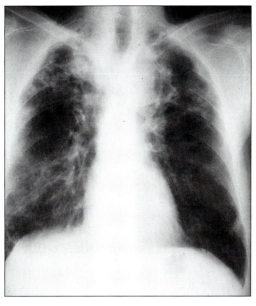

Figure 2-15. Radiograph showing chronic pneumonia. Chronic coccidioidal pneumonia is characterized by persistent symptoms and progressive pulmonary involvement. Patients have chronic cough, weight loss, and fever. Radiographically, both fibrosis and alveolar infiltrates are present, which often worsen in the apical regions.

Cutaneous Manifestations

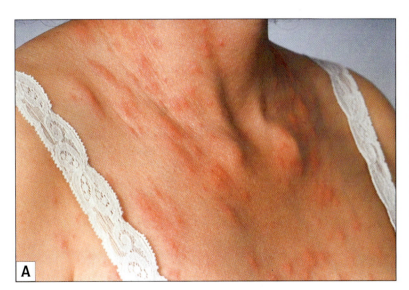

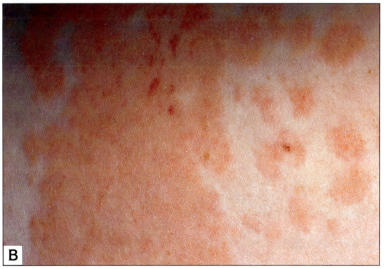

Figure 2-16. Erythema multiforme. During primary coccidioidal infection, three distinct cutaneous reactions may occur, including erythema multiforme. Frequently, these target lesions are distributed in the upper body, often in a "necklace" pattern.

A, Erythema multiforme in a patient whose reaction was not a result of natural infection but of a killed spherule vaccine.
B, Example of bullous erythema multiforme during coccidioidomycosis. (Panel B *courtesy of* Dr. Ronald Hansen.)

Fungal Infections

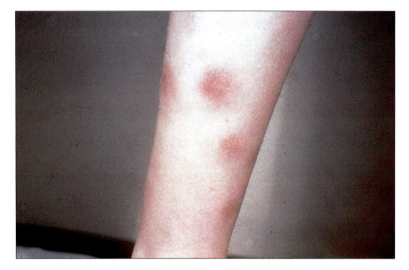

FIGURE 2-17. Erythema nodosum. Another common cutaneous manifestation of primary coccidioidomycosis is erythema nodosum. Patients present with painful erythematous nodules in the lower extremities. It most often occurs in women and is usually, but not always, associated with a good prognosis.

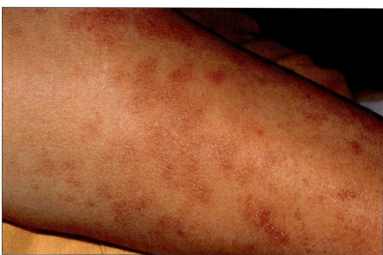

FIGURE 2-18. Sweet's syndrome and coccidioidomycosis. Sweet's syndrome, an erythematous reaction associated with neutrophilic infiltration of the skin, has been associated with pulmonary coccidioidomycosis. The figure shows a typical example on the arm of a patient. (*Courtesy of* Dr. Ronald Hansen.)

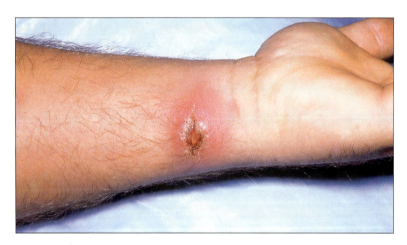

FIGURE 2-19. Primary cutaneous inoculation. Although most cases of coccidioidomycosis are acquired through inhalation, infection occasionally occurs through local inoculation of the skin. This patient sustained an injury with the thorn of an ocotillo plant, a spiny native of the Sonoran Desert. Note the intense local erythema with purulent drainage. Primary cutaneous inoculation often heals without antifungal therapy.

Extrathoracic Coccidioidomycosis Due to Dissemination

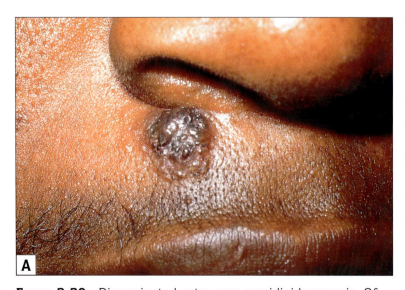

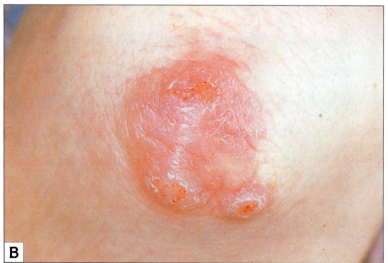

FIGURE 2-20. Disseminated cutaneous coccidioidomycosis. Of the various types of extrathoracic coccidioidomycosis, dissemination to the skin and underlying soft tissues is the most frequent manifestation. Although coccidioidal skin lesions may have a variety of appearances, they often become verrucous over time. For reasons not understood, skin involvement in coccidioidomycosis often occurs on the face. **A**, Verrucous papule is shown beneath the nose of a patient. **B**, A large, erythematous plaque is apparent on a patient's knee. (Panel A *courtesy of* Dr. Ronald Hansen.)

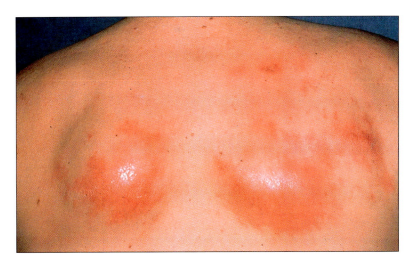

Figure 2-21. Subcutaneous abscess. Coccidioidomycosis may cause large, subcutaneous abscesses, like the two shown in the figure on the back of a patient. When aspirated, they have the gross appearance of pus and are full of polymorphonuclear leukocytes. *Coccidioides immitis* is easily isolated by culture.

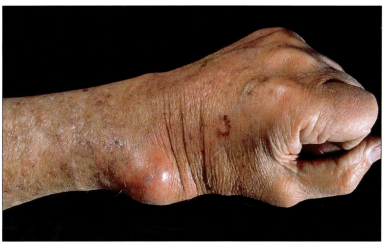

Figure 2-22. Coccidioidal synovitis of the tendon. The figure shows a Native American man with a chronic mass in his left wrist. Surgical débridement was required and showed involvement of the tendon synovium by *Coccidioides immitis*.

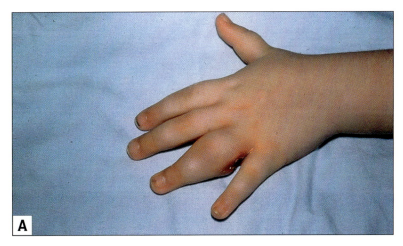
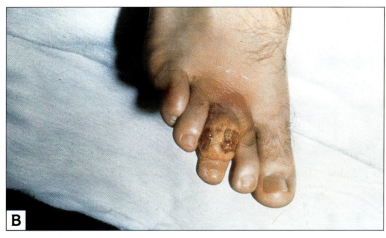

Figure 2-23. Coccidioidal osteomyelitis. **A**, The proximal phalangeal bone of the fourth finger is affected with coccidioidal osteomyelitis in a child. Overlying skin and soft tissue also can become involved with sinus track formation, subcutaneous abscesses, or frank skin involvement. **B**, Both cutaneous and bony infection due to *Coccidioides immitis* is shown.

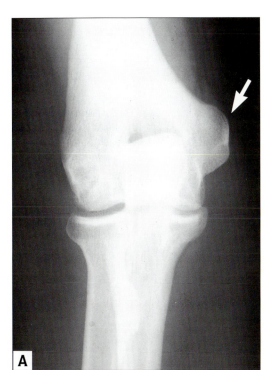
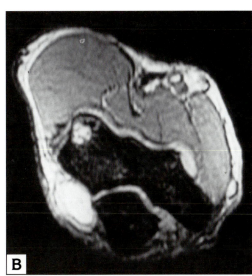

Figure 2-24. Radiographic assessment of coccidioidal osteomyelitis and synovitis of the elbow. This radiograph is from a 34-year-old man who complained of pain for 2 months, swelling, and redness of the right elbow. **A**, Anterioposterior radiograph shows a focal, well-defined lucency in the capitellum (*arrow*). **B**, Magnetic resonance image of the same elbow after intravenous gadolinium demonstrates focal enhancement at the site of the radiographic lucency as well as a focal area of enhancement within the synovium [7]. (*Courtesy of* Dr. Pamela Lund.)

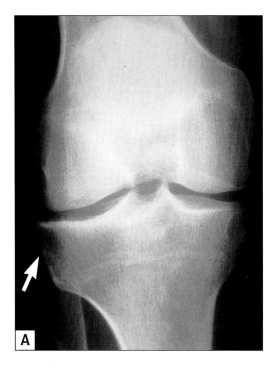
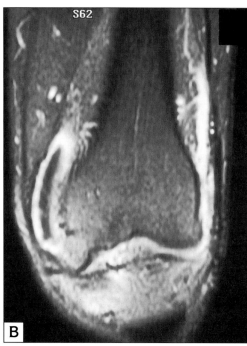

Figure 2-25. Radiographic assessment of coccidioidal osteomyelitis and synovitis of the knee. These radiographs were obtained from a 60-year-old man with a 2-year history of pain and swelling of the right knee. **A,** Anteroposterior radiograph shows erosion at the marginal borders of both the medial and lateral tibial condyles (*arrow*), which is a typical presentation of coccidioidal osteomyelitis. **B,** Coronal magnetic resonance image (MRI) obtained after intravenous gadolinium reveals diffuse enhancement and thickening of the synovium. Many cases of coccidioidal osteomyelitis also demonstrate synovial involvement when more sensitive techniques, such as MRI, are used. (*Courtesy of* Dr. Pamela Lund.)

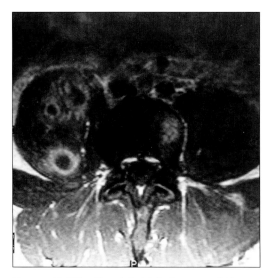

Figure 2-26. Coccidioidal abscess of the paraspinous muscles with vertebral involvement. Disseminated coccidioidomycosis may occur in multiple sites. In the magnetic resonance image shown in the figure, involvement of the body of the fourth vertebra as well as paraspinous muscles abscesses can be seen. Surgical therapy in addition to antifungal treatment usually is required. This complication is particularly common among black men. (*From* Galgiani [6]; with permission.)

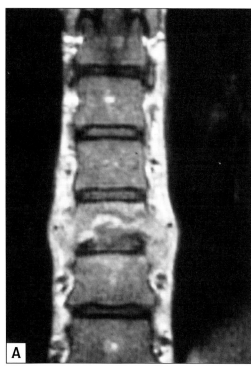
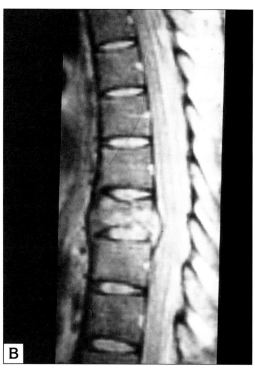

Figure 2-27. Coccidioidal spondylitis. Like tuberculosis, coccidioidomycosis may infect the vertebral bodies while sparing the intervertebral disks. Shown are magnetic resonance images with T1-weighting after intravenous gadolinium. The involvement of the T8 vertebra is clear in both the coronal (**A**) and sagittal (**B**) views. In *panel B*, compression of the spinal cord is evident. (*Courtesy of* Dr. William Erly.)

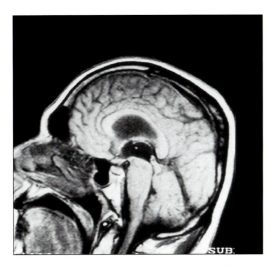

Figure 2-28. Coccidioidomycosis of the central nervous system. Coccidioidomycosis may present as a chronic lymphocytic meningitis with extensive inflammation of the basilar meninges. Both communicating and noncommunicating hydrocephalus may occur. In this magnetic resonance image, the Sylvian aqueduct is patent, whereas the third ventricle is enlarged, which is consistent with a communicating hydrocephalus. (*From* Galgiani [6]; with permission.)

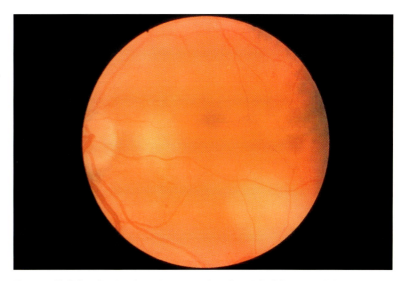

Figure 2-29. Ocular involvement by *Coccidioides immitis*. Although it is not common, coccidioidomycosis may be associated with a variety of ocular manifestations. Asymptomatic chorioretinal scars occur in as many as 10% of individuals with coccidioidal infection. No relationship exists between the degree of activity of disease elsewhere in the body and the presence of these scars. In most cases, they represent asymptomatic lesions. The figure shows two areas of well-circumscribed depigmentation in the retina. An additional scar is seen with increased pigmentation.

Diagnosis

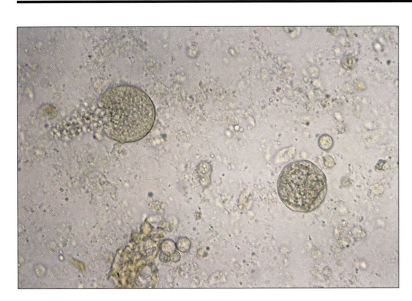

Figure 2-30. Potassium hydroxide (KOH) preparation of sputum. The chitin in the spherule cell wall is resistant to digestion by KOH, whereas host cells in sputum are not. Two mature spherules are evident in the figure, one of which has ruptured and is releasing endospores. Although KOH is not a sensitive test, the finding of spherules in a sputum specimen is diagnostic of coccidioidomycosis. Additionally, *Coccidioides immitis* grows readily on routine culture media. Unlike other dimorphic fungi, colonies usually are visually apparent within 3 to 5 days. On solid media, the fungus appears as a nonpigmented mold. Specific identification currently may be accomplished by genomic analysis using chemiluminescence. Unlike specimens obtained from patients, *C. immitis* growing in culture is highly infectious and represents an extreme laboratory hazard.

Application of Serologic Tests in Coccidioidomycosis

Serologic Test	Detection of	
	IgM	IgG
Tube precipitin	Yes	No
Latex particle agglutination	Yes	No (±)[†]
Immunodiffusion tube precipitin	Yes	No
Complement fixation	No (rare)*	Yes
Immunodiffusion complement fixation	No	Yes
Counterimmunoelectrophoresis	Yes	Yes
Enzyme-linked immunoassay	Yes	Yes

*Rarely positive complement fixation in presence of positive immunodiffusion tube precipitin (IgM and absence of detectable IgG by immunodiffusion complement fixation).
[†]Occasional positive latex particle agglutination in presence of detectable IgG but not IgM by immunodiffusion.

Figure 2-31. Uses of coccidioidal serologic tests. A variety of methods may be used to detect the major serologic antibodies used in the diagnosis of coccidioidomycosis. The first antibody detected during the course of disease is the tube precipitin antibody, which is now known to be a member of the IgM class. Later, a complement fixing antibody, which is a member of the IgG class, appears. Several techniques exist to detect these antibodies, from the original methods of tube precipitation and complement fixation, to immunodiffusion and enzyme-linked immunoassay. (*From* Pappagianis [8]; with permission.)

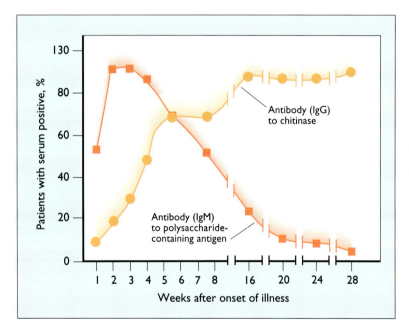

Figure 2-32. Early serologic response in coccidioidomycosis. The early serologic response in individuals recently infected with *Coccidioides immitis* is shown. The tube precipitin, or IgM antibody, is detected first and then disappears over several weeks. Complement fixation, or IgG antibody, follows and persists longer. The *lines* in the figure indicate the response seen with the older standard methods detecting the tube precipitin and complement fixation antibodies, and the *shaded areas* indicate the imprecisely defined sensitivity of immunodiffusion and enzyme-linked immunoassay methods for detecting IgM and IgG anticoccidioidal antibodies. (*From* Pappagianis [9]; with permission.)

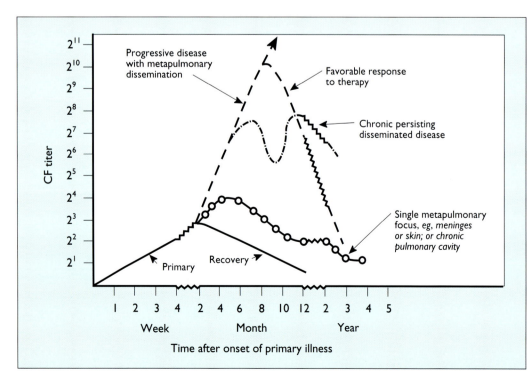

Figure 2-33. Patterns of complement fixation antibody response in different forms of coccidioidomycosis. The titer of complement fixation, or IgG antibody, in the serum is associated with the clinical stage of coccidioidomycosis and can be used to assess the risk of dissemination and the response to treatment. In primary infection, a transient rise in antibody occurs. This rise declines over time as the patient clinically improves. Chronically elevated serum titers occur with extrapulmonary disease in single sites or with chronic pulmonary disease (*open circles*). In patients with extensive dissemination (*dashed lines*), the IgG antibody titer rises precipitously. If therapy is successful, the antibody titer will decline. (*Adapted from* Pappagianis [10].)

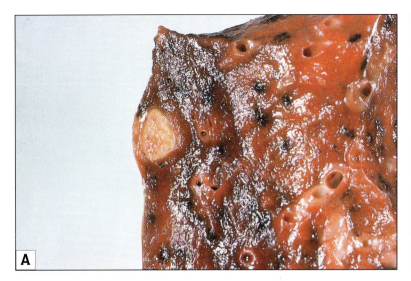
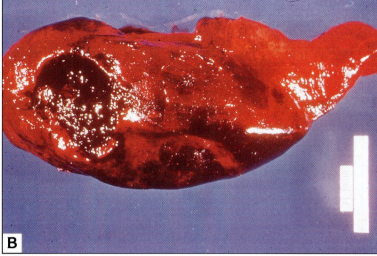

FIGURE 2-34. Gross pathologic appearance of coccidioidomycosis. **A**, Gross appearance of a coccidioidal nodule after surgical removal is shown. Note the well-circumscribed lesion. **B**, Hemorrhagic coccidioidal cavity is shown. Such cavities can be associated with severe hemoptysis requiring surgical removal. **C**, Multiple granulomatous lesions are revealed in the lung. (Panel C *courtesy of* Dr. James Byers.)

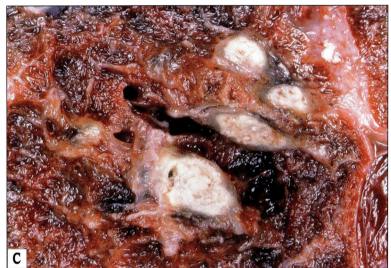

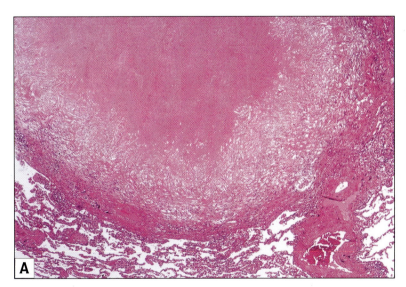
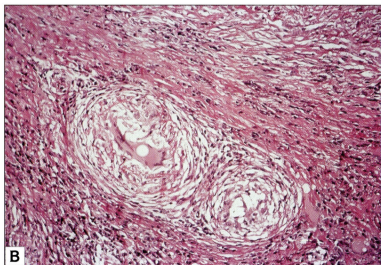

FIGURE 2-35. Histologic appearance of *Coccidioides immitis*. Coccidioidomycosis often is associated with an intense granulomatous response. **A**, Caseating granuloma in the lung. **B**, Noncaseating pulmonary granulomata containing spherules. The finding of a spherule is a classic stigmata of coccidioidomycosis.

(continued on next page)

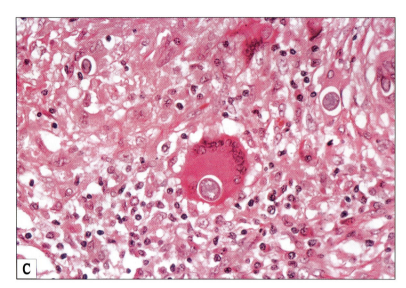
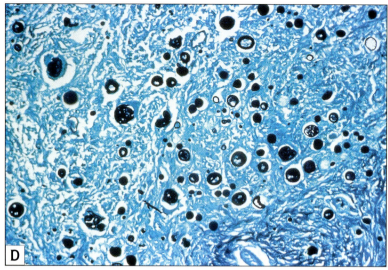

Figure 2-35. (*continued*) **C**, A spherule within a multinucleate giant cell is demonstrated. Spherules are more easily seen in tissue after silver staining, such as the Gomori methenamine silver stain (**D**). (Panels A and B *courtesy of* Dr. James Byers.)

Treatment

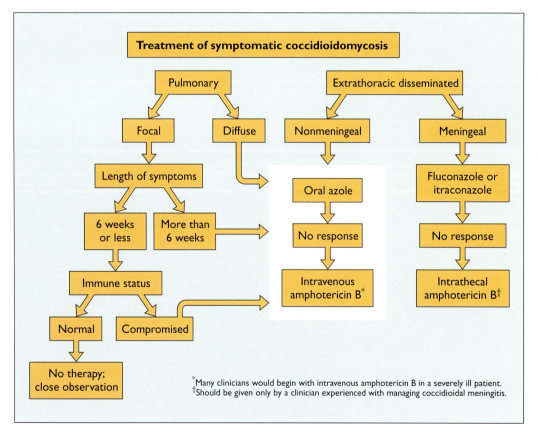

Figure 2-36. Treatment algorithm for coccidioidomycosis. The therapy of coccidioidomycosis is complex. For uncomplicated, primary pneumonia in a patient without any underlying immunodeficiency, close observation without specific antifungal therapy is often all that is required. Although amphotericin B was once the mainstay of therapy, it has been supplanted by the oral azoles, particularly the triazoles fluconazole and itraconazole, for many forms of disease. In particular, fluconazole and itraconazole essentially have replaced intrathecal injection of amphotericin B for the treatment of coccidioidal meningitis.

References

1. Pappagianis D: Epidemiology of coccidioidomycosis. In *Coccidioidomycosis*. Edited by Stevens DA. New York: Plenum Medical Book Company; 1980:63–85.
2. Edwards PQ, Palmer CE: Prevalence of sensitivity to coccidioidin, with special reference to specific and nonspecific reactions to coccidioidin and to histoplasmin. *Dis Chest* 1957, 13:35–60.
3. Ochoa AG: Coccidioidomycosis in Mexico. In *Coccidioidomycosis: Papers from the Second Symposium on Coccidioidomycosis*. Edited by Ajello L. Tucson, AZ: The University of Arizona Press; 1967:293–299.
4. Pappagianis D, Zimmer BL: Serology of coccidioidomycosis. *Clin Microbiol Rev* 1990, 3:247–268.
5. Snyder LS, Galgiani JN: Coccidioidomycosis: the initial pulmonary infection and beyond. *Semin Respir Crit Care Med* 1997, 18:235–246.
6. Galgiani JN: Coccidioidomycosis. *West J Med* 1993, 159:153–171.
7. Lund PJ, Chan KM, Unger EC, *et al.*: Magnetic resonance imaging in coccidioidal meningitis. *Skeletal Radiol* 1996, 25:661–665.
8. Pappagianis D: Current and future approaches to the diagnosis of coccidioidomycosis. In *Coccidioidomycosis: Proceedings of the 5th International Conference on Coccidioidomycosis*. Edited by Einstein HE, Catanzaro A. Washington, DC: National Foundation for Infectious Diseases; 1996:116–128.
9. Pappagianis D: Coccidioides immitis. In *Topley & Wilson's Microbiology and Microbial Infections* vol 4, edn 9. Edited by Ajello L, Hays RJ, Collier L, *et al*. London: Arnold; 1998:357–371.
10. Pappagianis D: Coccidioidomycosis. In *Laboratory Diagnosis of Infectious Diseases: Principles and Practice* vol 1. Edited by Balows A, Hausler WJ, Ohashi M, Turano A. New York: Springer Verlag; 1988:618.

Selected Bibliography

Drutz DJ, Catanzaro A: Coccidioidomycosis: parts I and II. *Am Rev Respir Dis* 1978, 117:559–585, 727–771.

Galgiani JN: Coccidioidomycosis. *West J Med* 1993, 159:153–171.

Pappagianis D: Epidemiology of coccidioidomycosis. *Curr Top Med Mycol* 1988, 2:199–238.

Pappagianis D, Zimmer BL: Serology of coccidioidomycosis. *Clin Microbiol Rev* 1990, 3:247–268.

Stevens DA: Coccidioidomycosis. *N Engl J Med* 1995, 332:1077–1082.

CHAPTER 3

Blastomycosis

Peter G. Pappas

Fungal Infections

Originally described in 1894 by Gilchrist [1], blastomycosis is an important pyogranulomatous systemic mycosis caused by *Blastomyces dermatitidis*. In his initial description, Gilchrist categorized the organism as a protozoan, but later recognized the organism as a fungus. Although it is now understood that most cases of blastomycosis result from inhalation of infectious spores, early cases were perceived to be a primary dermatologic disorder. It was not until the early 1950s that the concept of primary pulmonary blastomycosis with secondary dissemination to extrapulmonary sites was adopted, largely based on the clinical and pathologic observations of Schwartz and Baum [2].

Blastomycosis is endemic to much of the eastern United States, especially the south central and midwestern regions. It also occurs in Canada and has been reported in Central and South America, Western Europe, and Africa [3,4]. The spectrum of disease is quite broad. Primary infection usually occurs through inhalation of aerosolized infectious spores, which may lead to acute pneumonitis. Rarely, acute infection results in rapidly progressive pneumonia and respiratory compromise. In its chronic form, pneumonia is the most common clinical presentation of blastomycosis and may mimic neoplasms or other granulomatous infections clinically and radiographically [4,5]. Extrapulmonary involvement of the skin, bone, and male genitourinary tract are common, usually occurring with concomitant pulmonary involvement [4]. Itraconazole is the oral antifungal of choice for most cases of mild to moderate disease [6], whereas amphotericin B generally is given to patients with life-threatening disease and central nervous system involvement. Blastomycosis can be severe in immunocompromised patients, and early diagnosis and aggressive intervention are essential for a good outcome [7,8]. This chapter focuses on some of the important microbiologic, clinical, diagnostic, and therapeutic aspects of this disease.

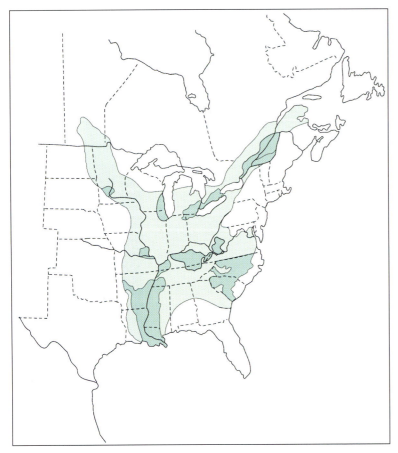

FIGURE 3-1. Map of areas endemic for blastomycosis. Blastomycosis, like the other endemic mycoses, is predominantly an infection of the western hemisphere. Some disease activity is seen in Africa, but the vast majority of cases come from the United States and Canada. Blastomycosis is coendemic with histoplasmosis over much of the central United States east of the Mississippi River. Disease activity extends northward across northern Wisconsin and Minnesota and into south central Canada. (*Darker shaded areas* denote higher disease activity.) (*Adapted from* Rippon [9].)

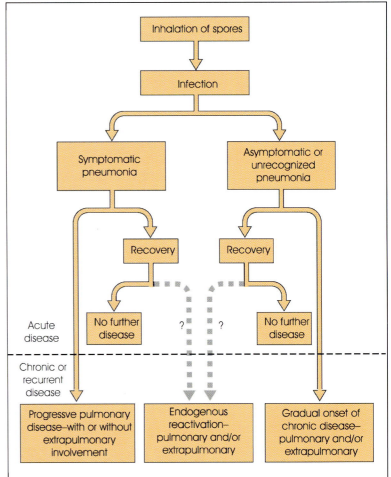

FIGURE 3-2. Clinical classification of blastomycosis. This is a schematic representation of the clinical course of blastomycosis following exposure to inhaled spores. The majority of patients have clinically inapparent primary infection. (*Adapted from* Sarosi and Davies [3].)

Clinical Manifestations of Blastomycosis	
Sites of Involvement	%
Pulmonary Lobar pneumonia, pulmonary masses, diffuse infiltrates	60–70
Cutaneous Ulcerations, nodules, subcutaneous abscesses	40–50
Osteoarticular Osteomyelitis, septic arthritis	10–15
Genitourinary Prostatitis, prostate abscess	10
Central nervous system Brain abscess, chronic meningitis	<10

FIGURE 3-3. Clinical manifestations of blastomycosis. In many patients, involvement of multiple organ systems (*eg*, lungs, skin, bone) is seen.

Diagnosis of Blastomycosis	
Histopathology	8–15-µm single budding yeast, with broad-based budding, multiple nuclei, doubly refractive cell wall
Special stains	Potassium chloride stain, Gomori's methenamine silver stain, periodic acid–Schiff stain
Culture	Saboraud's media; may require up to 6 wk for growth
Serology	Generally not helpful diagnostically; more specific and sensitive assays for protein A may be useful in the future
Skin tests	Unreliable, possibly useful in epidemiologic studies

FIGURE 3-4. Diagnosis of blastomycosis. The diagnosis of blastomycosis is usually suggested by finding characteristic yeast forms from clinical specimens. The diagnosis is confirmed once *Blastomycosis dermatitidis* has been isolated in culture.

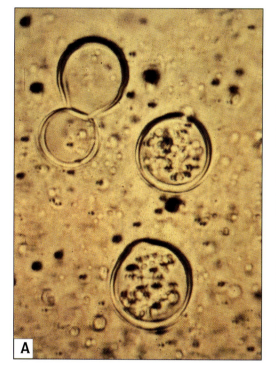
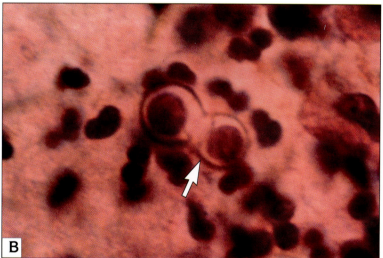
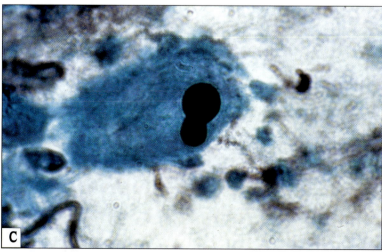

FIGURE 3-5. Histopathology of blastomycosis. **A,** Sputum potassium hydroxide (KOH) preparation showing the characteristic appearance of *Blastomyces dermatitidis*. Among patients producing purulent sputum, 60% to 70% will have positive sputum smears by KOH, Gomori's methenamine silver (GMS), or Periodic acid–Schiff (PAS) stains. Cultures are usually positive. The organism is large, 8 to 15 µm, and has a highly characteristic morphology on KOH and PAS stains. Budding is broad based, the cell wall is doubly refractive, and multiple nuclei are seen. These organisms can be seen in any involved site and are highly suggestive of blastomycosis. **B,** PAS stain of the sputum from a patient with pulmonary blastomycosis. Note the dense staining of the cell wall (*arrow*) and the multiple intracellular nuclei. **C,** GMS stain of bronchoalveolar lavage fluid in a patient with pulmonary blastomycosis. In this case, the GMS stain does not allow one to distinguish clearly from other budding yeasts such as *Candida* species and *Cryptococcus neoformans*. (Panel A *from* Sarosi and Davies [3]; with permission.)

PULMONARY BLASTOMYCOSIS

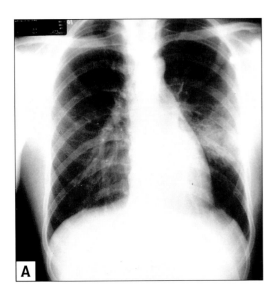
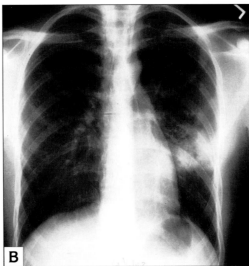
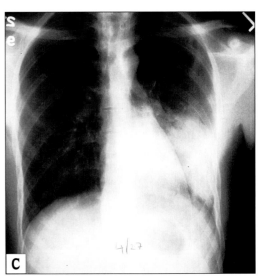
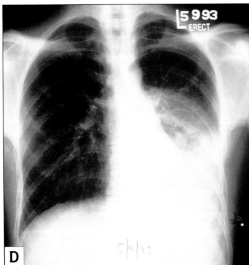
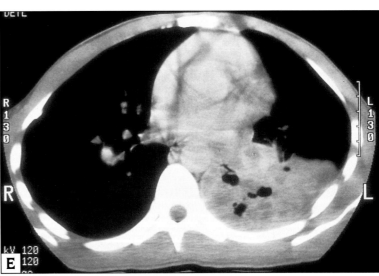

FIGURE 3-6. Series of chest radiographs and chest CT scan showing pulmonary blastomycosis. A 23-year-old man with chronic schizophrenia who rarely left his home developed a left lower lobe pneumonia, which was believed to be a result of aspiration but was unresponsive to conventional oral antimicrobial therapy. After several weeks of unsuccessful therapy, characterized by persistent fever, nonproductive cough, and progressive infiltrate on chest radiograph, he was admitted for evaluation and bronchoscopy. Yeast forms consistent with *Blastomyces dermatitidis* were seen on Gomori's methenamine silver stain, and cultures confirmed a diagnosis of blastomycosis. **A**, Chest radiograph from March 1993 reveals a superior segment left upper lobe infiltrate. **B** and **C**, Similar studies from April 1993 reveal progression of the infiltrate. **D**, Chest radiograph from May 1993 shows continued progression of infiltrate and suggests a left pleural effusion. **E**, CT scan of the chest from May 1993 confirms a dense left lower lobe infiltrate with multiple areas of necrosis and a small effusion.

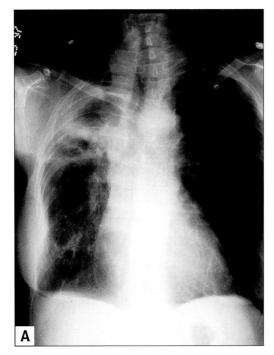
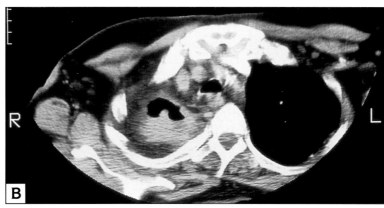

FIGURE 3-7. Pulmonary blastomycosis in a 35-year-old man with chronic cough, weight loss, and a right upper lobe cavitary infiltrate reminiscent of pulmonary tuberculosis. **A,** Radiograph showing pulmonary blastomycosis. The diagnosis of blastomycosis was suspected on the basis of a positive potassium hydroxide sputum sample and subsequently was confirmed with a positive culture. Blastomycosis may resemble tuberculosis clinically and radiographically. It also commonly resembles pulmonary malignancy with solitary or multiple mass lesions. Pleural effusion is uncommon among normal hosts. **B,** Chest computed tomography scan of the same patient demonstrates dense consolidation of the right upper lobe with significant necrosis and cavity formation. No other significant abnormalities were seen.

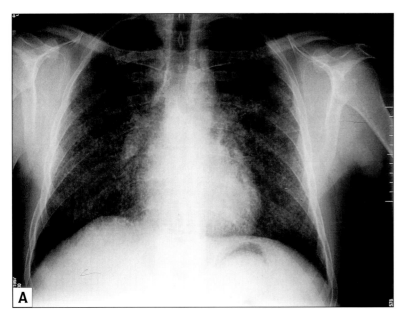
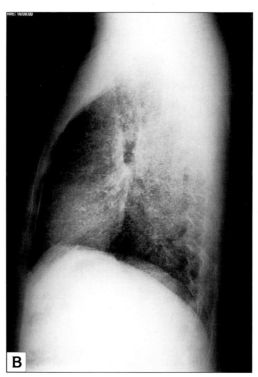

FIGURE 3-8. Posteroanterior (**A**) and lateral (**B**) chest radiographs showing miliary blastomycosis. A 38-year-old man, who was otherwise healthy, was complaining of increasing dyspnea, nonproductive cough, and fever. Findings revealed a miliary pattern most compatible with tuberculosis. Transbronchial biopsy and culture confirmed a diagnosis of blastomycosis. Miliary pulmonary disease with blastomycosis is rare among normal hosts, as is adult respiratory distress syndrome [10]. A high index of suspicion, early diagnosis, and early aggressive therapy are essential for a successful outcome.

CUTANEOUS BLASTOMYCOSIS

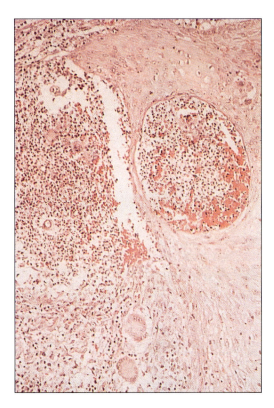

FIGURE 3-9. Histopathologic features of blastomycosis in skin biopsy. Blastomycosis causes a mixed pyogenic and granulomatous tissue response. The skin biopsy specimen shows giant cells but also small microabscesses containing neutrophils within both the epithelium and dermis. (Hematoxylin-eosin stain; original magnification, × 400.) (*From* Salfelder *et al.* [11]; with permission.)

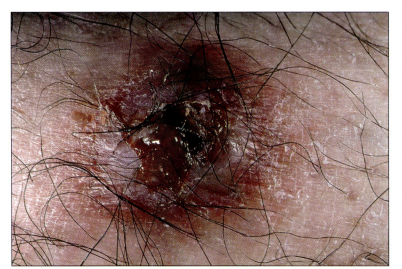

FIGURE 3-10. Dermatologic manifestations of cutaneous blastomycosis. Subcutaneous nodules with suppuration are one of the three main dermatologic manifestations of cutaneous blastomycosis. Most lesions are painful and may occur anywhere on the skin surface. Untreated nodules will suppurate, drain, and possibly develop into ulcerative lesions. Other clinical manifestations include proliferative, plaquelike lesions and chronic ulcerative lesions. Cutaneous lesions do not resolve spontaneously and tend to progress unless treated with systemic antifungal therapy.

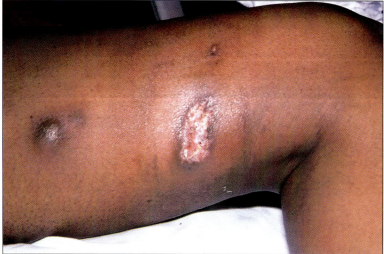

FIGURE 3-11. Subcutaneous nodular and ulcerative lesions. A subcutaneous nodular thigh lesion (proximal) and a lesion that has become ulcerative (distal) demonstrate the natural evolution of progressive cutaneous blastomycosis.

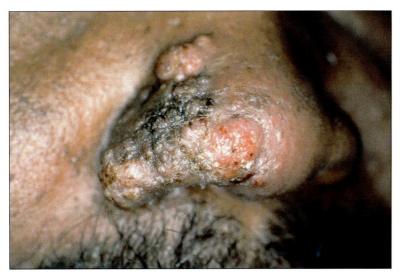

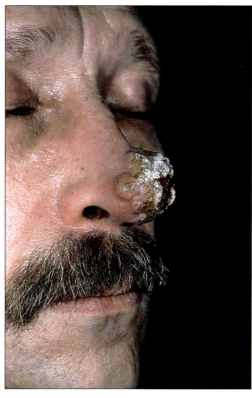

FIGURE 3-12. Verrucous lesions. Proliferative, verrucous lesions are a common manifestation of blastomycosis and typically occur on the face and other sun-exposed areas. Lesions frequently are misdiagnosed as cutaneous malignancies or common warts. Other deep mycoses, especially cryptococcosis, paracoccidioidomycosis, and coccidioidomycosis, can present similarly. Biopsy of the lesion is diagnostic on histopathology, and culture is almost always positive for *Blastomyces dermatitidis*.

FIGURE 3-13. Proliferative, verrucous nasal lesions of blastomycosis. This patient had concomitant pulmonary, bony, and prostatic involvement with *Blastomyces dermatitidis*.

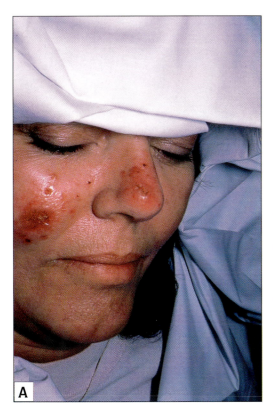

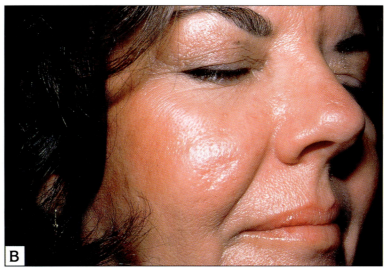

FIGURE 3-14. Lesions of the nose and malar region in a patient with blastomycosis. The patient is shown prior to therapy (**A**) and following completion of 6 months' therapy with itraconazole (**B**). Note that the lesions are ulcerative and erythematous and began as small pustules. These lesions were painful and originally believed to represent either bacterial cellulitis or rosacea.

Fungal Infections

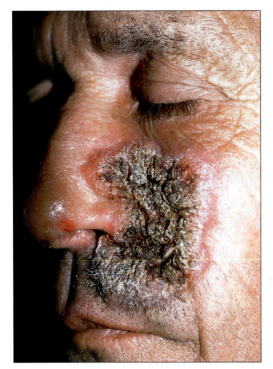

FIGURE 3-15. Proliferative, plaquelike facial lesion in a patient with pulmonary and cutaneous blastomycosis. The patient was originally believed to have squamous cell carcinoma. Biopsy of the lesion revealed findings of pyogranulomatous inflammation and organisms consistent with *Blastomyces dermatitidis*.

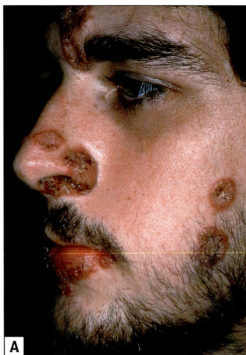 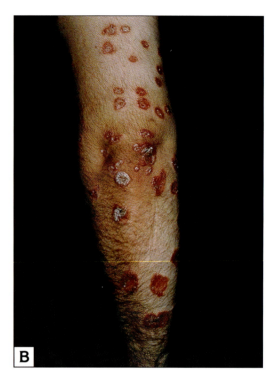

FIGURE 3-16. Disseminated cutaneous blastomycosis. Shallow ulcerations diffusely involved the face (**A**) and extremities (**B**). Lesions also were present on the trunk and abdomen. The patient initially was treated for varicella. Cutaneous blastomycosis often is mistaken for other disorders, especially pyoderma gangrenosum, nocardiosis, nontuberculous mycobacteria, and other invasive fungal diseases.

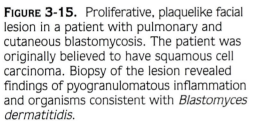

Differential Diagnosis of Cutaneous Blastomycosis

Sporotrichosis
Cryptococcosis
Histoplasmosis
Coccidioidomycosis
Paracoccidioidomycosis
Mycobacterium tuberculosis
Nontuberculous mycobacteria
  (esp. *Mycobacterium marinum, Mycobacterium chelonei*)
Nocardiosis (esp. *Nocardia brasiliensis*)
Actinomycosis
Bacillus anthracis (anthrax)
Francisella tularensis (tularemia)
Pyoderma gangrenosum
Cutaneous malignancy

FIGURE 3-17. Differential diagnosis of cutaneous blastomycosis. A number of other fungal, mycobacterial, and bacterial pathogens may mimic cutaneous blastomycosis. These disorders are often indistinguishable clinically, such that biopsy and culture of chronic skin lesions is especially helpful in confirming a specific diagnosis.

OSTEOARTICULAR BLASTOMYCOSIS

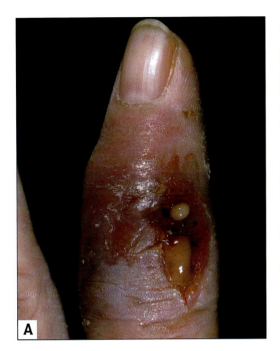
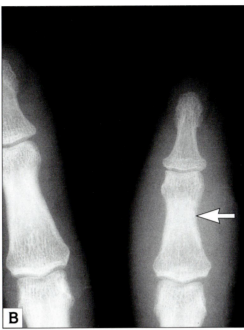

FIGURE 3-18. Osseous blastomycosis. The third most common site of involvement with *Blastomyces dermatitidis* are osseous sites. There is a predilection for long bones, vertebral bodies, and the skull, although any bone may be involved. A 43-year-old man has disseminated blastomycosis involving lung, skin, prostate, and bone. The middle phalanx of the left index finger is involved clinically (**A**) and radiographically (**B**). Note the subtle cortical bone erosion in the middle phalanx (*arrow*).

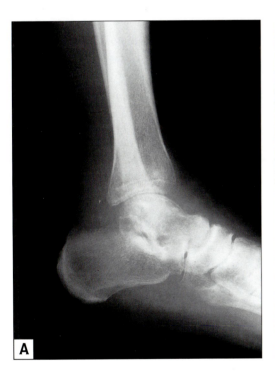
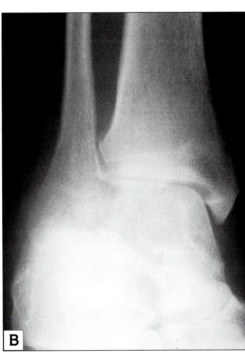

FIGURE 3-19. Destruction of the talus and a portion of the distal tibia due to osteoarticular blastomycosis. **A** and **B**, Articular involvement is demonstrated radiographically by the marked narrowing of the joint space. Also, note the osteopenia of the distal tibia. The patient required repeated surgical debridement and 1 year of antifungal therapy to achieve cure.

OTHER FORMS OF BLASTOMYCOSIS

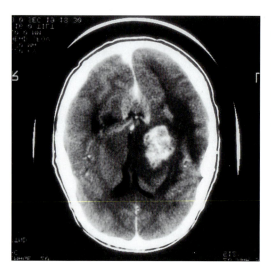

FIGURE 3-20. Central nervous system (CNS) blastomycosis. CNS blastomycosis is seen in less than 10% of otherwise normal patients [12,13]. In patients with significant underlying illness (*eg*, chronic glucocorticosteroids, AIDS), as many as 40% may have CNS involvement [7,8]. CNS blastomycosis generally presents with intraparenchymal brain lesions or chronic meningitis. The diagnosis of both forms requires histopathologic examination or culture unless the diagnosis can be established at a non-CNS site. This patient was a 50-year-old man who had diabetes mellitus and a history of pulmonary blastomycosis and was treated successfully with ketoconazole. Six months after completion of therapy with ketoconazole, the patient developed progressive right hemiparesis, and a mass lesion was discovered in the left basal ganglia. An open biopsy revealed organisms consistent with *Blastomyces dermatitidis*.

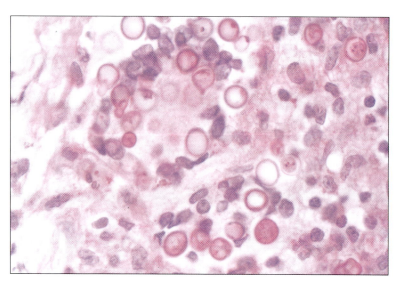

FIGURE 3-21. Meningeal biopsy results revealing *Blastomyces dermatitidis*. A 70-year-old woman with polymyalgia rheumatica who was receiving chronic steroids presented with headache, altered mental status, fever, and focal cranial nerve findings. The patient died despite receiving antifungal therapy. At autopsy, a small focus of pulmonary blastomycosis was found.

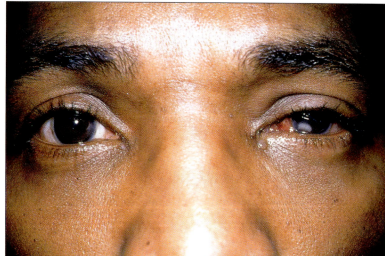

FIGURE 3-22. Ocular blastomycosis. A rare consequence of blastomycosis, ocular involvement has dire consequences often resulting in blindness. Definitive therapy may require enucleation in patients unresponsive to antifungal therapy. This 40-year-old man had a blastomycoma involving the left iris and left choroidal involvement in addition to pulmonary and cutaneous disease. His disease responded to intravenous and intravitreal antifungal therapy. (*From* Lopez *et al*. [14]; with permission.)

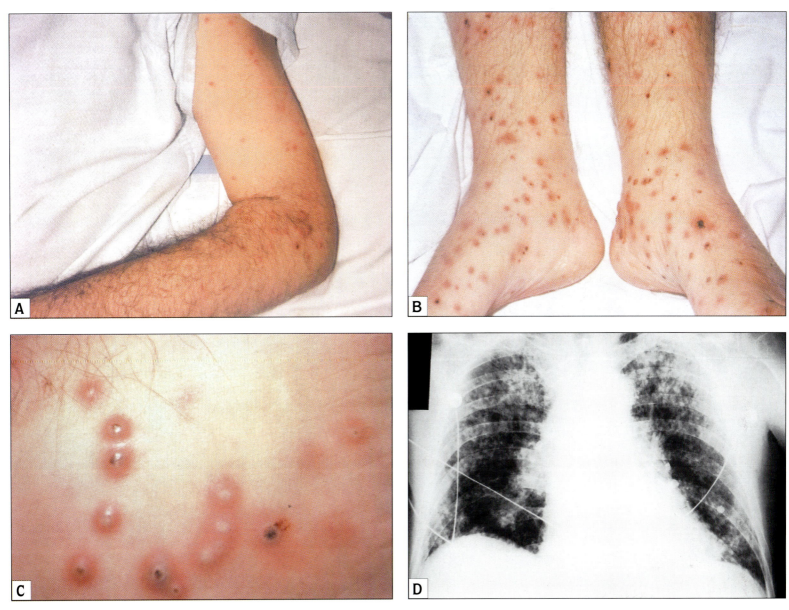

Figure 3-23. Disseminated blastomycosis is an immunocompromised patient. Although traditionally not closely associated with underlying defects of cell-mediated immunity, blastomycosis increasingly has been seen in patients with altered host immunity [8]. As many as 25% of patients in a recent series had some significant defect in host immunity. Patients with blastomycosis do less well than their otherwise healthy counterparts; mortality, multiple organ involvement, central nervous system involvement, and adult respiratory distress syndrome (ARDS) are all substantially more common in these patients. Early diagnosis and aggressive therapy are essential for a successful outcome in these patients. A patient who had underlying lymphoma on cytotoxic chemotherapy and glucocorticosteroids presented with disseminated cutaneous pustular lesions particularly involving the arms (**A**) and legs (**B**). **C**, A closer view of these lesions reveals vesiculopustular lesions, which are atypical for blastomycosis. **D**, A chest radiograph revealed diffuse interstitial infiltrates with ARDS. *Blastomyces dermatitidis* was isolated from skin lesions and sputum.

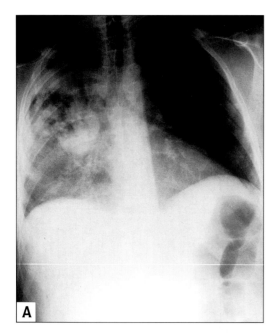
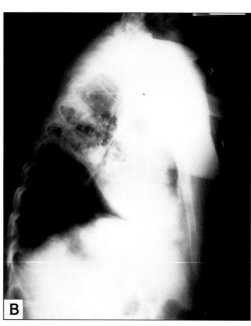
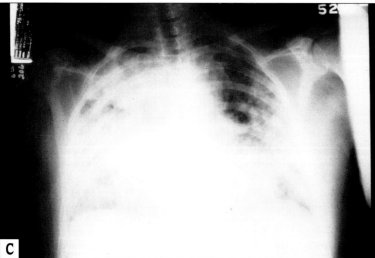

Figure 3-24. Pulmonary blastomycosis in an immunocompromised patient. One of the hallmarks of blastomycosis in immunocompromised patients is rapid progression of disease and development of respiratory failure from overwhelming disease and adult respiratory distress syndrome. This patient was a 20-year-old man with glioblastoma multiforme who had been receiving high-dose dexamethasone for months. Chest radiograph on admission revealed a right lung infiltrate (**A**), which on lateral radiograph appears to be localized to the right upper and right middle lobes (**B**). **C**, Within days, the process had progressed to involve both lungs diffusely, and the patient died despite receiving aggressive antimicrobial therapy. A diagnosis of diffuse pulmonary blastomycosis was made at autopsy.

Guidelines for Treatment of Various Forms of Blastomycosis

Type of Disease	Preferred Treatment	Alternative Treatment
Pulmonary*		
Life threatening	Amphotericin B, 1.5–2.5 g total	Initiate amphotericin and switch to itraconazole after patient's condition has stabilized
Non–life threatening	Itraconazole, 200–400 mg/d†	Ketoconazole, 400–800 mg/d *or* Fluconazole, 400–800 mg/d
Disseminated (CNS)	Amphotericin B, at least 2 g total	In patients unable to tolerate a full course of amphotericin B, consider fluconazole, 800 mg/d
Disseminated (non-CNS)		
Life threatening	Amphotericin B, 1.5–2.5 g total	Initiate amphotericin and switch to itraconazole after patient's condition has stabilized
Non–life threatening	Itraconazole, 200–400 mg/d‡	Ketoconazole, 400–800 mg/d *or* Fluconazole, 400–800 mg/d
Immunocompromised hosts	Amphotericin B, 1.5–2.5 g	After a primary course of amphotericin B, suppressive therapy should be continued with itraconazole, 200–400 mg/d. In patients who have CNS disease or are unable to tolerate itraconazole, consider fluconazole, 400–800 mg/d
Special circumstances		
Pregnant women	Amphotericin B, 1.5–2.5 g total	
Children	Amphotericin B, ≥30 mg/kg total *or* Itraconazole, 5–7 mg/kg	

*Some patients with acute pulmonary infection may have a spontaneous cure. Thus, patients with mild disease involving only the lungs may be monitored closely for resolution. Patients with progressive pulmonary disease should be treated.

†Treatment with an azole should be continued for a minimum of 6 mo.

‡Patients with bone disease should be treated with an azole for 12 mo.

CNS—central nervous system.

FIGURE 3-25. Guidelines for treatment of various forms of blastomycosis. Therapy for treatment of blastomycosis varies, depending on anatomic site of involvement and the underlying immunologic status of the patient [6,15–18].

REFERENCES

1. Gilchrist TC: Protozoan dermatitis. *J Cutan Gen Dis* 1984, 12:496–499.
2. Schwartz J, Baum GL: Blastomycosis. *Am J Clin Pathol* 1951, 21:999–1029.
3. Sarosi GA, Davies SF: Blastomycosis. *Am Rev Resp Dis* 1979, 120:911–938.
4. Bradsher RW: Blastomycosis. *Infect Dis Clin North Am* 1988, 2:877–898.
5. Abernathy RS: Clinical manifestations of pulmonary blastomycosis. *Ann Intern Med* 1959, 51:707–727.
6. Dismukes WE, Bradsher RW, Cloud GC, *et al.*: Itraconazole therapy for blastomycosis and histoplasmosis. *Am J Med* 1992, 93:489–497.
7. Pappas PG, Pottage JC, Powderly WG, *et al.*: Blastomycosis in patients with the acquired immunodeficiency syndrome. *Ann Intern Med* 1992, 116:847–853.
8. Pappas PG, Threlkeld MG, Bedsole GD, *et al.*: Blastomycosis in immunocompromised patients. *Medicine* 1993, 72:311–325.
9. Rippon JW: *Medical Mycology: The Pathogenic Fungi and the Pathogenic Actinomycetes*, edn 3. Philadelphia: WB Saunders; 1988.
10. Meyer KC, McManus EJ, Maki DG: Overwhelming pulmonary blastomycosis associated with the adult respiratory distress syndrome. *N Engl J Med* 1993, 329:1231–1236.
11. Salfeder K, deLiscano TR, Sauerteig E: *Atlas of Fungal Pathology*, vol 17. Boston: Kluwer Academic Publishers; 1990.
12. Gonyea EF: The spectrum of primary blastomycotic meningitis: a review of central nervous system blastomycosis. *Ann Neurol* 1978, 3:26–39.
13. Buechner HA, Clawson CM: Blastomycosis of the central nervous system, II: a report of nine cases from the Veterans Administration Cooperative Study. *Am Rev Respir Dis* 1967, 95:820–826.
14. Lopez R, Mason JO, Parker JS, Pappas PG: Intraocular blastomycosis: case report and review. *Clin Infect Dis* 1994, 18:805–807.
15. NIAID: Treatment of blastomycosis and histoplasmosis with ketoconazole: results of a prospective randomized clinical trial. *Ann Intern Med* 1985, 103:861–872.
16. Mangino JE, Pappas PG: Itraconazole for the treatment of histoplasmosis and blastomycosis. *Internat J Antimicrob Agents*, 1995, 5:219–225.
17. Pappas PG, Bradsher RW, Kauffman CA, *et al.*: Treatment of blastomycosis with higher dose fluconazole. *Clin Infect Dis* 1997, 25:200–205.
18. Chapman SW, Bradsher RW, Campbell GD, *et al.*: Practice guidelines for the management of patients with blastomycosis. *Clin Infect Dis* 2000, 30:679–683.

CHAPTER 4

Paracoccidioidomycosis

Arnaldo Lopes Colombo
Flavio Queiroz-Telles
John R. Graybill

Fungal Infections

Paracoccidioidomycosis, previously known as South American blastomycosis or Lutz, Splendore, and Almeida disease, is a subacute to chronic granulomatous fungal infection caused by *Paracoccidioides brasiliensis*, a thermally dimorphic fungus. Originally described in 1908 by Lutz [1], paracoccidioidomycosis is the most prevalent systemic endemic mycosis in many countries in Latin America. It is believed that the disease is acquired by respiratory route [2, 3]. The primary pulmonary infection in most of the cases is inapparent or olygosymptomatic, but later it can disseminate, involving many organs, especially mucous and cutaneous tissue, lymph nodes, adrenals, and the central nervous system [4, 5].

Geographic Distribution

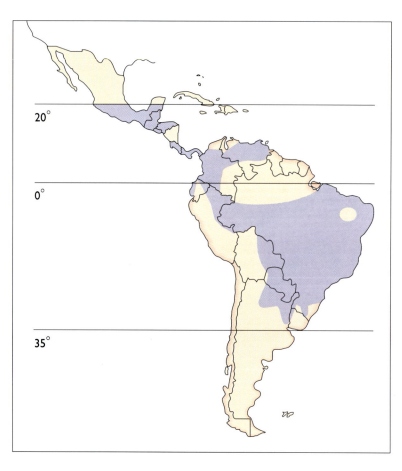

Figure 4-1. Geographic distribution of paracoccidioidomycosis (PCM). PCM, previously known as South American blastomycosis or Lutz disease, is the most frequent endemic systemic mycosis in Latin America. Except for Chile, Guyanas, Surinam, and some Caribbean islands, PCM has been reported from Mexico to Argentina [6]. Most of the cases have been reported in Brazil, Colombia, and Venezuela. Nonautochthonous cases have been reported outside the endemic area; however, all of these patients previously had lived in Latin America [7,8]. Therefore, PCM should be regarded as a disease of travelers who have lived for extended periods in endemic areas. (*Adapted from* Wanke and Londero [6].)

LIFE CYCLE AND ECOEPIDEMIOLOGY

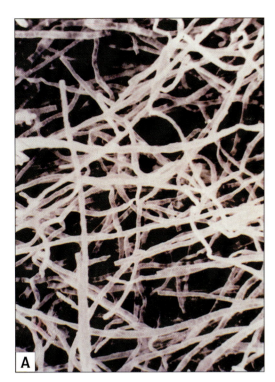 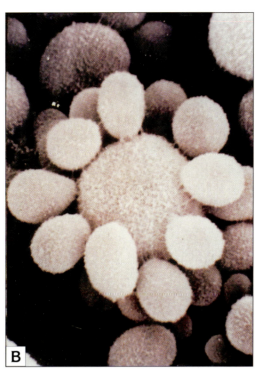

FIGURE 4-2. Mycology of paracoccidioidomycosis (PCM). PCM is caused by a dimorphic fungus, *Paracoccidioides brasiliensis*. Its perfect (sexual) phase has not been identified. Dimorphism of *P. brasiliensis* appears to be regulated by temperature, nutrients, and oxygen. **A,** In nature and in cultures maintained at room temperature, the fungus grows in the mycelial form, which is represented by septate and dychotomously branching hyalo hyphae [9]. Mycelia form different types of conidia, including arthroconidia, which are believed to be the infectious propagule. **B,** The yeast form (5 to 30 μm in diameter) is found in cultures incubated at 37°C as well as in tissue and body fluids. The characteristic morphology of the yeast phase of *P. brasiliensis* is a mother cell surrounded by several blastoconidia [9]. The outermost cell wall layer of the multiple budding cells is composed mainly of an α-1,3-glucan, in contrast to mycelial cell walls, which have an outer β-1,3-glucan layer. Earlier studies suggested that the α-1,3-glucan fibrils correlate with the fungal virulence and pathogenicity, playing an important role in the pathogenesis of PCM [10]. However, these conclusions have been challenged by other investigators, who suggest that other factors may be involved in the host–parasite relationship [4,11]. Until recently, humans were considered the natural host for *P. brasiliensis*. Evidence is mounting that armadillos may be naturally infected by *P. brasiliensis* in endemic areas [12]. The role of this finding in the ecoepidemiology of this mycosis is not yet completely understood. (*From* Queiroz-Telles [9]; with permission.)

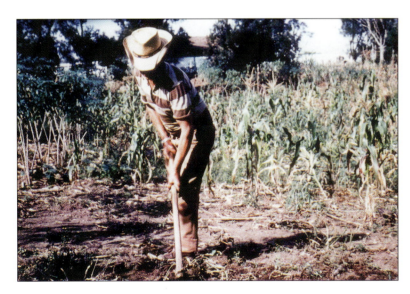

FIGURE 4-3. Risk groups for paracoccidioidomycosis (PCM). Rural workers have the greatest rate of infection with *Paracoccidioides brasiliensis*. The fungus has been sporadically isolated from soil of some endemic areas. In adults with chronic PCM, the disease is clearly prevalent among men between the ages of 30 and 60 years. Data collected from different countries show rates of incidence ranging from 10 to 70 men for each woman. β-Estradiol seems to protect infected women from the disease. Consequently, this difference of prevalence between genders is not reported among prepubescent individuals. PCM is contained by cell-mediated immunity, and cases rarely have been reported among patients with AIDS or cancer or those who have undergone organ transplantations [4,5,13].

Pathophysiology

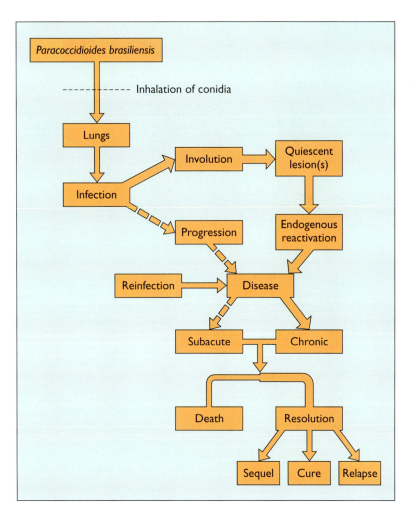

Figure 4-4. Natural history of paracoccidioidomycosis. Experimental and clinical data support the inhalation route of infection as the main portal of entry for *P. brasiliensis*, although entry of organism through the skin, mucous membranes, and gastrointestinal tract has also been suggested. After infection, the progression to clinically apparent disease depends on virulence of the strain, inoculum size, and the status of the host defense mechanisms. In a competent host, fungal growth is contained, and resolution of the infection usually occurs without any signs or symptoms. In this situation, scars formed at the primary and methastatic focus may contain viable quiescent forms of the fungus. After a long period of time, following changes in the host–parasite balance due to conditions not clearly defined, the infection may progress and give rise to full-blown disease. Less frequently, the disease also may arise from a primary focus without a latency period or by reinfection of the host in an endemic area. Once established, acute or chronic clinical forms may develop. Most patients respond to therapy, but incapacitating residual lesions and relapses frequently occur. *Solid arrows* indicate most common course; *dashed arrows* indicate less common course [3,5,14].

Clinical Manifestations

Classification of Clinical Forms

Paracoccidioidomycosis infection
Paracoccidioidomycosis disease
   Acute or subacute form (juvenile type)
   Chronic form (adult type)
      Unifocal
      Multifocal
Residual forms (sequel)

Figure 4-5. Classification of clinical forms. The primary infection, almost always devoid of clinical manifestations, is recognized by a positive paracoccidioidin intradermal test or by finding *Paracoccidioides brasiliensis* in partially calcified lesions from patients with no clinical evidence of this mycosis. The disease may evolve into two different clinical patterns: the acute (or subacute) form and the chronic form. The acute form usually is seen in children and young adults under 30 years of age (juvenile type) and represents not more than 5% to 10% of all cases of paracoccidioidomycosis. Involvement of the monocytic phagocytic system results in the most common clinical manifestation: systemic superficial and deep lymph node enlargement, sometimes accompanied by hepatosplenomegaly and bone marrow dysfunction. Eventually, skin involvement and multiple osteolytic lesions also are reported. In contrast, lung involvement with the chronic form rarely is seen. Signs and symptoms of the disease rapidly progress, and within weeks to a few months the patient's general condition is seriously impaired. This form also is seen in patients with AIDS. The chronic form affects mostly adult men. Signs and symptoms usually progress slowly, and the patients do not ask for health assistance until several months after the onset of the disease. Symptoms may be related to a single organ or system (unifocal) or to several organs (multifocal). The lungs, mucosa of the upper airway and digestive pathway, skin, lymph nodes, gut, adrenal glands, central nervous system organs, bones, and joints are usually involved. Other sites, such as the genital organs, eyes, thyroid, and organs of the cardiovascular system, are rarely compromised. The two most common sequels of the disease are chronic respiratory insufficiency and Addison's disease. Patients with AIDS may develop meningitis [3–5,14,15].

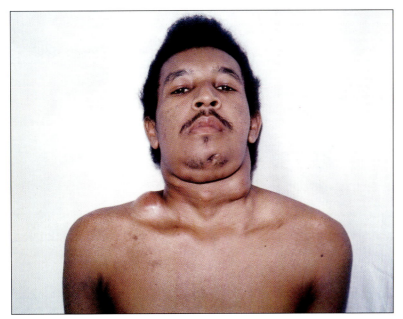

Figure 4-6. Cervical lymph node enlargement. This patient, a 23-year-old man, was admitted to the hospital with a 2-month history of fever, weight loss, and cervical, axillary, and inguinal lymph node enlargement. In the acute form of paracoccidioidomycosis, the patient may exhibit generalized remarkable lymphadenopathy. At the onset, lymph nodes are tender and have a fibroelastic consistency. As the disease progresses, the lymph nodes become necrotic, forming a coalescent inflammatory tumor as shown in the figure. Skin fistulas of the adjacent lymph nodes are also a common finding.

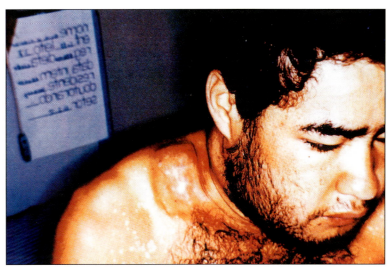

Figure 4-7. Syndrome of upper vena cava compression by paracoccidioidomycosis (PCM). Deep lymph node enlargement may cause compression of important surrounding structures, such as the bile duct or vena cava, inducing obstructive jaundice or syndrome of upper vena cava compression. This patient, a 27-year-old man, had an acute form of PCM that exhibited a supraclavicular, facial, and thoracic edema related to superior vena cava compression of lymph nodes. The macular hypochromic skin lesions were caused by *Malassezia furfur*.

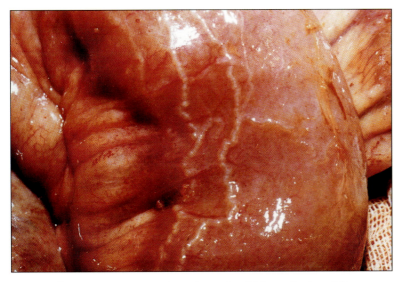

Figure 4-8. Intestinal lymphangiectasia. This patient, a 32-year-old man, had a clinical history of fever, weight loss, abdominal pain, vomiting, jaundice, and diarrhea for 3 months. This case was unusual because the patient's jaundice was related to a stenosis of the biliary tract caused by paracoccidioidomycosis (PCM). Jaundice in PCM is usually a consequence of biliary tract obstruction caused by enlarged surrounding lymph nodes. The patient's diarrhea (note the intense intestinal lymphangiectasia) was due to obstruction of the mesenteric lymphatic circulation. Laboratory investigation revealed hypoalbuminemia and reduced immunoglobulin and lymphocyte levels in the blood.

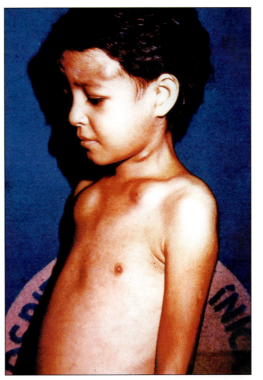

Figure 4-9. Paracoccidioidomycosis (PCM) in a 10-year-old boy. The patient presented with enlargement of multiple lymph nodes, fever, and weight loss. PCM rarely has been reported among patients less than 14 years of age; up to 3% of the patients in most of the studies are children. The disease occurs with equal frequency in both genders [16,17].

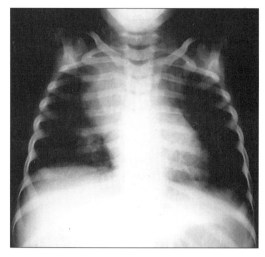

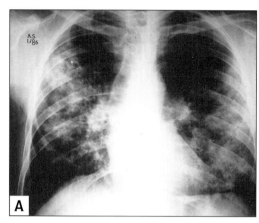
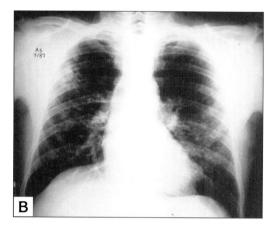

FIGURE 4-10. Chest radiograph from a 5-year-old patient with paracoccidioidomycosis (PCM). This patient showed striking mediastinal lymphadenopathy with no pulmonary infiltrates. In contrast to the chronic form of PCM, patients with the acute form of the disease rarely have clinical or radiographic evidence of lung involvement.

FIGURE 4-11. Radiographs showing lung involvement in paracoccidioidomycosis (PCM). Pulmonary disease is the most frequent manifestation of chronic PCM. Radiologic studies usually show bilateral lung involvement, frequently in the middle or lower lung fields. Bilateral reticulonodular or interstitial infiltrates, frequently involving nodular, micronodular, consolidated, and cavitary lesions may also be observed. Pleural effusions are very rare. Despite the severity of lung involvement documented by chest radiographs, patients usually have few symptoms. At first, some patients complain of dry or productive cough and dyspnea. Patients with advanced-stage disease may progress to respiratory insufficiency and cor pulmonale. Resolution of pulmonary lesions may lead to formation of bilateral fibrotic scars, which cause an obstructive or mixed pattern of pulmonary dysfunction with hypoxemia [18,19]. **A,** Chest radiograph of a patient with PCM taken before therapy was started. Areas of pneumonic infiltrate pattern of lung involvement can be seen. **B,** Chest radiograph from the same patient taken after 16 months of therapy. Residual fibrosis of the lungs is observed after treatment.

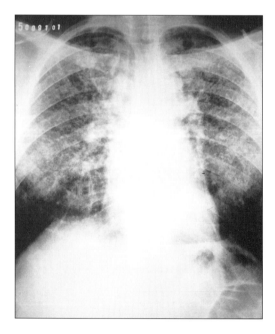

FIGURE 4-12. Reticulonodular pattern of lung paracoccidioidomycosis. Diffuse reticulonodular lung infiltrate due to paracoccidioidomycosis is shown.

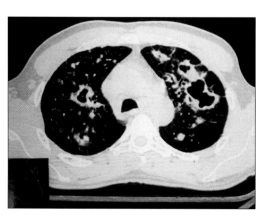

FIGURE 4-13. Chest CT scan from a 50-year-old man with cavitary lesions of both lungs. Differential diagnosis should include tuberculosis.

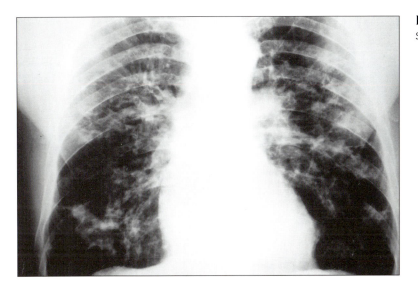

Figure 4-14. Fibrotic scars and areas of air retention (emphysema) as sequelae of paracoccidioidomycosis.

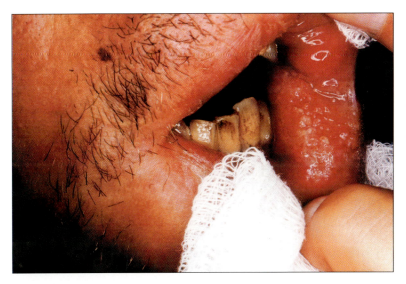

Figure 4-15. "Mulberry-like" stomatitis. Oropharyngeal lesions from hematogenous spreading of the fungus are very common in paracoccidioidomycosis (PCM). They were found in 50% of our 150 cases studied between 1986 and 1996. It is believed higher local pO_2 and lower temperature of the oropharyngeal mucosa provide better conditions for fungal growth. These environmental characteristics are probably more similar to those supporting saprobic growth of *Paracoccidioides brasiliensis*. Mucosal lesions also can be linked to transitory fungemia during systemic infections, when yeast cells can attach to previously damaged tissues in the oropharyngeal mucosa. Bacterial infections (caries, gingivitis, gingivostomatites), local trauma (dental prosthesis, plants fragments for tooth cleaning), and smoking all may cause local damage to the oral mucosa. Shown is an ulcerated lesion with fine granulation resembling a mulberry ("mulberry-like stomatitis"). These lesions are commonly found in patients with the chronic form of PCM, evolve slowly, and are painful.

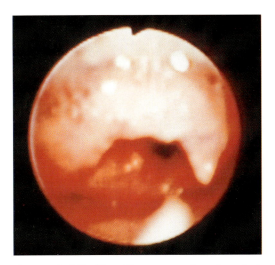

Figure 4-16. Nasofibroscopy showing destruction of the epiglottis. This patient had an extensive lesion of the hypopharynx and partial destruction of the epiglottis. Ulcerative mucous lesions may involve the oral cavity, tongue, oropharynx, hypopharynx, and larynx. Involvement of the pharynx usually causes pain on swallowing, which induces patients to decrease their food intake.

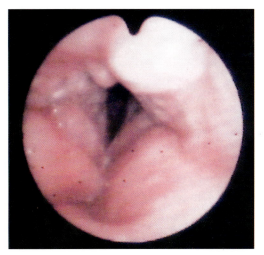

Figure 4-17. Nasofibroscopy showing a larynx lesion. This 34-year-old patient, had a history of 6 months of respiratory symptoms and 3 months of progressive dysphonia and dysphagia. Nasofibroscopy showed two nodular lesions of the vocal cords caused by paracoccidioidomycosis. Ulcerative mucous lesions of the larynx may damage the vocal cords, causing severe dysphonia. Potentially life-threatening upper respiratory tract obstruction may occur due to fibrosis after antifungal treatment.

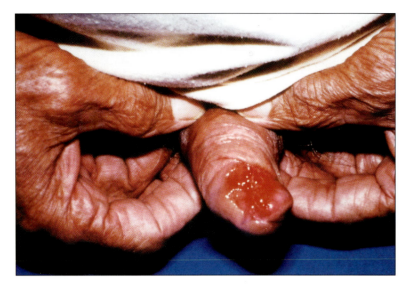

FIGURE 4-18. Genital lesion. Genital lesions are rare but focal lesions between the prostate and the penis have been reported. An ulcerated mucous membrane lesion in the glans of a 65-year-old man is shown. The lesion cleared completely after 3 months of therapy.

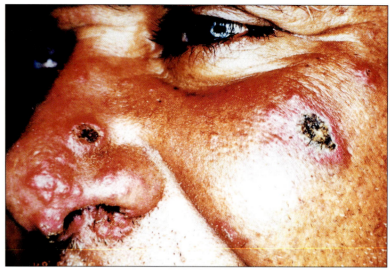

FIGURE 4-19. Papuloerythematous and ulcerated facial lesions in a 42-year-old. As many as 30% to 50% of patients with paracoccidiodomycosis have cutaneous lesions. The face is the most frequently affected. Skin lesions result from hematogenous spreading of *Paracoccidioides brasiliensis*. The lesions are polymorphic; papules, nodules, plaques, tumors, and ulcers may occur. Surfaces of the lesions may be erythematous, scaling, verrucous, or ulcerated. Some lesions may be secondarily infected by bacteria, resulting in purulent discharge.

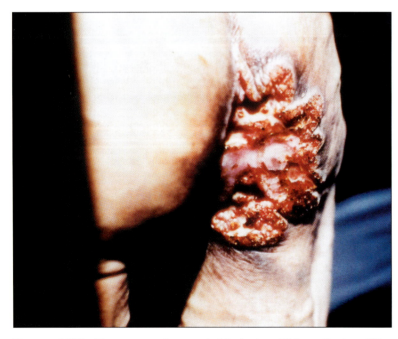

FIGURE 4-20. Tumorous ulcerated skin lesion. This patient, a 62-year-old man, presented with a large, ulcerated, tumorous lesion involving the buttocks and perineal area with severe bacterial superinfection.

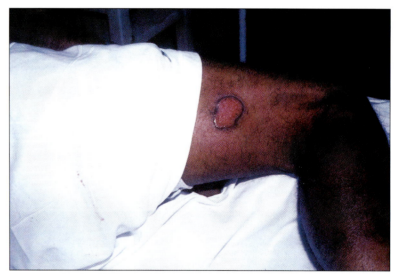

FIGURE 4-21. Plaque skin lesion. This figure shows a slightly ulcerated plaque-like lesion on the thigh of a 34-year-old male agricultural worker.

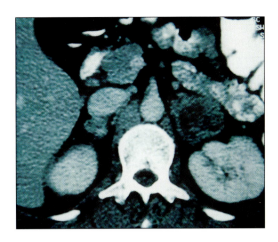

FIGURE 4-22. Abdominal CT scan of a patient with paracoccidioidomycosis (PCM), showing bilateral adrenal enlargement with clinical evidence of Addison's disease. Adrenal involvement is frequently documented in PCM. Postmortem studies report adrenal abnormalities in 40% to 80% of patients. Addison's disease has been reported as a common sequela of PCM. Sometimes, adrenal insufficiency may be the only clinical evidence of this systemic mycosis. Depending on the methodology applied by the investigator, the partial reduction of adrenocortical function among patients with PCM has ranged between 15% and 45% [20].

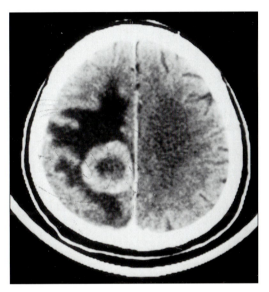

FIGURE 4-23. Cranial CT scan from a 45-year-old man with a progressive left hemiplegia due to a pseudotumoral form of neuroparacoccidioidomycosis. Involvement of the central nervous system by paracoccidioidomycosis (PCM) may be manifested by meningitis or, more frequently, parenchymal lesions. Clinical evidence of PCM in other organs or systems may be absent. Central nervous system lesions have been reported in up to 20% of patients in necropsy series. However, less than 5% of patients in clinical series have central nervous system involvement. Paracoccidioidomycotic meningitis has a chronic course. Neuroparacoccidioidomycosis most commonly occurs in the pseudotumoral form, with single or multiple lesions with mass effect causing sensory or motor deficits, seizures, mental status changes, and intracranial hypertension. Involvement of the brain stem, cerebellum, and spinal cord are less frequently reported than hemispheric lesions [21].

Differential Diagnosis of Paracoccidioidomycosis
Tuberculosis
Leishmaniasis
Cutaneous sporotrichosis
Chromoblastomycosis
Leprosy
Histoplasmosis
Malignant diseases

FIGURE 4-24. Differential diagnosis of paracoccidioidomycosis (PCM). PCM is a systemic disease with multiple manifestations. As a result, the differential diagnoses may vary according to the organ or system affected by *Paracoccidioides brasiliensis*. Pulmonary disease frequently is misinterpreted as tuberculosis. Depending on the pattern of skin lesions, the differential diagnosis should include leishmaniasis, cutaneous sporotrichosis, chromoblastomycosis, tuberculosis, leprosy, histoplasmosis, or neoplastic processes. Oropharyngeal PCM must be differentiated from leishmaniasis, tuberculosis, histoplasmosis, syphilis, and malignant diseases. The acute form of the disease is frequently misdiagnosed as a hematologic malignancy.

LABORATORY DIAGNOSIS

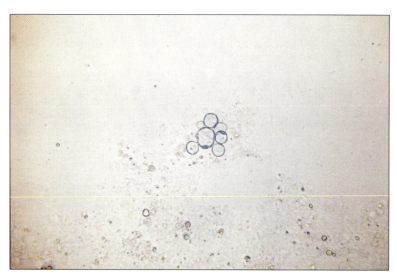

FIGURE 4-25. Fresh specimen examination of paracoccidioidomycosis (PCM). The diagnosis of PCM is based on positive cultures for *Paracoccidioides brasiliensis* or demonstration of characteristic yeast forms in tissue or body fluids. The mother cell surrounded by multiple narrow-necked buds may be recognized during direct examination of specimens (*shown*) from skin or mucosal lesions, sputum, and pus from draining lymph nodes. Fresh specimens are examined after digestion of potassium hydroxide. Specimens include cultured yeast extract and Sabouraud agars containing antibacterial agents and inhibitors of suprophytic molds. Specific serology may aid in the diagnosis of PCM, but its main clinical usefulness is in evaluating the clinical response of therapy [22].

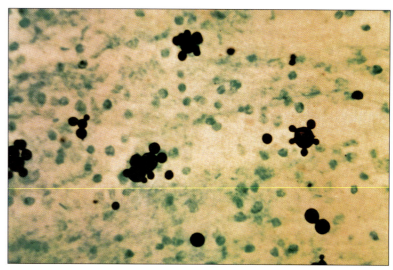

FIGURE 4-26. Histopathology of paracoccidioidomycosis. Histopathologic examination of tissues with hematoxylin-eosin, methanamine silver, and periodic acid–Schiff stains reveals a pyogranulomatous process with yeast elements. This figure shows yeasts with multiple buds stained by methanamine silver, exhibiting the characteristic "pilot wheel" appearance of *Paracoccidioides brasiliensis*.

Treatment of Paracoccidioidomycosis

Initial Treatment

Drug	Dosage	Duration of Treatment, *mo*
Itraconazole	200 mg/d	3
Ketoconazole	400 mg/d	6
Cotrimoxazole	Trimethoprim, 160 mg Sulfamethoxazole, 800 mg (orally or intravenously, 2 or 3 times a day)	6–9
Amphotericin B	1.5–2.0 g total dose	1–3

Maintenance Treatment

Drug	Dosage	Duration of Treatment
Itraconazole	100 mg/d	Variable
Ketoconazole	200 mg/d	Variable
Cotrimoxazole	Trimethoprim, 80 mg Sulfamethoxazole, 400 mg (orally, 2 times a day)	Variable

FIGURE 4-27. Treatment of paracoccidioidomycosis. Each of the drugs listed as therapeutic alternatives for the initial treatment of paracoccidioidomycosis are associated with good clinical response. The duration of initial treatment varies according to the severity of the case and the antifungal drug chosen. A significant remission of the clinical picture, failure to demonstrate fungal evidence in clinical specimens, and a decrease in the initial serologic titers are desired. Unfortunately, there is no randomized comparative study to evaluate the relative safety and efficacy of alternative regimens. However, data from open studies indicate that itraconazole has a remarkable therapeutic efficacy [23–24]. There is no clear scientific evidence to define the optimum duration of therapy. Treatment is continued until the criteria for cure have been met: clinical criteria include disappearance of signs and symptoms, except those resulting from sequelae; mycologic criteria include failure to isolate or observe the fungus in the clinical specimens; radiologic criteria include stabilization of the radiologic pattern (fibrosis) in a series of films periodically taken during maintenance therapy; and immunologic criteria include the conversion of the immunodiffusion test to negative or a decline to stable, low levels during maintenance therapy.

REFERENCES

1. Lutz A: Uma micose pseudococcídica localisada na boca e observada no Brasil. Contribuição ao conhecimento das hifoblastomicoses americanas. *Brasil Médico* 1908, 22: 141–44.

2. Londero AT, Ramos CD, Lopes JOS: The gamut of progressive pulmonary paracoccidioidomycosis. *Mycopathol* 1981. 75: 65–74.

3. McEwen JG, Bedoya V, Patino MM, *et al.*: Experimental murine paracoccidioidomycosis induced by the inhalation of conidia. *J Med Vet Mycol* 1987, 25:165.

4. Brummer E, Castaneda E, Restrepo A: Paracoccidioidomycosis: an update. *Clin Microbiol Rev* 1993, 6:89–117.

5. Negroni R: Paracoccidioidomycosis (South American blastomycosis, Lutz's mycosis). *Int J Dermatol* 1993, 32:847–859.

6. Wanke B, Londero AT: Epidemiology and Paracoccidioidomycosis infection. In *Paracoccidioidomycosis*. Edited by Franco M. Boca Raton: CRC Press; 1994:109–120.

7. Fujio J, Nishimura K, Miyaji M: Epidemiological survey of the imported mycoses in Japan. *Nippon Ishinkin Gakkai Zasshi* 1999, 40:103–109.

8. Silletti RP, Glezerov V, Schwartz IS: Pulmonary paracoccidioidomycosis misdiagnosed as Pneumocystis pneumonia in an immunocompromised host. *J Clin Microbiol* 1996, 34:2328–2330.

9. Queiroz-Telles F: *Paracoccidioides brasiliensis*. Ultrastructural findings. In Franco, M. *Paracoccidioidomycosis*. Edited by Franco M. Boca Raton: CRC Press;1994: 27–47.

10. San-Blas G, San-Blas F: *Paracoccidioides brasiliensis*: Cell wall and virulence: a review. *Mycopathologia* 1977, 62:77–86.

11. Zacharias D, Ueda A, Moscardi-Bacchi M, *et al.*: A comparative histopathological, immunological, and biochemical study of experimental intravenous paracoccidioidomycosis induced in mice by three *Paracoccidioides brasiliensis* isolates. *J Med Vet Mycol* 1986, 24:445–454.

12. Vergara ML, Martinez R: Role of the armadillo Dasypus novemcinctus in the epidemiology of paracoccidioidomycosis. *Mycopathologia* 1998-99, 144:131–133.

13. Restrepo A, Salazar ME, Cano LE, *et al.*: Estrogens inhibit mycelium-to-yeast transformation in the fungus *Paracoccidioides brasiliensis*: implications for resistance of females to paracoccidioidomycosis. *Infect Immun* 1984, 46:346–353.

14. Franco M., Mendes RP, Moscardi-Bacchi M, *et al.*: Paracoccidioidomycosis. In *Bailliere's Clinical Tropical Medicine and Comunicable Diseases. Tropical Fungal Infections*. London: Bailliere Tindall; 1989:185–220.

15. Goldani LZ, Sugar AM: Paracoccidioidomycosis and AIDS: an overview. *Clin Infect Dis* 1995, 21:1275–1281.

16. Londero AT, Melo IS: Paracoccidioidomycosis in childhood. A critical review. *Mycopathologia* 1983,82:49–55.

17. Fonseca ER, Pardal PP, Severo LC: Paracoccidioidomycosis in children in Belem, Para. *Rev Soc Bras Med Trop* 1999, 32:31–33.

18. Londero AT, Severo LC: The gamut of progressive pulmonary paracoccidioidomycosis. *Arch Med Res* 1995, 26:305–306.

19. Funari M, Kavakama J, Shikanai-Yasuda MA, *et al>*: Chronic pulmonary paracoccidioidomycosis (South American blastomycosis): high-resolution CT findings in 41 patients. *Am J Roentgenol* 1999, 173:59–64.

20. Colombo AL, Faical S, Kater CE: Systematic evaluation of the adrenocortical function in patients with paracoccidioidomycosis. *Mycopathologia* 1994, 127:89–93.

21. de Castro CC, Benard G, Ygaki Y, *et al.*: MRI of head and neck paracoccidioidomycosis. *Br J Radiol* 1999, 72:717–722.

22. Del Negro GM, Pereira CN, Andrade HF, *et al.*: Evaluation of tests for antibody response in the follow-up of patients with acute and chronic forms of paracoccidioidomycosis *J Med Microbiol* 2000, 49:37–46.

23. Restrepo A, Gomez I, Robledo J, Patino MM, Cano LE: Itraconazole in the treatment of paracoccidioidomycosis a preliminary report. *Reviews of Infectious Diseases* 1987, 9: 851–856.

24. Queiroz-Telles F, Nucci M: Comparative Efficacy of Cotrimoxazole and Itraconazole in the Treatment of Paracoccidioidomycosis. ICAAC, San Diego, September, 1998.

CHAPTER 5

Sporotrichosis

Carol A. Kauffman

Sporotrichosis is a subacute to chronic infection of cutaneous and subcutaneous tissues caused by *Sporothrix schenckii*, a fungus that exhibits temperature dimorphism and is found worldwide in temperate and tropical climates. Infection usually follows local inoculation of the organism, although patients with pulmonary involvement presumably develop infection after inhalation of *S. schenckii*. Infection is most frequent in persons who have vocations or avocations, such as landscaping, Christmas tree farming, rose gardening, or topiary production, that expose them to the organism. Infections involving osteoarticular structures, lungs, and other organs occur most often in individuals with underlying illnesses, especially alcoholism, diabetes mellitus, chronic obstructive pulmonary disease, and AIDS.

Patients with lymphocutaneous sporotrichosis develop a primary ulcerated nodule at the site of inoculation, followed by the development of similar lesions along the local lymphatics. Less commonly, a chronic cutaneous lesion without lymphatic spread may develop. Pulmonary sporotrichosis occurs typically in those with chronic obstructive pulmonary disease or alcoholism. Symptoms and radiographic findings mimic those of tuberculosis. Osteoarticular sporotrichosis may be manifest as unifocal or multifocal septic arthritis, osteomyelitis, or tenosynovitis. Disseminated sporotrichosis is very uncommon, occurring primarily in patients with AIDS.

The diagnosis of sporotrichosis is readily made when a patient presents with classic lymphocutaneous lesions; however, diagnosis of other, less well known forms of sporotrichosis is frequently delayed. The most definitive diagnostic test is growth of the organism from material aspirated from a lesion or a tissue biopsy. Growth of *S. schenckii* usually occurs within several days to weeks.

Treatment of sporotrichosis varies with the type of disease. Oral itraconazole is the preferred treatment for lymphocutaneous sporotrichosis. Saturated solution of potassium iodide can also be used for treatment, but side effects are common. Patients with osteoarticular sporotrichosis also can be treated with itraconazole, as the infection usually is chronic and localized. Even if the infection is cured, functional outcome following sporotrichal arthritis is poor. Patients with life-threatening pulmonary or disseminated infection should be treated with amphotericin B initially; therapy can be changed to itraconazole after the patient's condition has stabilized. If the patient is not acutely ill, itraconazole can be given as primary treatment for these forms of sporotrichosis.

CAUSATIVE ORGANISM AND EPIDEMIOLOGY

Sporotrichosis

Causative organism is *Sporothrix schenckii*
Organism exhibits temperature dimorphism
At 25°–30°C in the environment, organism is a mold
  Off-white to brown-black with fuzzy mycelium
  Thin, septate, branching hyphae with right-angle
    conidiophores topped by tiny oval conidia in flowerlike
    arrangement
At 35°–37°C in vitro and in vivo, organism is a yeast
  Off-white, smooth, moist colony
  Tiny oval or cigar-shaped yeast forms
Worldwide distribution of the organism in the soil; most cases
    reported from the temperate and tropical regions of the
    Americas

FIGURE 5-1. Characteristics of *Sporothrix schenckii*, the fungus that causes sporotrichosis.

Epidemiology of Sporotrichosis

Environmental acquisition
  Inoculation of conidia
    Sources: sphagnum moss, soil, wood, hay, etc
    Activities: rose gardening, tree farming, hay baling, topiary
      production, outdoor sports, motor vehicle accidents,
      mining, etc
  Inhalation of conidia
    Activities: construction work or landscaping
Zoonotic acquisition
  Sources: lesions in infected cats; cat, dog, rodent,
    armadillo bites or scratches; bird pecks; insect stings
Laboratory acquisition
  Inoculation or aerosolization of culture material

FIGURE 5-2. Epidemiology of sporotrichosis. Infection with *Sporothrix schenckii* can usually be traced back to outdoor activities or animal exposure.

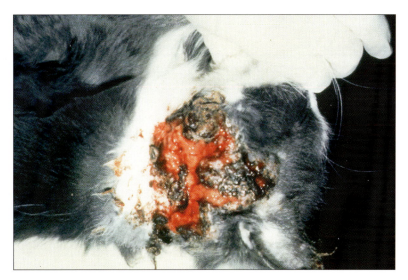

FIGURE 5-3. Irregular ulcerated lesion on the side of the face and neck of a cat with sporotrichosis. The cat did not respond to therapy with ketoconazole and was ultimately subjected to euthanasia. (*Adapted from* Reed [1].)

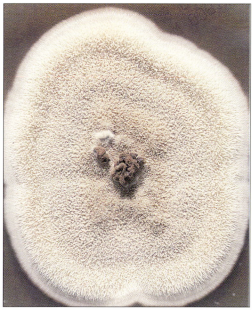

FIGURE 5-4. Typical appearance of *Sporothrix schenckii* growing in vitro at 25°C on malt extract agar. (*From* Kauffman [2].)

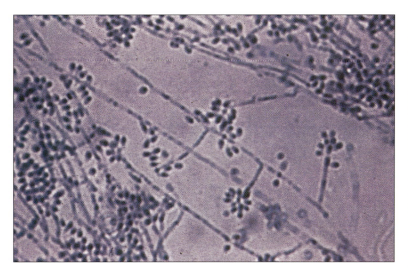

FIGURE 5-5. *Sporothrix schenckii* growing at 25° to 30°C. At 25° to 30°C, the colony is composed of septate hyphae. Slender conidiophores branch off at right angles and bear clusters of oval conidia. (*From* Raugi [3].)

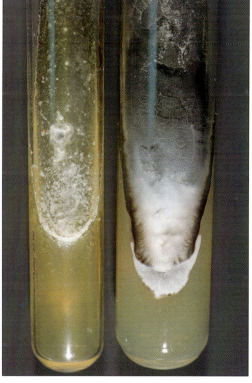

FIGURE 5-6. *Sporothrix schenckii*. The tube on the *left* shows growth at 35° to 37°C. At this temperature, the organism grows in the yeast phase as creamy, off-white colonies. The tube on the *right* shows the same organism grown at room temperature, showing the growth of the mold form of *S. Schenckii*.

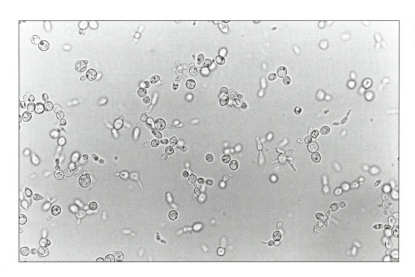

FIGURE 5-7. Microscopic morphology of *Sporothrix schenckii* yeast phase growth at 35° to 37°C showing spherical to oval blastoconidia.

Manifestations

Manifestations of Sporotrichosis

Lymphocutaneous
  Fixed cutaneous
  Cutaneous with lymphangitic spread
Pulmonary
  Acute pneumonia
  Chronic cavitary
Osteoarticular
  Septic arthritis
  Osteomyelitis
  Bursitis
  Tenosynovitis
Meningitis
Disseminated
  Cutaneous ± osteoarticular
  Visceral involvement
Other localized infection (rare)
  Eye, breast, larynx, pericardium, epididymis

Figure 5-8. Manifestations of sporotrichosis.

Lymphocutaneous Sporotrichosis

Lymphocutaneous Sporotrichosis

Localized to skin, subcutaneous tissues, and lymphatics
Initial lesion develops at site of inoculation in several days to weeks; followed by subsequent lesions along lymphatic distribution
Lesions are nodular or ulcerative; drain seropurulent material; mild-to-moderate pain may be present
Some patients have only a single lesion that remains localized to skin with no lymphatic involvement

Figure 5-9. Clinical manifestations of lymphocutaneous sporotrichosis, the most common form of infection.

Differential Diagnosis of Lymphocutaneous Sporotrichosis

Nontuberculous mycobacterial infections
  Mycobacterium marinum especially; less commonly *Mycobacterium chelonei*, *Mycobacterium fortuitum*, etc
Nocardial infections
  Nocardia brasiliensis usually; rarely *Nocardia asteroides*
Tularemia
Cutaneous leishmaniasis
  Leishmania brasiliensis usually; rarely other *Leishmania* spp.

Figure 5-10. Differential diagnosis of lymphocutaneous sporotrichosis. Other infections can mimic the classic findings of lymphocutaneous sporotrichosis.

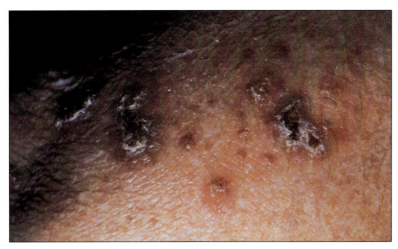

FIGURE 5-11. Fixed cutaneous sporotrichosis. Grouped reddish-brown dermal papules and ulcers consistent with granulomatous dermal inflammation were seen in a patient who never developed nodular lymphangitis. (*From* Raugi [3]; *courtesy of* Dr. K. Abson.)

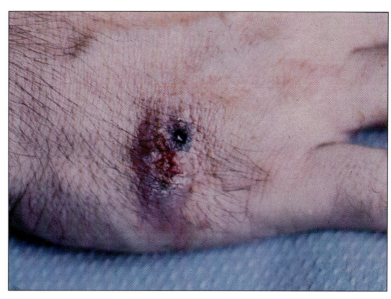

FIGURE 5-12. Primary lesion of sporotrichosis at site of inoculation of the organism. Lymphangitic spread and development of new lesions has not yet occurred. (*From* Everett [4].)

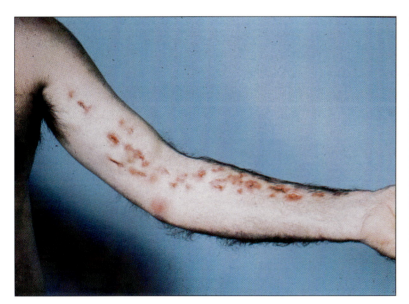

FIGURE 5-13. Lymphangitic spread of sporotrichosis proximally along the forearm following inoculation of *Sporothrix schenckii* into one of the digits of the hand. (*From* Everett [4].)

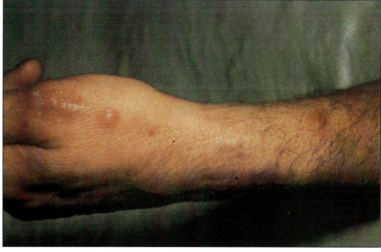

FIGURE 5-14. Nodular lymphangitis from sporotrichosis. Note the nearly linear distribution of dermal or subcutaneous papules and nodules on the forearm. (*From* Raugi [3]; *courtesy of* Dr. K. Abson.)

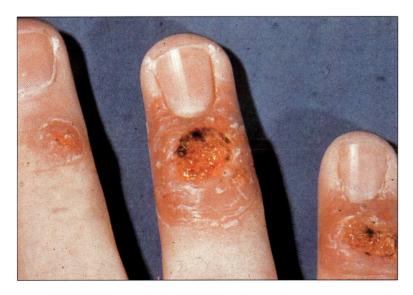

FIGURE 5-15. Multiple primary lesions of *Sporothrix schenckii* infection. Multiple primary lesions, each representing a separate site of inoculation of *S. schenckii*, were observed in this patient who sustained many cutaneous wounds from packing holly plants in sphagnum moss contaminated with the fungus. (*From* Raugi [3].)

Fungal Infections

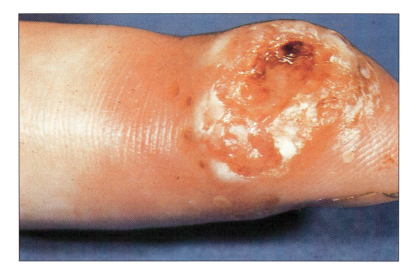

FIGURE 5-16. Ulcerated nodule of *Sporothrix schenckii* infection. An ulcerated nodule with satellite pustules developed on the distal digit of this patient who was involved in gardening. The nodule was accompanied by nodular lymphangitis. (*From* Raugi [3].)

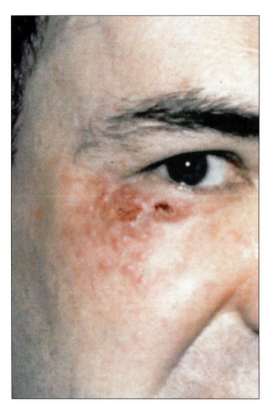

FIGURE 5-17. Ulceratied lesions present under the left eye on a veterinarian who had treated a cat with sporotrichosis 3 weeks previously. He had cleaned, debrided, and sutured the cat's lesion and had worn no gloves during the procedure. *Sporothrix schenckii* grew from the lesion, which resolved with potassium iodide. (*Adapted from* Reed [1].)

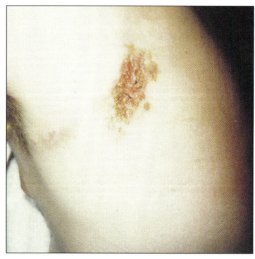

FIGURE 5-18. Nodular, ulcerating skin lesions of sporotrichosis. A man aged 27 years was involved in a motor vehicle accident, in which he scraped his back on the dirt. Several weeks later, several lesions developed. The posterior lesion drained serous material, the anterior lesion became nodular, and both were painful. The lesions gradually enlarged over the course of the month. Culture yielded *Sporothrix schenckii*. (*From* Kauffman [5]; with permission.)

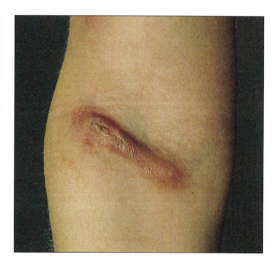

FIGURE 5-19. Multiple nodular cutaneous lesions of sporotrichosis. Multiple cutaneous lesions arose in a young woman several weeks after she walked through a recently harvested corn field. These lesions were slightly tender, gradually increased in size over the course of 4 weeks, and were present on both arms and legs. Biopsy revealed granulomatous inflammation but no organisms. *Sporothrix schenckii* was found on culture of the biopsy specimen. (*From* Kauffman [2].)

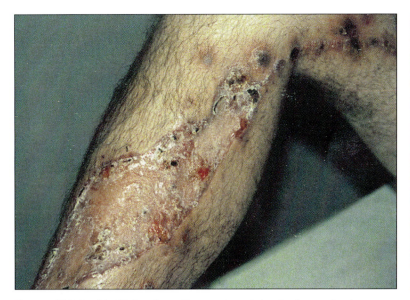

FIGURE 5-20. Multiple ulcerating and nodular lesions of cutaneous sporotrichosis on the lower leg. Multiple cutaneous lesions developed after a dirt bike accident in a 22-year-old man. The lesion on the lower leg had received a skin graft several weeks previously, and then new lesions arose at the borders of the graft. Culture of the material removed at operation yielded *Sporothrix schenckii*, and the patient ultimately responded to oral azole therapy. (*From* Kauffman [2].)

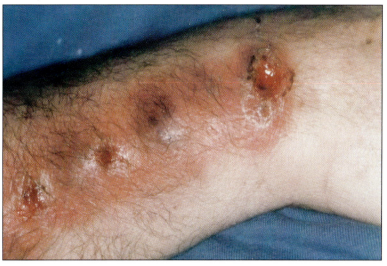

FIGURE 5-21. Sporotrichosis. A man aged 46 years, who owned a nursery, developed a pimple on the wrist 1 month before presentation. Over the course of 2 weeks, it became nodular, painful, and ulcerated. Over the subsequent 2 weeks, several more nodules developed along a red streak extending up his forearm. Culture yielded *Sporothrix schenckii*. The patient responded to itraconazole therapy. (*From* Watanakunakorn [6]; with permission.)

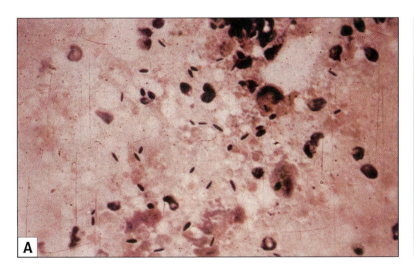
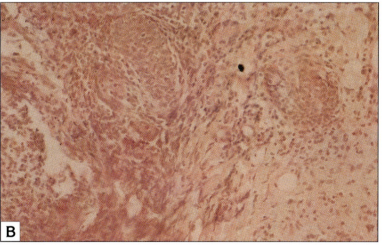

FIGURE 5-22. Varying tissue responses with lymphocutaneous sporotrichosis. **A,** Exudate from ulcerated lesion shows abundant yeast forms of *Sporothrix schenckii* stained with methenamine silver stain. **B,** A more typical pattern observed in biopsies of cutaneous lesions of sporotrichosis involves granulomatous inflammatory response. A single yeast cell is seen on periodic acid–Schiff stain of the tissue. (*From* Raugi [3]; *courtesy of* Dr. K. Abson.)

Pulmonary Sporotrichosis

Pulmonary Sporotrichosis

Uncommon manifestation of sporotrichosis
Pathogenesis involves inhalation of *Sporothrix schenckii* conidia from the environment
Acute pulmonary sporotrichosis rarely seen; most likely asymptomatic infection or diagnosis is missed
Usual picture is that of chronic pulmonary disease
Most common in middle-aged men, especially those with underlying chronic obstructive pulmonary disease and alcoholism
Symptoms include fever, weight loss, fatigue, productive cough, hemoptysis, dyspnea
Chest radiograph usually shows upper lobe cavitary fibronodular infiltrates

FIGURE 5-23. Underlying risk factors, pathogenesis, and clinical features of pulmonary sporotrichosis.

Differential Diagnosis of Pulmonary Sporotrichosis

Tuberculosis
Nontuberculous mycobacterial infection
Fungal pneumonia
  Histoplasmosis
  Blastomycosis
  Coccidioidomycosis
  Chronic necrotizing aspergillosis
Sarcoidosis

FIGURE 5-24. Differential diagnosis of pulmonary sporotrichosis includes mycobacterial and fungal infections and occasionally sarcoidosis.

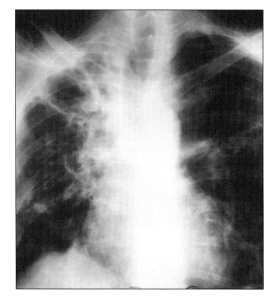

FIGURE 5-25. Chest radiograph from a patient with pulmonary and osteoarticular sporotrichosis. The patient also had chronic obstructive pulmonary disease. Extensive bilateral infiltrates with upper lobe cavitary lesions were due to sporotrichosis. (*From* Kauffman [2].)

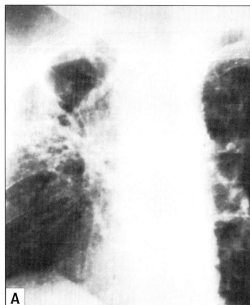

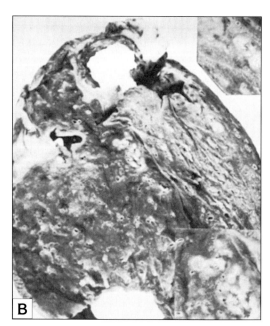

FIGURE 5-26. Pulmonary sporotrichosis. **A**, Chest radiograph of a patient presenting with a history of cough, fever, and weight loss and found to be infected with *Sporothrix schenckii*. Radiographically, primary pulmonary sporotrichosis closely resembles postprimary tuberculosis. Findings include isolated nodular masses that may cavitate, hilar lymph node enlargement, and, occasionally, a diffuse reticulonodular pattern. **B**, Gross pathologic specimen from the lung demonstrates the apical cavity and the granulomatous foci in the superior portion of the lingula and superior segment of the lower lobe. (*From* McGarran *et al.* [7]; with permission.)

OSTEOARTICULAR SPOROTRICHOSIS

Osteoarticular Sporotrichosis

Unusual manifestation of sporotrichosis
Pathogenesis involves direct inoculation or hematogenous spread to bony structures
Most common in middle-aged men, especially those with alcoholism
Septic arthritis more common than osteomyelitis
Isolated tenosynovitis presenting as a nerve entrapment syndrome may occur
Arthritis is chronic, destructive, leading to decreased function and contiguous osteomyelitis

FIGURE 5-27. Osteoarticular sporotrichosis. Osteoarticular manifestations of sporotrichosis are uncommon and occur mostly in middle-aged men who are alcoholics.

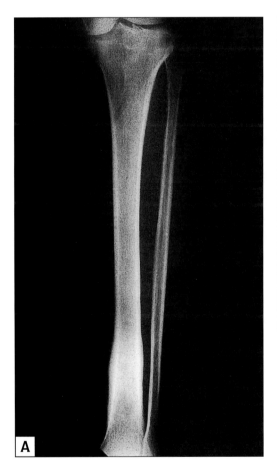
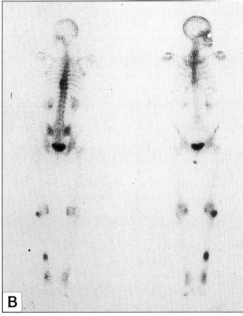

FIGURE 5-28. Osteomyelitis of the leg caused by *Sporothrix schenckii*. **A,** Anteroposterior radiograph of the left leg in a woman aged 32 years shows a punched-out lesion in the proximal tibia and sclerotic changes in the distal tibia. *Sporothrix schenckii* was isolated from a bone biopsy specimen of the proximal tibia. The woman grew roses in her garden, where she probably acquired the infection. She presented with left leg swelling and inguinal lymphadenopathy. **B,** Three-hour total-body ^{99m}Tc-methyldiphosphonate scans show increased uptake in the proximal and distal tibia. (*From* Mader *et al.* [8].)

Fungal Infections

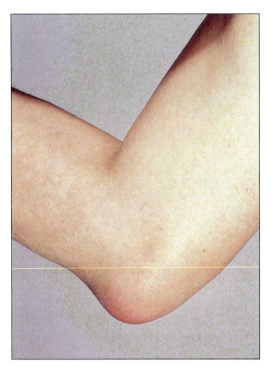

Figure 5-29. Swollen olecranon bursa in osteoarticular sporotrichosis. The elbow was red, warm, tender to touch, and had limitation of movement. Aspirated bursal fluid revealed many neutrophils but no organisms; culture yielded *Sporothrix schenckii*. The patient, a 45-year-old man with chronic alcohol abuse, ultimately developed osteomyelitis and severe limitation of joint movement. (*From* Kauffman [2].)

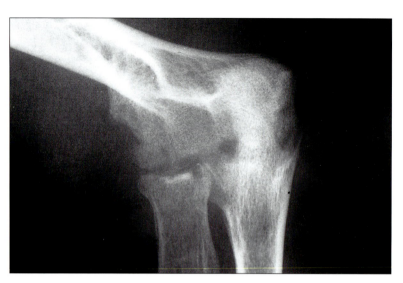

Figure 5-30. Osteoarticular sporotrichosis. Radiograph of the elbow from the patient in Fig. 5-29 is shown. Extensive bony changes are noted in the distal humerus, proximal ulna, and radius. The patient had loss of motion in the joint despite therapy with amphotericin B. (*From* Lesperance *et al.* [9]; with permission.)

SPOROTRICHOSIS IN HIV INFECTION

Disseminated Sporotrichosis

Uncommon manifestation of infection

May have dissemination to multiple cutaneous sites only, multiple joints involved with or without cutaneous lesions, or dissemination to viscera in addition to cutaneous lesions

Described most often in individuals with AIDS

Poor response to therapy with high mortality rate in patients with AIDS and disseminated sporotrichosis

Figure 5-31. Disseminated sporotrichosis. Dissemination of *sporothrix schenckii* to multiple cutaneous or osteoarticular sites is uncommon but does occur rarely in persons who do not have overt immunosuppression. Spread to viscera other than the lungs is exceedingly uncommon and has been described mostly in persons with HIV infection.

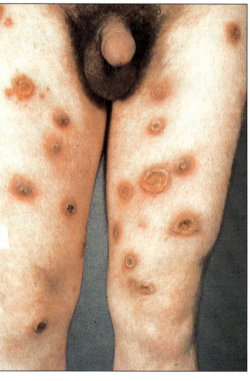

Figure 5-32. Sporotrichosis in a patient who worked as a horticulturist and who was known to be HIV positive for several years. The patient sustained cuts on his hand from rose thorns. Within a few days, he developed local inflammation on his left hand along with lymphangitis extending up his arm and axillary lymphadenopathy. By the next week, multiple large, tender, nodular red lesions developed all over his skin, and some of the lesions became ulcerated. A biopsy of one of these lesions revealed granulomatous inflammation with the organism readily detectable in the tissue. A culture also was taken, which was positive for *Sporothrix schenckii*. (*From* Friedman-Kien [10].)

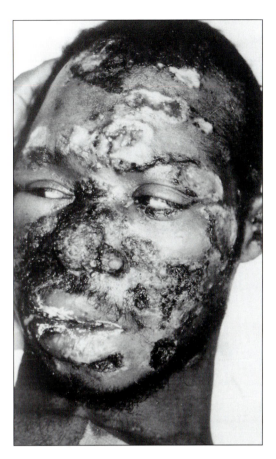

Figure 5-33. Sporotrichosis in a patient with HIV infection. This 22-year-old man who had advanced HIV infection (CD4 count, 17/mm^3) developed painful ulcerated lesions on his face, trunk, and extremities; infiltrative lesions of the palate and tongue; and multiple central nervous system lesions seen on magnetic resonance imaging scan. Despite antifungal therapy, the patient died. Necropsy showed widespread infection with *Sporothrix schenckii*. (*From* Donabedian *et al.* [11]; with permission.)

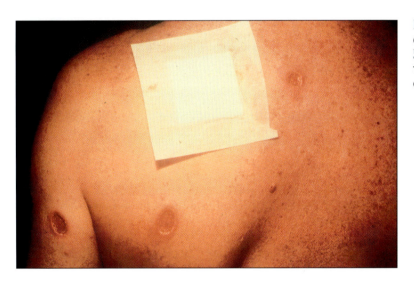

Figure 5-34. Sporotrichosis in a patient with AIDS. Large ulcers developed in this 43-year-old man who had AIDS (CD4 count, 56/mm^3). There was minimal host response noted in the biopsy tissue. Despite antifungal therapy, dissemination to the meninges occurred, and the patient died. (*Courtesy of* Dr. Elliot Goldstein.)

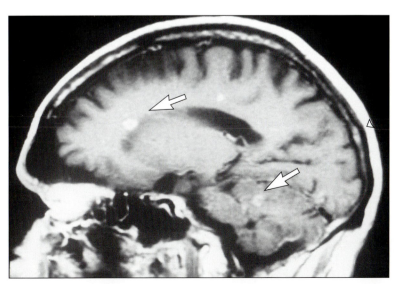

Figure 5-35. Magnetic resonance imaging scan showing sporotrichosis. Magnetic resonance imaging scan of the brain of a patient aged 40 years with AIDS (CD4 count, 80/mm^3), who developed vomiting and dysequilibrium. Cerebrospinal fluid culture yielded *Sporothrix schenckii*. The scan shows multiple enhancing intracranial lesions (*arrows*) and enhancement of the meninges (*arrowhead*). The patient died of the infection. (*Courtesy of* Dr. Elliot Goldstein.)

Diagnosis

Diagnosis of Sporotrichosis

Evokes mixed granulomatous and pyogenic inflammatory response in tissues; organisms can be stained with silver or periodic acid–Schiff stains, but often difficult to visualize in tissues

Diagnosis established by culture of *Sporothrix schenckii* from aspirates of lesions, biopsies of tissues, or fluids from sterile body sites; generally easy to grow from all sites, except central nervous system

Serology of uncertain use for diagnosis; agglutination tests and enzyme immunoassays available through reference laboratories

Figure 5-36. Diagnosis of sporotrichosis. The diagnosis of sporotrichosis is usually made by culture of material taken from cutaneous lesions, sputum, synovial fluid, or biopsy material.

Treatment

Treatment of Sporotrichosis

Type of disease	Preferred treatment	Alternate treatment	Comments
Lymphocutaneous	Itraconazole 100–200 mg daily × 3–6 mo	Saturated solution of potassium iodide, titrated dose	Poorly tolerated at higher doses
		Fluconazole 400 mg	Not as effective as itraconazole
		Terbinafine	No established dose
		Hyperthermia	Effective for fixed cutaneous lesions
Pulmonary	Itraconazole 400 mg daily × 1–2 yr	Amphotericin B 1–2 g	Amphotericin B is first-line therapy for severe infection; resection useful if patient can tolerate
Osteoarticular	Itraconazole 400 mg daily × 1–2 y	Amphotericin B 1–2 g	Treat 6–12 mo for tenosynovitis
		Fluconazole 800 mg	Minimal usefulness
Meningitis	Amphotericin B 1–2 g	Itraconazole 400 mg	Itraconazole may have role in maintenance therapy
Disseminated	Amphotericin B 1–2 g	Itraconazole 400 mg	Severe infection requires amphotericin B, but for less severe disease, can use itraconazole

Figure 5-37. Treatment of sporotrichosis.

References

1. Reed KD, Moore FM, Geiger GE, Stemper ME: Zoonotic transmission of sporotrichosis: case report and review. *Clin Infect Dis* 1993, 16:383–387.

2. Kauffman CA: Systemic fungal infections. In *Atlas of Infectious Diseases*, vol 8. Edited by Mandell GL, Fekety R. Philadelphia: Current Medicine; 1997:11.1–11.18.

3. Raugi GJ: Fungal and yeast infections of the skin, appendages, and subcutaneous tissues. In *Atlas of Infectious Diseases*, vol 2. Edited by Mandell GL, Stevens DL. Philadelphia: Current Medicine; 1995:6.1–6.28.

4. Everett ED: Infections associated with animal contact. In *Atlas of Infectious Diseases*, vol 2. Edited by Mandell GL, Stevens DL. Philadelphia: Current Medicine; 1995:5.1–5.8.

5. Kauffman CA: Fungal infections in the elderly. *Emerg Med* 1993, 25:24–32.

6. Watanakunakorn C: Photo quiz. *Clin Infect Dis* 1996, 22:765.

7. McGarran MH, Koboyaski G, Newmark L, *et al.*: Pulmonary sporotrichosis. *Dis Chest* 1969, 56:547–549.

8. Mader JT, Kumar R, Simmons D, Calhoun J: Osteomyelitis. In *Atlas of Infectious Diseases*, vol 2. Edited by Mandell GL, Stevens DL. Philadelphia: Current Medicine; 1995:14.1–14.34.

9. Lesperance M, Baumgartner D, Kauffman CA: Polyarticular arthritis due to *Sporothrix schenckii*. *Mycoses* 1988, 31:599–603.

10. Friedman-Kien AE: Cutaneous manifestations. In *Atlas of Infectious Diseases*, vol 1, 2nd ed. Edited by Mandell GL, Mildvan D. Philadelphia: Current Medicine; 1997:5.1–5.18.

11. Donabedian H, O'Donnell E, Olszewski C, *et al.*: Disseminated cutaneous and meningeal sporotrichosis in an AIDS patient. *Diagn Microbiol Infect Dis* 1994, 18:111–115.

CHAPTER 6

Cryptococcosis

John R. Perfect

Cryptococcus neoformans is an encapsulated yeast that causes cryptococcosis. Cryptococcosis has changed from a relatively obscure fungal pathogen that infects immunocompetent patients to a leading cause of central nervous system infection in the world's enlarging immunocompromised populations [1–4].

C. neoformans is divided into two varieties, *C. neoformans* var. *neoformans* (serotype a, d), and *C. neoformans* var. *gattii* (serotype b, c). Both varieties have geographic and clinical differences. The species has a teleomorph state called *Filobasidiella neoformans*, which has been identified under certain nutritionally deprived conditions in vitro, but its significance to human disease, including production of possible infectious propagules such as basidiospores, remains undefined. However, in clinical microbiology, yeast cells are the primary pathogenic form of this fungus and grow as spherical, budding encapsulated yeasts. The yeasts produce white- to cream-colored colonies, which vary in their colonial mucosity, depending on their capsule sizes. Most routine fungal media support growth of this urease-producing and inositol-utilizing yeast, and colonies generally appear after 3 to 10 days of specimen incubation.

Cryptococcosis has a worldwide occurrence but is not evenly distributed throughout certain locations within North America and sub-Sahara Africa, which have recorded extremely high numbers of cases. Although *C. neoformans* var. *gattii* has been found to have a natural association with flowering eucalyptus trees, *C. neoformans* var. *neoformans* does not have a proven natural environment, but it is frequently associated with bird guano. There is no proven animal-to-human or human-to-human transmission of cryptococcosis. Also, unlike certain endemic mycoses, outbreaks of cryptococcosis in which patients acquire clinical infection at the same time and place from an exposure to a common source have not been documented. Unfortunately, a standardized skin test is not available as an epidemiologic marker for subclinical infections, and thus the magnitude of infection with this yeast has not been accurately determined [5].

The three possible factors that initially determine the outcome of infection are 1) the status of the host defenses, 2) the virulence of the strain, 3) the size of the inoculum. Cell-mediated immunity with its $CD4^+$ and $CD8^+$ lymphocytes, natural killer cells, activated macrophages, and polymorphonuclear cells represents an important effector mechanism against *C. neoformans*. However, humoral immunity with both specific antibodies and complement factors also may add to the protective immunity of the host [6]. Several virulence factors have been identified for *C. neoformans*, with the classic group identified as capsule, melanin, and growth at 37°C [7,8]. However, many other virulence factors remain to be defined, because strains with all these characteristics still vary in their virulence within standardized animal models. Finally, it is likely that the disease can be initiated in healthy hosts when they are exposed to an unusually high inoculum of yeasts.

Clinical diagnosis is confirmed by cultures from blood, cerebrospinal fluid, peritoneal fluid, urine, or tissue. Histopathologic characteristics are helpful in diagnosis, and India ink examination on fluids such as cerebrospinal fluid can make a rapid diagnosis. A serologic test for the detection of cryptococcal polysaccharide antigen is excellent, with more than 90% sensitivity and specificity. It also may be used to estimate burden of organisms and help in prognosis, but this test is more difficult to use in specific therapeutic decisions [9].

Cryptococcal meningitis that was once uniformly fatal is now a curable infection. Success rates for treatment regimens depend heavily on the patient's prognostic factors and particularly on control of underlying diseases. Present regimens for disseminated infection use concepts of induction therapy with amphotericin B plus flucytosine and consolidation therapy with an azole such as fluconazole or itraconazole. For patients with AIDS, suppressive therapy is continued with fluconazole indefinitely [10–12]. However, with improved antiretroviral therapy for the underlying disease, it is hoped that further definition of optimal lengths of therapy in this population can be made. Complications such as increased intracranial pressure need to be defined in symptomatic patients and may respond to cerebrospinal fluid withdrawal for outflow obstruction or a V-P shunt for development of standard hydrocephalus. Future studies will be required to define the success of new antifungal agents, cytokine augmentation, and serotherapy for cryptococcosis.

Life Cycle and Distribution

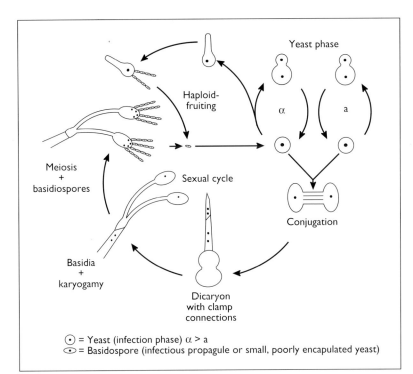

FIGURE 6-1. Life cycle of *Cryptococcus neoformans*.

Species of Mammals and Birds Reported to Have Natural Infections of Cryptococcosis			
Bat	Dog	Kiwi	Pig
Camel	Dolphin	Koala	Pigeon
Cat	Ferret	Macaw	Rat
Cheetah	Fox	Mangabey	Shrew
Cockatoo	Goat	Monkey	
Columbiforme	Guinea pig	Mouse	
Cow	Horse	Parrot	

FIGURE 6-2. Species of mammals and birds reported to have natural infections of cryptococcosis.

Yeast Characteristics

Comparison of the Two Varieties of *Cryptococcus neoformans*

Nomenclature (yeast)	*Cryptococcus neoformans* var. *neoformans/grubii*	*Cryptococcus neoformans* var. *gattii*
Teleomorph	*Filobasidiella neoformans* var. *neoformans*	*Filobasidiella neoformans* var. *bacillispora*
Serotype	A, D, or AD	B or C
Ecology	Soil and avian guano	Eucalyptus trees
Geographic distribution (natural isolates)	Worldwide	Tropical (southern California, Australia, southeast Asia, Africa)
Phenoloxidase (melanin production)	Yes	Yes
Capsule	Yes	Yes
Malate assimilation	No	Yes
$NH_3 \downarrow$ creatinine deaminase	Yes	No
Canavanine susceptibility	Yes	No
Glycine assimilation	10%–20%	100%
Clinical properties		
Risk groups	Majority immunocompromised host	Nonimmunocompromised host
HIV infection	Common (serotype a)	Rare
CNS parenchymal lesions and hydrocephalus	Occasional	Common
Length of infection	Subacute	Chronic
Common sites of infection	Lung, CNS, skin	Lung, CNS

Figure 6-3. Comparison of the two varieties of *Cryptococcus neoformans* [13].

Molecular Biology of *Cryptococcus neoformans*

Epidemiology and pathogenesis can be studied with
  Karotypes
  Restriction fragment length polymorphism with repetitive elements or mitochondria DNA
  Random amplified polymorphic DNAs or polymerase chain reaction fingerprints
Variety of gene cloning techniques in use
Transformation systems:
  DNA delivery: electroporation, biolistics
  Complementation of auxotrophs, dominant selection
  Homologous recombination
Heterologous gene expression systems (beta-glucuronidase, beta-galactosidase, aminoglycosides, green fluorescent protein)

Figure 6-4. Molecular biology of *Cryptococcus neoformans*.

Potential and Proved Specific Virulence Phenotypes for *Cryptococcus neoformans*

Capsule	Protease	Signal transductions: through calcineurin, alpha subunit G-protein, and RAS
Melanin	Phospholipase	
MAT α locus	Myristoylation	
Growth at 37°C	Urease	
Mannitol	Auxotrophy (purine/pyrimidine)	

Figure 6-5. Potential and proved specific virulence phenotypes for *Cryptococcus neoformans*.

CLINICAL EPIDEMIOLOGY

Risk Groups for Cryptococcosis

Groups	Frequency (importance)
HIV infection	++++
Corticosteroids (≥20 mg of prednisone)	++++
Transplants (solid organ)	+++
Diabetes*	++
Chronic pulmonary disease (chronic obstructive pulmonary disease, lung cancer)*	++
Lymphoma*	++
Chronic leukemias*	++
Sarcoidosis	+
Cirrhosis	+
Connective tissue disease (systemic lupus erythematosus, rheumatoid arthritis)*	+
Pregnancy	+

*Steroid treatment adds to the risk.

++++—must always consider in differential diagnosis of infection or fever; +++—a complicating infectious disease factor; ++—major risk groups without severe immunosuppression; +—more than a dozen cases reported.

FIGURE 6-6. Risk groups for cryptococcosis [5].

Comparison of Cryptococcosis in Patients With or Without AIDS

	Patients With AIDS	Patients Without AIDS
Laboratory findings		
Initial direct examination (India ink) of clinical material	Often positive (>80%) with numerous yeasts	May be positive for sparse numbers of encapsulated yeasts
Culture of clinical specimens for *Cryptococcus neoformans*	Frequently positive cultures (blood, CSF, urine)	CSF cultures are usually positive; blood and urine are rarely positive
Prognostic value of latex agglutination test for capsular antigen	Antigen in serum and CSF may persist at very high titers for long periods, even after treatment	Antigen titers in CSF at start of therapy tend to reflect prognosis; serum titer is usually negative or low
Lymphocyte subpopulations	CD4 <100 cells/µL	CD4 >200 cells/µL
Pathology		
Sites of involvement	Lung, CNS, skin, prostate, more sites of extraneural dissemination	CNS, lung, occasionally bone or skin
Histopathology	Many yeast cells, few inflammatory cells	Fewer yeasts; inflammation active with granulomas
Serology	A and D	A, B, C, D
Treatment	Amphotericin B and flucytosine with suppressive fluconazole	Amphotericin B and flucytosine
Prognosis	Good if suppressive therapy is used	Good to poor, depending on control of underlying disease

CNS—central nervous system; CSF—cerebrospinal fluid.

FIGURE 6-7. Comparison of cryptococcosis in patients with or without AIDS [14–18].

Initiation and Dissemination

A. Clinical Manifestations of Cryptococcosis: Major Site for Dissemination*

Central nervous system
  Acute, subacute, chronic meningitis
  Cryptococcomas of brain (abscess)
  Subdural effusion
  Spinal granuloma
  Dementia

*Most common and serious.

B. Clinical Manifestations of Cryptococcosis: Major Site for Initiation [19–23]

Lung (entry site for infection)*
  Nodules (single or multiple)
  Lobar infiltrates
  Interstitial infiltrates
  Cavities
  Endobronchial masses
  Tumor-like projections
  Allergy
  Colonization
  Adult respiratory distress syndrome
  Concomitant opportunistic infection
  Bronchiolitis obliterans with organizing pneumonia
  Mediastinal masses
  Hilar adenopathy
  Pneumothorax
  Pleural effusions/empyema
  Miliary pattern

*Wide range of symptoms, from severe pulmonary symptoms to asymptomatic.

C. Clinical Manifestations of Cryptococcosis: Intermediate Sites for Dissemination*

Skin (essentially every type of skin lesion has been described)
  Papules
  Tumorlike projections
  Acneiform
  Draining sinuses
  Ulcers
  Bullae
  Herpetiformis-like
  Molluscum contagiosum–like
  Concomitant tumor or infection
  Vesicles
  Plaques
  Abscesses
  Cellulitis
  Purpura
Ocular and bone (represents disseminated sites of infection in 5%–20% of cases)
Eye
  Extraocular muscle paresis
  Keratitis
  Choroiditis
  Endophthalmitis
  Optic nerve atrophy
Bone and joints
  Osteomyelitis (chronic) single or multiple sites
  Arthritis (acute/chronic)

*May occur with or without simultaneous central nervous system involvement.

Figure 6-8. Clinical manifestations of cryptococcosis [7,9,24]. **A,** The central nervous system is the major site for dissemination. **B,** The lung is the major site for initiation. **C,** The skin, ocular and bone, eye, and bone and joints are the intermediate sites for dissemination.

(continued on next page)

D. Clinical Manifestations of Cryptococcosis: Rare Sites for Dissemination*	
Genitourinary tract	Thyroid
Prostatitis	Thyroiditis
Pyelonephritis	Thyroid mass
Genital lesions	Adrenal gland
Muscle	Adrenal insufficiency
Myositis	Cushing's disease
Heart	Adrenal mass
Cryptococcemia	Head and neck
Endocarditis (native and prosthetic)	Gingivitis
Mycotic aneurysm	Sinusitis
Myocarditis	Salivary gland involvement
Pericarditis	Larynx
Vascular foreign body	Neck mass

*Except for cryptococcemia, prostatitis, and peritonitis, these sites represent well-described but rare cases of cryptococcosis (>12 reported cases).

FIGURE 6-8. *(continued)* **D**, The genitourinary tract, muscle, heart, thyroid, adrenal gland, and head and neck are rare sites for dissemination.

TREATMENT

Treatment of Cryptococcosis*	
Lung	**CNS**[†]
Mild to moderate symptoms and/or culture positive specimen from this site	Induction[‡]
Fluconazole, 200–400 mg/d x 6–12 mo	Amphotericin B, 0.7 mg/kg/d + flucytosine, 100 mg/kg/d x 2 wk
Severe symptoms—treat like CNS disease	Consolidation
	Fluconazole, 400–800 mg/d x 8 wk
	Suppression[§]
	Fluconazole, 200 mg/d
Alternatives	Alternatives
Low-dose amphotericin B, 0.3–0.5 mg/kg/d	Amphotericin, 0.7 mg/kg/d x 2 wk[‡]
Ketoconazole, 200–400 mg/d	Amphotericin B, 0.3 mg/kg/d + flucytosine, 150 mg/kg/d x 6 wk[†]
Itraconazole, 200–400 mg/d	Fluconazole, 400–800 mg/d x 10 wk
Flucytosine, 100 mg/kg/d	Flucytosine, 100–150 mg/kg/d[†]
	Intrathecal amphotericin B, rarely necessary as adjunct therapy

*Infection in other body sites must be judged by a clinician to follow either lung therapeutic regimen or CNS (disseminated) regimen. When other disseminated sites of infection are noted, it is important to rule out CNS disease.

[†]Best studied in non-AIDS patients.

[‡]Initial therapy, which is followed by consolidation therapy.

[§]If patient is HIV-positive, administer indefinite length of treatment; if patient is HIV-negative, administer treatment for 6–12 mo.

CNS—central nervous system.

FIGURE 6-9. Treatment of cryptococcosis [7,9–12].

Prognostic Factors for Failure of Treatment for Cryptococcal Meningitis		
Categories	High risk	Low risk
Underlying disease [25]	Neoplasia, AIDS	None
Burden of organisms	Positive India ink >10^6 CFU/mL Antigen ≥1:1024	Positive culture only
Host inflammatory response [26]	CSF ≤20 cells/mm^3 High doses of prednisone >20 mg/d	CSF ≥20 cells/mm^3
Mental status	Stupor, coma	Lucid
Intracranial pressure	Increased	Normal

CFU—colony-forming units; CSF—cerebrospinal fluid.

FIGURE 6-10. Prognostic factors for failure of treatment for cryptococcal meningitis.

Antifungal Drug Resistance With *Cryptococcus neoformans*			
Drug	Target	Clinical frequency	MIC*
Amphotericin B	↓↓ Drug flux† Sterol $\Delta^8 \rightarrow ^7$ isomerase	+	≥2 µg/mL
Flucytosine	Mutations in cytosine deaminase/permease or UMP pyrophosphorylase	+++	≥64 µg/mL
Fluconazole	↓↓ Drug flux P450$_{14dm}$‡	++	≥16–32 µg/mL

*NCCLS methods.

†↓↓ Drug flux associated with probable drug-resistant pumps.

‡Abnormal 14-lanosterol demethylase

+—Rare (< 6 cases); ++—≈12–24 cases; +++—common occurrence when used alone.

FIGURE 6-11. Antifungal drug resistance with *Cryptococcus neoformans*.

Culture and Histopathology

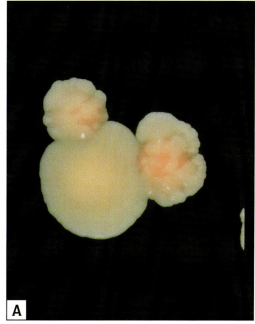
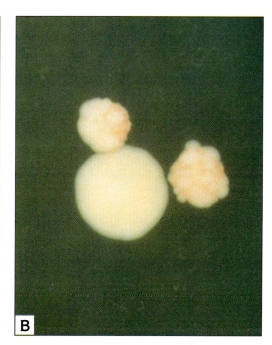

Figure 6-13. *Cryptococcus neoformans* strains demonstrating colony morphology differences within a single strain. **A** and **B**, In these figures, both smooth and rough colonies are seen, which are similar to other yeasts. *C. neoformans* apparently has a switching mechanism for changing between these various colony morphologies.

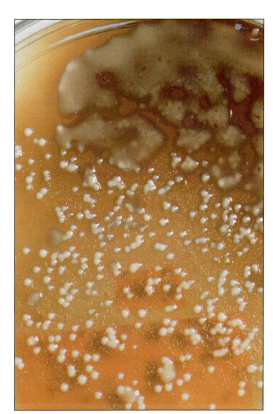

Figure 6-12. Mixed culture of candida and cryptococcus on Sabouraud dextrose agar. The mucoid appearance of *Cryptococcus neoformans* is shown on the right side of this plate. Although strains can vary, a mucoid colony of *C. neoformans* demonstrates the encapsulation of this yeast with a polysaccharide capsule composed of high molecular weight alpha 1-3 linked polymannose back bone with monomeric branches of xylose and glucuronic acid.

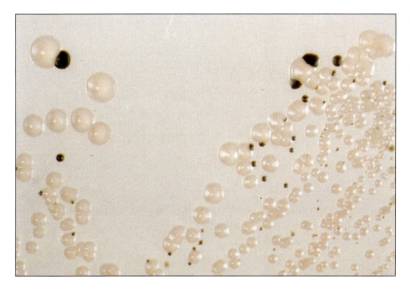

Figure 6-14. Mixed culture of *Candida albicans* and *Cryptococcus neoformans* grown on a caffeic acid agar. The dark colonies represent *C. neoformans* colonies, which possess a laccase gene that produces a phenoloxidase enzyme to metabolize diphenolic compounds to melanin. Media that allow melanin production are used to identify *C. neoformans* colonies within contaminated specimens.

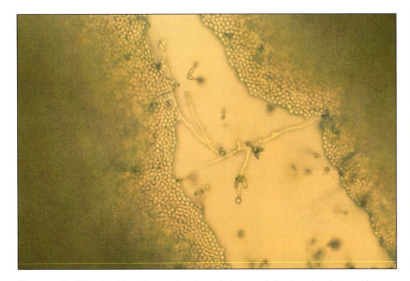

Figure 6-15. Mating type strains alpha and A streaked together onto V-8 juice agar. From the edge of the streaks hypha have begun to develop. These structures represent the beginnings of the sexual stage (teleomorph), which will end in the formation of basidia and terminal basidiospores. The hypha are formed in response to secreted pheromones.

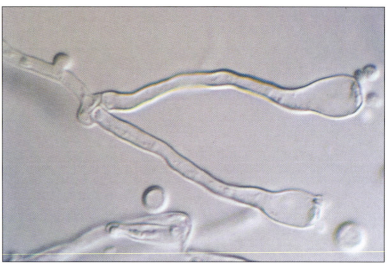

Figure 6-16. *Filobasidiella neoformans* var. *neoformans*. *Filobasidiella neoformans* var. *neoformans* demonstrated with its filamentous branches and globular basidia at the end, where meiosis occurs to form the terminal basidiospores. These basidiospores can be seen attached to the basidium. The clinical significance of the perfect stage or the ability to produce haploid fruiting, both of which produce basidiospores, remains undefined.

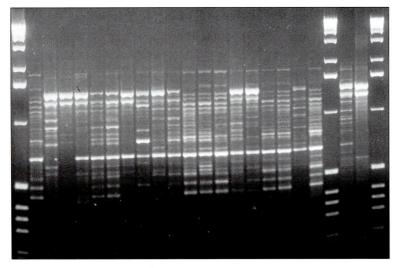

Figure 6-17. PCR fingerprinting. Molecular epidemiologic studies for cryptococcosis can be aided by a series of molecular techniques, such as restriction fragment length polymorphisms with repetitive elements, random amplified polymorphic DNAs, and karyotypes. This gel is an example of polymerase chain reaction fingerprinting in which short oligonucleotides are used to amplify multiple fragments (bands) within the genome. If carefully performed with quality controls, each strain will have a different banding pattern identified by the ethidium bromide staining.

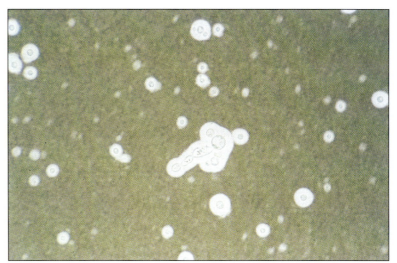

Figure 6-18. Budding encapsulated yeasts seen on India ink examination. An India ink examination is a rapid test performed on cerebrospinal fluid to diagnose cryptococcal meningitis when these budding encapsulated yeasts are seen. The test is positive in 80% to 90% of patients with AIDS and cryptococcal meningitis, but is only 40% to 50% positive in patients with other risk factors. A heavily positive test, such as the one shown in this figure, illustrates the large burden of yeasts in some patients and possibly predicts a more difficult treatment course.

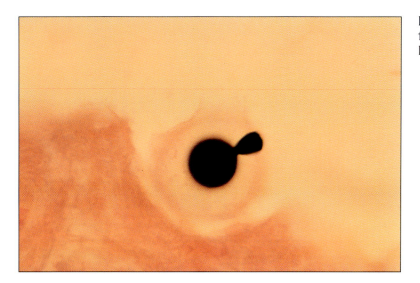

FIGURE 6-19. Gomori-methenamine silver stain of cerebrospinal fluid specimen showing the narrow-based budding yeast and a light-pale-pink capsule surrounding the yeast.

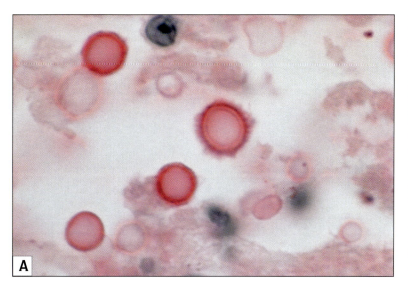 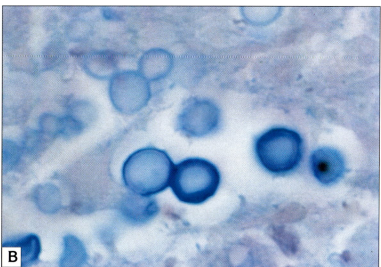

FIGURE 6-20. A and **B,** *Cryptococcus neoformans* in lung tissue stained with either mucicarmine (*panel A*) or alcian blue (*panel B*). In these histopathologic slides, the stains are particularly helpful to the pathologist because they will identify the polysaccharide capsule around the yeast (red stain for mucicarmine, blue for alcian blue).

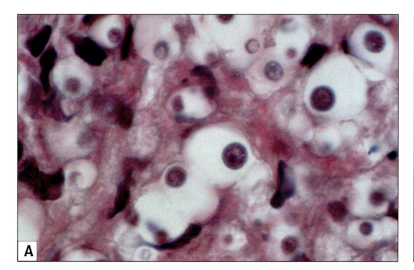 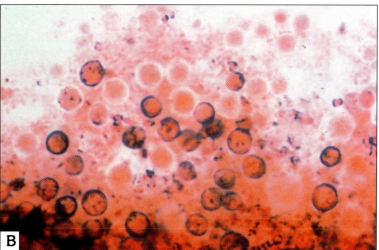

FIGURE 6-21. A, Hematoxylin-eosin stain showing yeasts in tissue with clear surroundings, which represent the capsule. **B,** Gram stain of *Cryptococcus neoformans* cells illustrating that it poorly stains positive.

Clinical Manifestations

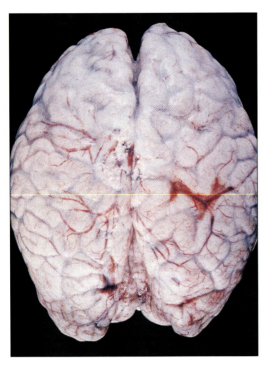

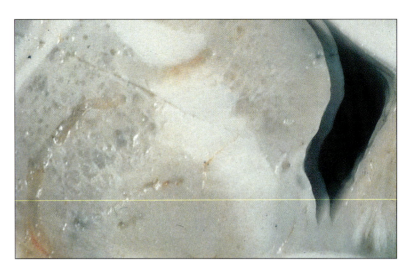

Figure 6-22. Leptomeningitis in cryptococcal meningitis. Leptomeningitis is the primary feature of central nervous system cryptococcosis. The leptomeningitis is usually devoid of a thick exudate-like bacterial meningitis. Slight clouding of the leptomeninges is shown in this dorsal view of the cerebral hemisphere in a patient with cryptococcal meningitis. (*From* Okazaki and Scheithauer [27]; with permission.)

Figure 6-23. Brain parenchymal involvement in cryptococcal meningitis. Radiographic brain parenchymal involvement is a much less common clinical manifestation of *Cryptococcus neoformans* than meningitis. However, a characteristic feature of cryptococcal meningitis is its extension into the brain parenchyma along Virchow-Robin spaces in the basal ganglia or cerebral cortex. Here, multiple, tiny bubbles can be seen with the naked eye or detected with sensitive radiographic methods such as magnetic resonance imaging scans. (*From* Okazaki and Scheithauer [27]; with permission.)

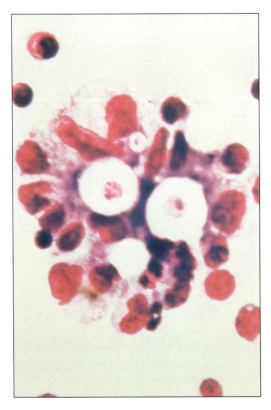

Figure 6-24. Hematoxylin-eosin–stained cytologic preparation. This hematoxylin-eosin–stained cytologic preparation from a cerebrospinal fluid specimen demonstrates the importance of an active inflammatory process, including the role of macrophages and lymphocytes in the killing of the encapsulated yeasts within the center of this host response.

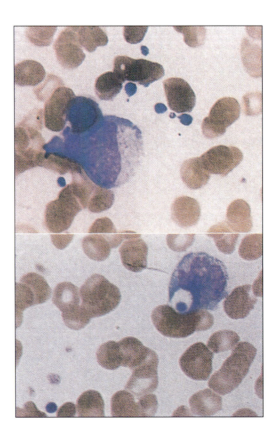

Figure 6-25. Disseminated cryptococcosis. The diagnosis of disseminated cryptococcosis was made by the demonstration of encapsulated yeast forms within a blood monocyte (Giemsa stain $\times$ 1000). Cryptococcemia may be the first infectious site clinically detected. It is particularly common in patients infected with HIV or those with a high burden of yeasts in tissue. However, despite positive blood cultures, this yeast only rarely causes endocarditis. (*From* Yao *et al.* [28]; with permission.)

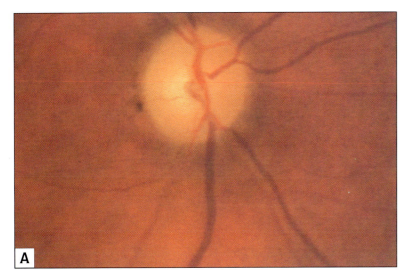
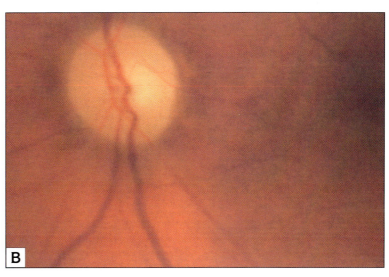

Figure 6-26. Cryptococcal optic neuropathy. **A** and **B**, Cryptococcal optic neuropathy presented with light perception in the right eye (*panel A*) and no light perception in the left eye (*panel B*). Direct infiltration of the optic nerves may be responsible for these findings.

Ocular signs and symptoms can be found in up to 45% of patients with disseminated cryptococcosis. Manifestations range from ocular palsies to chorioretinitis. (*From* Davis and Palestine [29].)

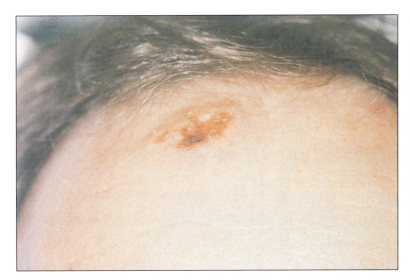
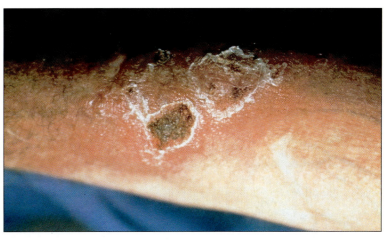

Figure 6-28. Cryptococcal cellulitis. Cryptococcal cellulitis in a patient receiving corticosteroid therapy, which appears similar to a bacterial cellulitis. This case illustrates that *Cryptococcus neoformans* can mimic both viral and bacterial infections.

Figure 6-27. Cryptococcal ulcer on the forehead of a patient with HIV infection and concomitant cryptococcal meningitis. No specific characteristics exist for skin lesions, and biopsy is required for diagnosis of cryptococcosis.

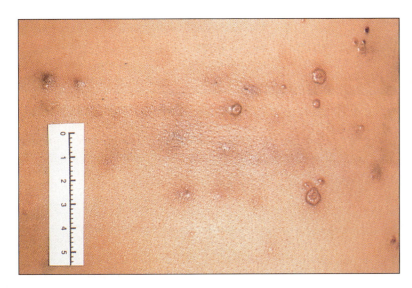

Figure 6-29. Unusual skin manifestations. *Cryptococcus neoformans* can produce raised, punctate lesions measuring 2 to 8 mm. This skin manifestation also may be found in patients with AIDS and histoplasmosis and pencillinosis. *C. neoformans* may be found concurrently on the skin with these mycotic pathogens or may appear like other pathogens such as molluscum contagiosum. In severely immunosuppressed patients, biopsies of different-appearing skin lesions should be performed separately. (*From* Dore and Cooper [30].

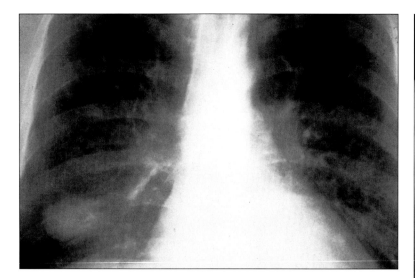

FIGURE 6-30. Chest radiograph showing a solitary nodule in right lung. There are many chest radiographic presentations for cryptococcosis, and asymptomatic nodules in the lung on a routine radiograph that mimics a neoplasm is a common presentation.

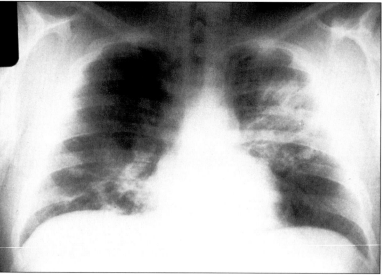

FIGURE 6-31. Chest radiograph identifying a left upper lobar pneumonitis. This radiograph, combined with symptoms of a lower respiratory infection, may be clinically confused with a bacterial pneumonia. If *Cryptococcus neoformans* is considered a cause of the pneumonia, sputum cultures must be observed for a longer period than routine bacterial cultures to detect the fungus.

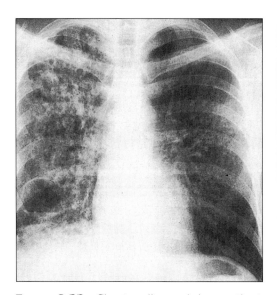

FIGURE 6-32. Chest radiograph in a patient infected with HIV demonstrating bilateral diffuse infiltrates. This radiograph could be confused with a variety of disease states, including infections with *Pneumocystis carinii*. (*From* Rosen [31].)

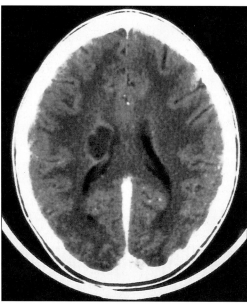

FIGURE 6-33. Computed tomogram showing cryptococcoma. Cryptococcoma may present as a single mass lesion. In this computed tomogram, a large cystic-appearing periventricular mass is shown with only minimal enhancement. When aspirated, the mass revealed *Cryptococcus neoformans*. However, it should be emphasized that in severely immunosuppressed patients such as those with AIDS, even with cryptococcal meningitis, solitary brain masses may represent a second etiologic infection, such as toxoplasmosis or nocardiosis.

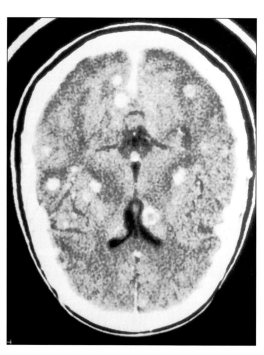

FIGURE 6-34. CT scan of the brain demonstrates multiple, enhanced nodules throughout the brain parenchyma caused by cryptococcus. Brain lesions can be either multiple or single and appear to be more common in CNS infections with *Cryptococcus neoformans* var. *gattii* while *Cryptococcus neoformans* var. *neoformans* commonly produces a meningitis syndrome.

REFERENCES

1. Aberg JA, Powderly WG: Cryptococcosis. *Adv Pharmacol* 1997, 37:215–251.

2. Diamond RD: *Cryptococcus neoformans*. In *Mandell, Douglas and Bennett's Principles and Practice of Infectious Diseases*, 4th ed. Edited by Mandell GL, Bennett JH, Dolin R. New York: Churchill Livingstone; 1995:2331–2340.

3. Sabetta JR, Andriole VT: Cryptococcal infection of the central nervous system. *Med Clin North Am* 1985, 69:333–344.

4. White MH, Armstrong D: Cryptococcosis. *Infect Dis Clin North Am* 1994, 8:383–398.

5. Levitz SM: The ecology of *Cryptococcus neoformans* and the epidemiology of cryptococcosis. *Rev Infect Dis* 1991, 13:1163–1169.

6. Murphy JW: Cryptococcal immunity and immunostimulation. *Adv Exp Med Biol* 1992, 319:225–230.

7. Casadevall A, Perfect JR: *Cryptococcus neoformans*. ASM Press; 1998:1–544.

8. Kwon-Chung KJ, Bennett JE: Cryptococcosis. In *Medical Mycology*. Edited by Kwon-Chung KJ, Bennett JE. Philadelphia. Lea & Febiger; 1992:397–446.

9. Mitchell TG, Perfect JR: Cryptococcosis in the era of AIDS 100 years after the discovery of *Cryptococcus neoformans*. *Clin Microbiol Rev* 1995, 8:515–548.

10. Dismukes WE: Management of cryptococcosis. *Clin Infect Dis* 1993, 17:507–512.

11. Bennett JE, Dismukes W, Duma RJ, *et al.*: A comparison of amphotericin B alone and combined with flucytosine in the treatment of cryptococcal meningitis. *N Engl J Med* 1979, 301:126–131.

12. van der Horst C, Saag MS, Cloud GA, *et al*: Treatment of cryptococcal meningitis associated with the acquired immunodeficiency syndrome. *N Engl J Med* 1997, 337:15–21.

13. Speed B, Dunt D: Clinical and host differences between infections with the two varieties of *Cryptococcus neoformans*. *Clin Infect Dis* 1995, 21:28–34.

14. Zuger A, Louie E, Holzman RS, *et al.*: Cryptococcal disease in patients with acquired immunodeficiency syndrome: diagnostic features and outcome of treatment. *Ann Intern Med* 1986, 104:234–240.

15. Chuck SL, Sande MA: Infections with *Cryptococcus neoformans* in the acquired immunodeficiency syndrome. *N Engl J Med* 1989, 321:794–799.

16. Eng RH, Bishburg E, Smith SM: Cryptococcal infections in patients with acquired immune deficiency syndrome. *Am J Med* 1986, 81:19–23.

17. Kovacs JA, Kovacs AA, Polis M, *et al.*: Cryptococcosis in the acquired immunodeficiency syndrome. *Ann Intern Med* 1985, 103:533–538.

18. Powderly WG: Cryptococcal meningitis and AIDS. *Clin Infect Dis* 1993, 17:837–842.

19. Perfect JR, Cameron ML: Pulmonary Cryptococcosis: Pathophysiological and Clinical Characteristics. In *Infectious Agents and Pathogenesis: Pulmonary Infections and Immunity*. Edited by Friedman and Chmel. 1993:249–279.

20. Campbell GD: Primary pulmonary cryptococcosis. *Am Rev Respir Dis* 1966, 94:236–243.

21. Duperval R, Hermans PE, Brewer NS, *et al.*: Cryptococcosis, with emphasis on the significance of isolation of *Cryptococcus neoformans* from the respiratory tract. *Chest* 1977, 72:13–19.

22. Cameron ML, Bartlett JA, Gallis HA, *et al.*: Manifestations of pulmonary cryptococcosis in patients with acquired immunodeficiency syndrome. *Rev Infect Dis* 1991, 13:64–67.

23. Kerkering TM, Duma RJ, Shadomy S: The evolution of pulmonary cryptococcosis: clinical implications from a study of 41 patients with and without compromising host factors. *Ann Intern Med* 1981, 94:611–616.

24. Lewis JL, Rabinovich S: The wide spectrum of cryptococcal infections. *Am J Med* 1972, 53:315–322.

25. White M, Cirrincione C, Blevins A, *et al.*: Cryptococcal meningitis with AIDS and patients with neoplastic disease. *J Infect Dis* 1992, 165:960–966.

26. Diamond RD, Bennett JE: Prognostic factors in cryptococcal meningitis. a study of 111 cases. *Ann Intern Med* 1974, 80:176–181.

27. Okazaki H, Scheithauer BW, eds.: *Atlas of Neuropathology*. London: Gower Medical Publishing; 1988.

28. Yao JDC, Arkin CF, Doweiko JP, Hammer SM: Disseminated cryptococcosis diagnosed on peripheral blood smear in a patient with aquired immunodeficiency syndrome. *Am J Med* 1990, 89:100–102.

29. Davis JL, Palestine AG: Ophthalmic manifestations. In *Atlas of Infectious Diseases*, vol 1, 2nd ed. Edited by Mandell GL, Mildvan D. Philadelphia: Current Medicine; 1997:6.1–6.15.

30. Dore GJ, Cooper DA: Classification and spectrum. In *Atlas of Infectious Diseases*, vol 1, 2nd ed. Edited by Mandell GL, Mildvan D. Philadelphia: Current Medicine; 1997:4.1–4.11.

31. Rosen MJ: Pulmonary complications. In *Atlas of Infectious Diseases*, vol 1, 2nd ed. Edited by Mandell GL, Mildvan D. Philadelphia: Current Medicine; 1997:8.1–8.10.

CHAPTER 7

Systemic Candidiasis

Laurie Anne Chu
Scott G. Filler

Despite the widespread use of amphotericin B and azole antifungal agents, hematogenously disseminated infections caused by *Candida* species are a serious problem in hospitalized patients. *Candida* species continue to be the fourth most common cause of nosocomial septicemia, accounting for 5% to 10% of all nosocomial bloodstream infections. This incidence of candidemia surpasses the incidence of bacteremia caused by *Escherechia coli* or *Klebsiella* species. Furthermore, *Candida* species are the most common cause of deep-seated fungal infections in patients who have extensive burns or who have undergone orthotopic liver or bone marrow transplantation. In many cases, an indwelling vascular catheter is considered to be the portal of entry. In fact, *Candida* species are the third most common cause of catheter-related infections, causing 11% of these infections.

Besides being common, nosocomial candidemia has an attributable mortality of 22% to 38%, even with therapy. *Candida*-related mortality is even higher in certain types of patients. For example, the mortality of patients who develop a disseminated candidal infection during bone marrow transplantation is 73%.

An additional concern is the development of antifungal resistance. *Candida albicans* remains the most common species isolated, accounting for approximately 50% of cases of deep-seated candidal infections. Although fluconazole resistance is relatively common in strains of *C. albicans* isolated from AIDS patients with oropharyngeal or esophageal infections, it continues to be uncommon in nosocomial isolates of this organism. However, possibly as a result of heavy usage of fluconazole in patients at risk for disseminated candidal infections, there is an increasing incidence of infections caused by *Candida glabrata, Candida tropicalis, Candida parapsilosis,* and *Candida krusei*. The rising number of infections caused by *C. glabrata* and *C. krusei* is especially worrisome, as these species are frequently resistant to fluconazole.

Because Candida fungemia is low grade and intermittent, hematogenously disseminated candidiasis is particularly difficult to diagnose. A sterile blood culture does not rule out the presence of this infection. The diagnosis of hematogenously disseminated candidiasis should be entertained in any patient who remains febrile despite broad-spectrum antibiotics and has one or more risk factors for this infection.

All patients with candidemia should receive antifungal therapy. In addition, all vascular catheters should be changed, whenever possible. Currently, fluconazole, itraconazole, and the deoxycholate or lipid formulations of amphotericin B are the standard therapies for hematogenously disseminated candidiasis. In the near future, other agents, may be released for this indication.

Epidemiology

Risk factors for hematogenously disseminated candidiasis

Immunosuppression
  Neutropenia >1 wk
  Adrenocorticosteroids
Broad-spectrum antibiotics
Colonization
Central intravascular catheters
Hyperalimentation
Abdominal surgery
Injection drug use (especially heroin)
Prosthetic intravascular implants (cardiac valves, vascular grafts)
Severe burns
Candiduria

Figure 7-1. Risk factors for hematogenously disseminated candidiasis. Patients with immunosuppression are particularly susceptible to infection with *Candida* species because their normal host defenses are compromised. However, *Candida* infections also are seen in patients with no identifiable defect in their immune system. The increasing frequency of nosocomial *Candida* infections is due in part to the advent of invasive therapeutic modalities. For example, broad-spectrum antibiotics suppress normal bacterial flora and allow *Candida* species to overgrow in the gastrointestinal tract. Central venous catheters provide a direct route for *Candida* species into the vascular system. The importance of colonization is well documented, because most patients become infected with the same strain with which they are colonized [1].

Species implicated in human disease

Common species	Rare species
Candida albicans	*C. ciferrii*
Candida dubliniensis	*C. haemulonii*
C. glabrata (previously *Torulopsis glabrata*)	*C. lipolytica*
C. guilliermondii	*C. norvegensis*
C. krusei	*C. pulcherrima*
C. lusitaniae	*C. rugosa*
C. parapsilosis	*C. utilis*
C. pseudotropicalis	*C. zeylanoides*
Candida stellatoidea	
C. tropicalis	

Figure 7-2. *Candida* species implicated in human disease. There are more than 100 types of *Candida* species. *Candida albicans* is the most common species isolated in human infection; however, other species are being identified with increasing frequency. The species that are rarely implicated in human disease have been isolated as pathogens in case reports [2].

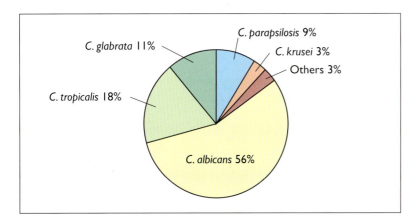

Figure 7-3. Distribution of *Candida* species isolated from the bloodstream in hematogenously disseminated candidiasis. In recent series of patients with hematogenously disseminated candidiasis, *Candida albicans* remains the most common pathogen isolated; however, non-*albicans* species are being isolated with increasing frequency. The reason for the emergence and the apparent shift toward isolation of non-*albicans* species is unclear. Selective pressure by use of fluconazole has been suggested as a contributing factor; however, insufficient data are available at this time [3–5].

Microbiology

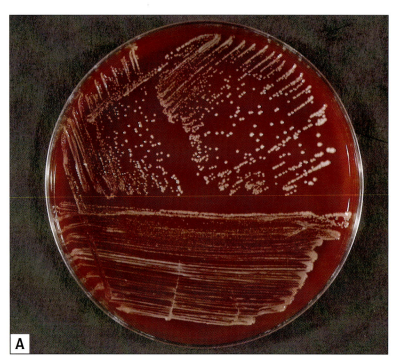
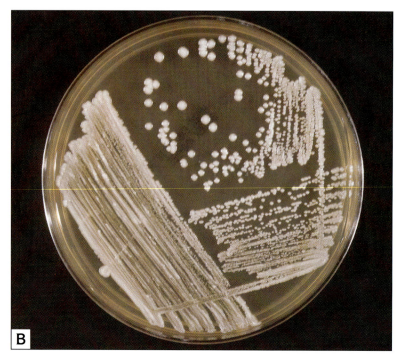

Figure 7-4. Colony appearance of *Candida albicans*. **A**, *C. albicans* colonies on blood agar. *Candida* organisms are not fastidious. They grow on routine blood agar plates and form smooth, creamy white, small colonies, which resemble colonies of *Staphylococcus* species. They grow well aerobically on minimal media at temperatures of 20° to 38°C. **B**, *C. albicans* colonies on Sabouraud's dextrose media.

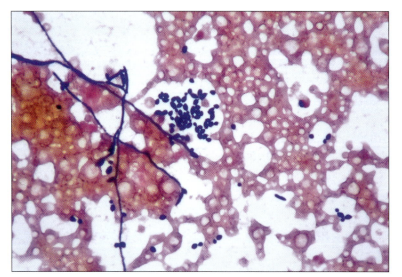

Figure 7-5. Gram stain of *Candida albicans* from BACTEC blood culture bottle. Blood cultures were obtained from a woman aged 61 years with primary pulmonary hypertension who remained febrile while on broad-spectrum antibiotics 14 days after right hemicolectomy for cecal volvulus. The yeasts appear Gram positive. Budding can be seen at the polar ends. Mycelia formation is also visible. Retrospective reviews reveal that in all patients with hematogenously disseminated candidiasis at autopsy, only 15% to 40% grow *Candida* species in antemortem blood cultures [6]. BACTEC radiometric blood culture detection systems and lysis centrifugation blood culture systems have improved the yield somewhat.

Profiles of common *Candida* species

Candida species	Laboratory tests
C. albicans	Germ tube formation is diagnostic. However, a few *C. albicans* strains are germ tube negative. Chlamydospore formation on cornmeal–Tween 80 agar. Carbohydrate assimilations are useful when germ tubes and chlamydospores are not demonstrable.
C. tropicalis	Germ tube negative. Carbohydrate assimilation when characteristic cornmeal–Tween 80 morphology is not observed.
C. glabrata	Germ tube negative. Assimilates only trehalose and glucose. Rapid trehalose assimilation is positive. Grows poorly on blood agar.
C. parapsilosis	Characteristic carbohydrate assimilation when characteristic cornmeal–Tween 80 morphology is not observed. Direct enzyme detection tests are useful.
C. krusei	Carbohydrate assimilation study when characteristic corn meal–Tween 80 morphology is not observed. Direct enzyme detection tests are useful. Some strains are urease positive, unlike most *Candida* spp.
C. kefyr	Carbohydrate assimilation study when characteristic cornmeal–Tween 80 morphology is not observed. Lactose assimilation positive. Direct enzyme detection tests are useful.
C. guilliermondii	Carbohydrate assimilation studies positive for galactose, D-arabinose, and raffinose. Enzyme detection tests are useful.
C. lusitaniae	Carbohydrate assimilation studies positive for rhamnose.

FIGURE 7-6. Differentiation of common *Candida* species. The common *Candida* species are easily differentiated by colonial morphology, various microscopic means, or characteristic carbohydrate assimilations. *Candida albicans* can be differentiated from the other *Candida* species by demonstration of germ tube formation after growth in serum at 37°C for 2 hours. (*Adapted from* Krissy *et al.* [7]; with permission.)

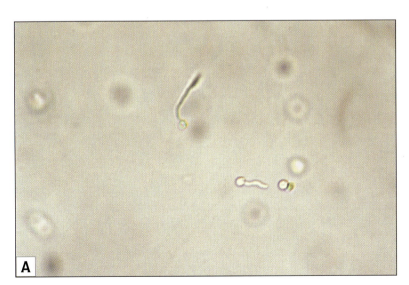

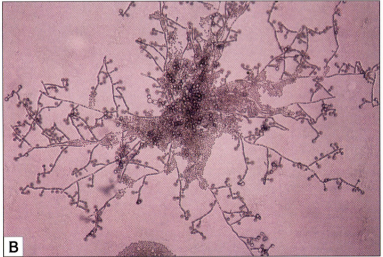

FIGURE 7-7. Identification of *Candida albicans*. **A,** Identification of *C. albicans* by germ tube formation. Yeast-phase organisms (called *blastospores* or *blastoconidia*) change to mycelia by forming germ tubes. To germinate, *C. albicans* blastospores require the correct nutrient state, an inducer (*ie*, serum), temperature greater than 33°C, and a near neutral pH. Other non-*albicans* species may form germ tubes if they are incubated longer than 3 hours.

B, Identification of *C. albicans* by chlamydospore formation on cornmeal–Tween 80 agar. Growth on cornmeal agar under a coverslide promotes formation of chlamydospores (or chlamydoconidia), which are large, thick-walled resting bodies. Other non-*albicans* species may rarely form chlamydospores; however, the morphology of their chlamydospores is different from those of *C. albicans*.

(*continued on next page*)

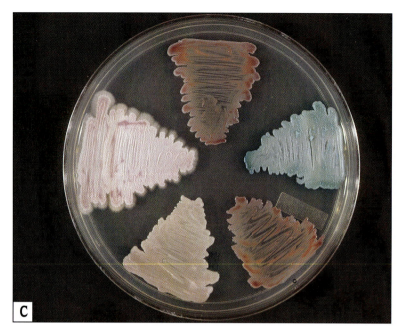

Figure 7-7. *(continued)* **C,** Identification of *C. albicans* by growth on CHROMagar Candida. Selective isolation of fungi and simultaneous presumptive identification of *C. albicans*, *Candida tropicalis*, *Candida glabrata*, and *Candida krusei* is possible by growth on CHROMagar. *C. albicans* forms colonies that are yellow-green to blue-green. *C. tropicalis* forms colonies that are dark blue-gray with a brown-purple agar halo. *C. glabrata* forms colonies that are dark pink with pale edges. *C. krusei* forms pale pink rough colonies [8]. Other *Candida* species (including *Candida parapsilosis*) form white, pale pink, or grayish purple colonies, which are not easily distinguished from one another [9]. (Panel B *courtesy of* Dr. Robert Yoshimori.)

Pathology

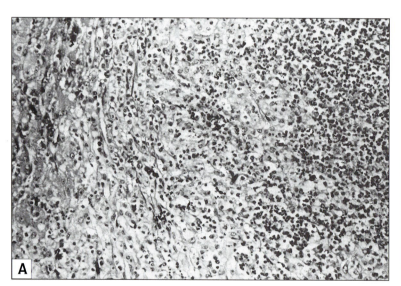
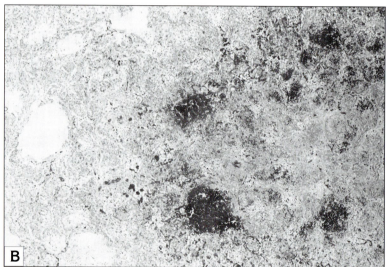

Figure 7-8. *Candida* species microabscess in an immunocompetent patient. **A,** In an immunocompetent patient, there is an initial polymorphonuclear response, followed by the appearance of histiocytes, giant cells, and epitheloid cells, which form a typical granuloma. Normal parenchyma is observed between the microabscesses. Both yeast and hyphal forms (for most *Candida* species) are present in the tissue. **B,** *Candida* species microabscess in an immunocompromised patient. The host inflammatory response is minimal and only the organisms and necrotic tissue is seen. (*From* Bodey [2]; with permission.)

Hepatosplenic Candidiasis

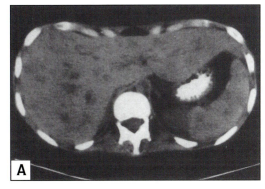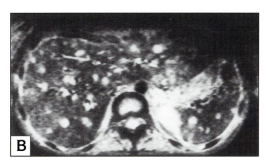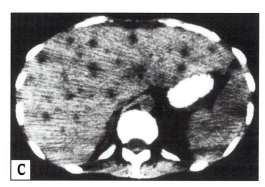

Figure 7-9. Computed tomogram and magnetic resonance imaging of hepatosplenic candidiasis. **A,** Magnetic resonance imaging of patient with hepatosplenic candidiasis. The lesions are seen as areas of decreased attenuation scattered throughout the liver and spleen. **B,** T2-weighted images of the same scan showing lesions with high-signal intensity. **C,** Computed tomogram of the same patient showing nonspecific lesions of low attenuation. Radiographic findings are nonspecific, and the diagnosis requires histologic or microbiologic confirmation. (*From* Thaler *et al.* [10]; with permission.)

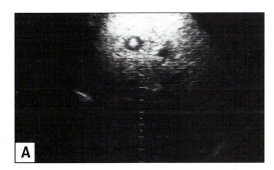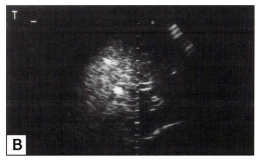

Figure 7-10. Ultrasound findings in hepatosplenic candidiasis. Four patterns of hepatosplenic candidiasis have been described. The first pattern is described as the "wheel within a wheel." This pattern usually is observed early in the course of the disease. Histologically, the central hypoechoic area corresponds to the inflammatory nidus and the outer hypoechoic rim corresponds to a ring of fibrosis. The second pattern is the typical bull's eye, or target, lesion. The third pattern is a hypoechoic lesion. The latter finding is the most common and frequently is seen on computed tomography as well. The fourth pattern is seen late in the disease and consists of areas of increased attenuation, which corresponds to calcification that occurs with healing [3]. **A,** Typical bull's eye lesion seen in hepatosplenic candidiasis. **B,** Later in the course of the disease, the lesions become more echogenic as healing occurs. (*From* Thaler *et al.* [10]; with permission.)

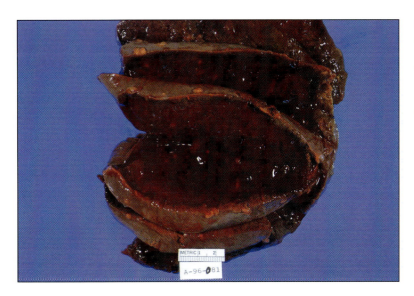

Figure 7-11. Postmortem findings. Cut surface of the spleen in a patient with hepatosplenic candidiasis. Hepatosplenic candidiasis occurs in patients who are severely immunocompromised and typically becomes manifest upon recovery from neutropenia. Gross examination shows multiple yellow to white nodules ranging from 1 mm to 2 cm in size that are scattered throughout the parenchyma in a miliary fashion.

Fungal Infections

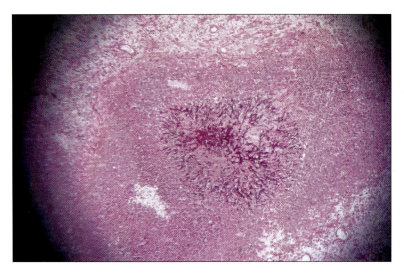

FIGURE 7-12. Microscopic section of *Candida* species liver abscess shown on periodic acid–Schiff stain. This postmortem microscopic section was taken from a patient aged 39 years with acute lymphocytic leukemia complicated by hematogenously disseminated candidiasis. On pathologic section, the organisms are found only in the center of the lesions. There is little inflammatory reaction seen due to the patient's immunocompromised state from his leukemia and chemotherapy. The morphology of a typical lesion is either that of a microabscess or a granuloma, depending on the status of the host immune system.

HEMATOGENOUS *CANDIDA* ENDOPHTHALMITIS

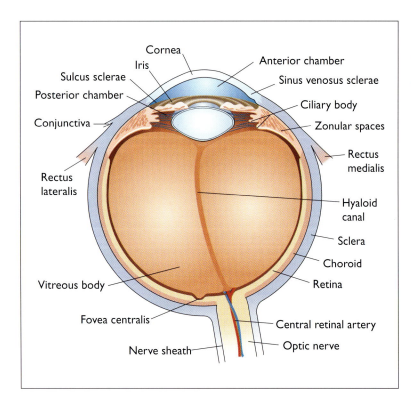

FIGURE 7-13. Horizontal section of the eyeball. In hematogenous *Candida* endophthalmitis, the blood-borne organisms become lodged in the chorioretinal capillaries. They then grow through the vessel walls into the retina and the vitreous. (*Adapted from* Clemente [11].)

Summary of predisposing factors for hematogenous *Candida* endophthalmitis	
Most common clinical settings	Most common predisposing factors
Patients with malignancy	Multiple antibiotics
Postoperative patients	IV catheters and needles
Patients with severe illness not related to malignancy or surgery	Parenteral hyperalimentation
	Immunosuppressive therapy
Normal women with vaginal candidiasis	Corticosteriod therapy
Seriously ill neonates	
Heroin addicts	

Figure 7-14. Summary of predisposing factors for hematogenous *Candida* endophthalmitis. Patients with endophthalmitis may complain of ocular pain, blurred vision, scotomas, photophobia, or visual "floaters." However, many patients at risk for hematogenous *Candida* endophthalmitis are too ill to communicate, thus a high degree of suspicion is required when caring for patients with the risk factors shown in the figure. Frequent ocular examinations by an experienced clinician is optimal. In patients with documented candidemia, the delay between identification of candidemia and the development of ocular lesions typically ranges from 3 days to several weeks. The infecting species is also an important determinant for the development of hematogenous *Candida* endophthalmitis. The majority of these infections are caused by *Candida albicans*; however, *Candida tropicalis*, *Candida parapsilosis*, and *Candida glabrata* also may cause endophthalmitis. Endophthalmitis in the presence of candidemia is pathognomonic of hematogenously disseminated candidiasis. (*From* Edwards [12]; with permission.)

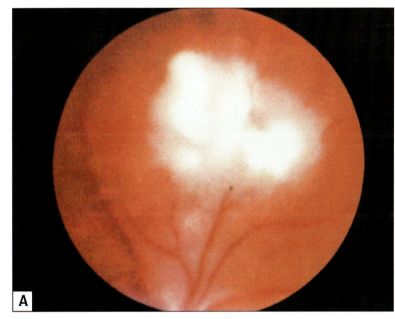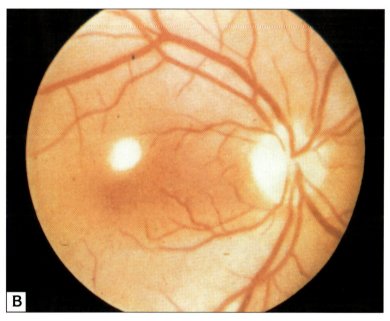

Figure 7-15. Fundoscopic findings of *Candida* endophthalmitis. The classic description of hematogenous *Candida* endophthalmitis is of a large, off-white, cottonball lesion with indistinct borders and associated vitreous haze. Because the lesions are extending into the vitreous, they have a three-dimensional quality. Lesions may be single, multiple, unilateral, or bilateral. They may extend to involve the entire vitreous. Early lesions may appear as an off-white "pinhead," extending only slightly into the vitreous. Lesions may be associated with hemorrhage giving the appearance of a Roth's spot. **A,** Multiple chorioretinal foci are seen with overlying vitreous haze from inflammation. **B,** Solitary parafoveal focus.

(continued on next page)

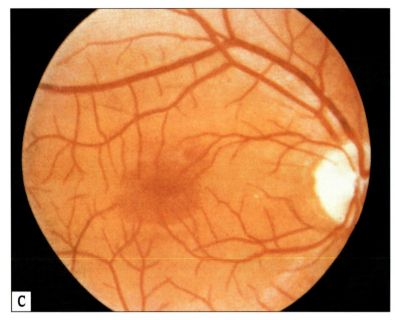
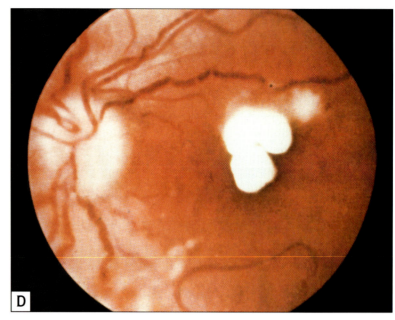

FIGURE 7-15. *(continued)* **C**, After treatment, the patient in *panel B* was left with a translucent gliotic scar. **D**, Large, white, lobulated macular mass, which extends into the vitreous. (*From* Fishman *et al*. [13]; with permission.)

Complications and variations of hematogenous *Candida* endophthalmitis
Adjacent hemorrhage
Papillitis
Iritis
Retinal detachment
Hypopyon
Ciliary body abscess
Conjunctivitis
Corneal perforation
Nonspecific panophthalmitis
Vitreous traction bands
Vitreous scarring
Chronic uveitis
Iris abscess
Vitreal detachment
Roth's spots
Vitreous "string of pearls"
Small pinhead lesions
Satellite buds

FIGURE 7-16. Complications and variations of hematogenous *Candida* endophthalmitis.

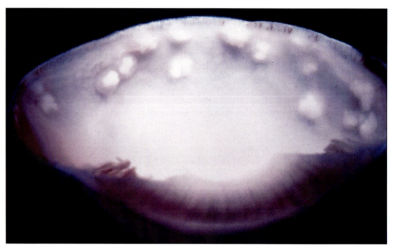

FIGURE 7-17. Hemisectioned eye at necropsy. On pathologic dissection, the lesion of hematogenous *Candida* endophthalmitis is a retinal or vitreous abscess. The predominant cells within the lesions are polymorphonuclear and mononuclear cells; only a few organisms are present. The lesion of hematogenous *Candida* endophthalmitis is not seen as often in patients with neutropenia, presumably because they lack enough inflammatory cells to develop a visible lesion. (*Courtesy of* Dr. John E. Edwards, Jr.)

Cutaneous Lesions

Cutaneous lesions of hematogenously disseminated candidiasis	
Adults	**Neonates**
Macronodular lesions	Superficial erythematous maculopapular lesions around mouth and perineum
Ecthyma gangrenosum	
Purpura fulminans	
	Subcutaneous abscesses
	Nonspecific erythematous lesions resembling erythema multiforme
	Diffuse burnlike lesions

FIGURE 7-18. Cutaneous lesions of hematogenously disseminated candidiasis. The macronodular lesions are the most commonly seen lesions. Definitive diagnosis is made via punch biopsy and demonstration of the organisms either histologically or on culture. The presence of macronodular skin lesions is pathognomonic of hematogenously disseminated candidiasis.

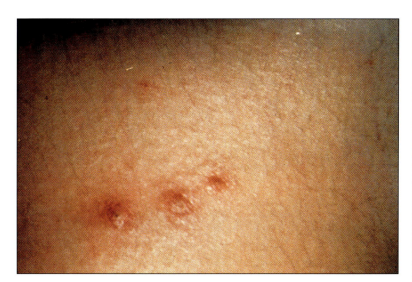

FIGURE 7-19. Macronodular skin lesions in hematogenously are disseminated candidiasis. Macronodular skin lesions are the most common skin finding in hematogenously disseminated candidiasis. They are seen in an estimated 10% of patients with hematogenously disseminated candidiasis. Macronodular skin lesions are 0.5 to 1.0 cm in diameter, vary in color from pink to red to purple, and can be either single or scattered. They are typically firm and nontender with discrete borders. They do not blanche with pressure and may have a pustular or necrotic central area. (*From* Edwards [6]; with permission.)

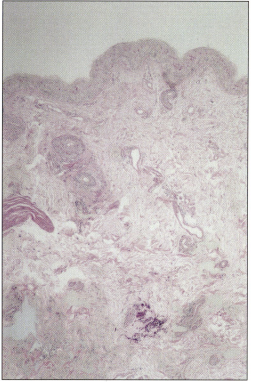

FIGURE 7-20. Punch biospy specimen of skin lesion stained with periodic acid–Schiff. The biopsy specimen shows yeasts and pseudohyphal forms consistent with *Candida* organisms in the dermis.

CANDIDA ENDOCARDITIS

Risk factors for *Candida* endocarditis
Underlying valvular heart disease
Heroin addiction
Cancer chemotherapy
Prosthetic heart valve
Prolonged use of IV catheters
Pre-existing bacterial endocarditis

FIGURE 7-21. Risk factors for acquiring *Candida* endocarditis. Of the risk factors listed in the figure, previous heart surgery is the most highly associated with *Candida* endocarditis. One explanation for this strong association is that many of these patients have damage to their endocardium plus implantation of prosthetic material and prolonged administration of multiple antibiotics and fluids via intravenous catheters. *Candida albicans* is the species implicated in more than half of the cases. Notably, *Candida parapsilosis* most often is associated with injection drug use. When *Candida* endocarditis is superimposed on pre-existing bacterial endocarditis, staphylococcus has been the most common bacterial pathogen [6].

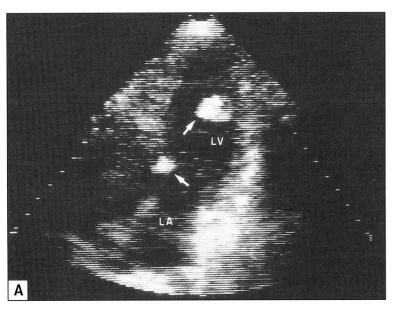
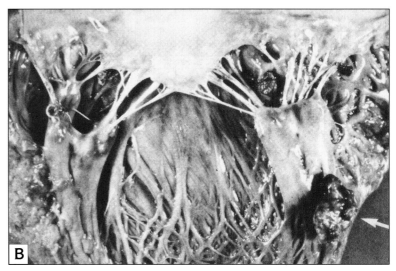

FIGURE 7-22. Endocardiographic and gross pathologic findings of *candida* endocarditis. **A**, Four-chamber view on two-dimensional transthoracic echocardiography showing two left ventricular (LV) mural vegetations (*arrows*) in a patient with systemic lupus erythematosus treated with prednisone and azathioprine. The patient initially was admitted for *Listeria monocytogenes* meningitis. Her hospital course was complicated by bacteremia with coagulase-negative staphylococi and *Klebsiella pneumoniae* along with candidemia. The patient died despite appropriate antibiotics. **B**, Gross pathologic section. At the time of autopsy, three LV masses were found: in the apex of the LV, associated with the posterior papillary muscle (*arrow*), and behind the anterior leaflet of the mitral valve. On microscopic examination, masses of fungal elements were seen and a pure culture of *Candida albicans* was grown. LA—left atrium. (*From* Herzog *et al.* [14]; with permission.)

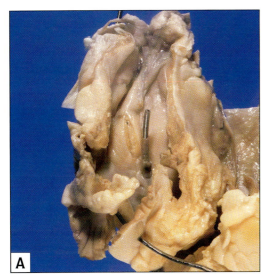
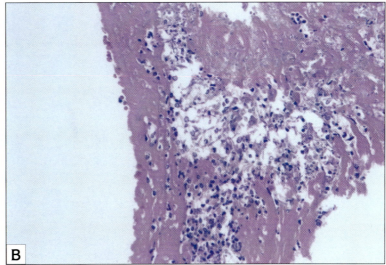

Figure 7-23. Postmortem findings. **A,** Postmortem findings in *Candida* pacemaker endocarditis. A vegetation is seen at the tip of the pacemaker lead from a patient aged 88 years who initially was admitted for repair of an abdominal aortic pseudoaneurysm. The patient's postoperative course was complicated by a nosocomial pneumonia with respiratory failure, renal failure, and catheter-related candidemia. At the time of autopsy, the vegetation was found with evidence of septic emboli to lungs and kidneys. **B,** Hematoxylin-eosin stain of a postmortem microscopic section of a vegetation found at the end of a pacemaker lead in the right ventricle. Antemortem blood culture and postmortem heart blood culture grew *Candida albicans*. Transthoracic echocardiogram performed prior to death was negative.

CANDIDA MYOCARDITIS

Nonspecific electrocardiogram findings seen in *Candida* myocarditis
Supraventricular arrhythmias
QRS changes mimicking infarction
Pronounced T wave changes

Figure 7-24. Nonspecific electrocardiogram findings seen in *Candida* myocarditis. *Candida* myocarditis without associated valvular involvement is found surprisingly often at autopsy. Retrospective autopsy reviews found myocardial involvement with *Candida* species in 8.4% to 93% of patients with disseminated candidiasis. These nonspecific electrocardiogram findings have been identified in patients with myocarditis, along with hypotension and shock.

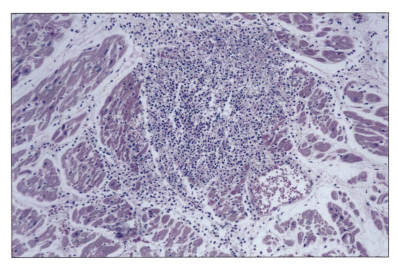

Figure 7-25. *Candida albicans* myocardial microabscesses shown on hematoxylin-eosin stain. On microscopic examination, diffuse myocardial microabscesses are seen scattered throughout the heart with normal myocardium intervening.

GENITOURINARY CANDIDIASIS

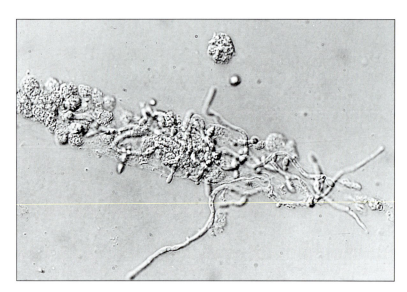

FIGURE 7-26. Light microscopy of renal tubular cast with *Candida albicans* blastospores and mycelia. Isolation of *Candida* species from the urine is a very frequent finding. However, the incidence of invasive urinary tract candidiasis is very low. Finding a renal tubular cast with *Candida* species on routine urinalysis can help localize the infection to the upper tract. Unfortunately, this is a rare finding. Upper urinary tract infection occurs via two routes: ascending infection from the bladder or as a result of hematogenous spread. (*Courtesy of* Dr. T. Walsh; *from* Gallis and Sobel [15].)

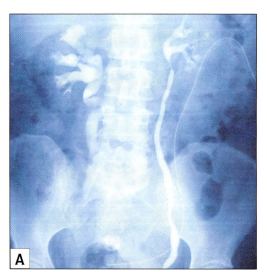
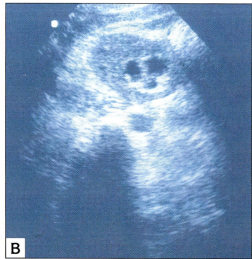
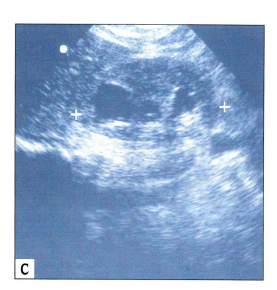
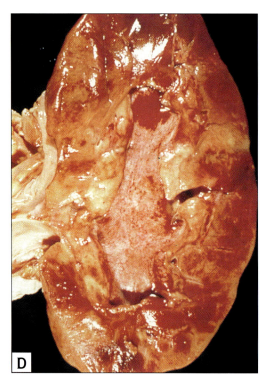

FIGURE 7-27. Ascending infections of the upper urinary tract. Ascending infections of the upper urinary tract typically occur in patients with some pre-existing abnormality of the kidney or ureter, such as urinary tract obstruction, kidney stones, diabetes mellitus, nephrostomy tubes, or ureteral stents. Patients may have intermittent urinary tract obstruction due to fungal ball formation. Radiographic findings are nonspecific, and intravenous pyelogram results may be falsely negative in up to 33% of patients. **A,** Retrograde pyelogram showing filling defect from fungus ball with papillary necrosis. **B** and **C,** Ultrasound scans of ascending pyelonephritis showing fungus ball. **D,** Large fungus ball seen in the dilated pelvis on gross pathologic section of the kidney.

(continued on next page)

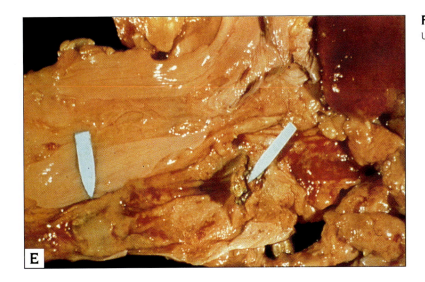

FIGURE 7-27. *(continued)* **E,** Large fungus ball seen in the dilated ureter. *(Courtesy of* Dr. Jack Sobel; *from* Gallis and Sobel [15].)

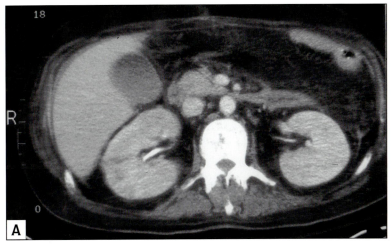

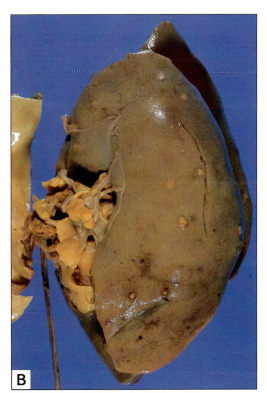

FIGURE 7-28. A, Computed tomogram from a patient with hematogenously disseminated candidiasis with renal involvement. Note the hypodense lesions seen especially in the right kidney. **B,** Postmortem findings from the same patient. Hematogenously acquired renal candidiasis typically leads to multiple micro- or macroabscesses scattered diffusely throughout the kidneys. This is the most common form of upper urinary tract candidiasis. When *Candida* species does disseminate, the kidney is one of the most common organs affected. Patients frequently present with candiduria, fever, chills, rigors, and shock, which are unresponsive to broad-spectrum antibiotics.

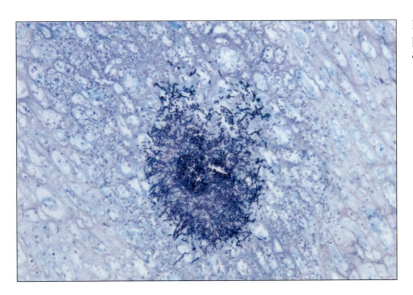

FIGURE 7-29. Methanamine silver stain of kidney specimen from a patient with disseminated candidiasis. Numerous microabscesses are seen with hyphal elements.

CENTRAL NERVOUS SYSTEM CANDIDIASIS

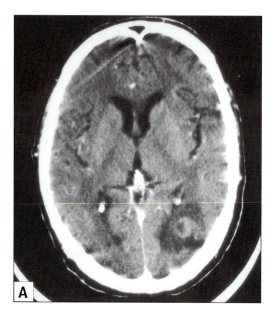
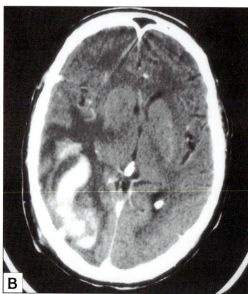

FIGURE 7-30. Computed tomograms (CTs) of patient with *Candida* brain abscess. **A**, CT from a patient aged 39 years with hematogenously disseminated candidiasis and acute lymphocytic leukemia who was undergoing chemotherapy. It is estimated that almost half of patients with disseminated candidiasis have central nervous system involvement. The lesions reported include meningitis, microabscesses, macroabscesses, vasculitis with thrombosis and infarction, mycotic aneurysm, subdural spinal fungal granuloma, demyelination and tranverse myelitis, fungus ball, and hemorrhage or hemorrhagic necrosis. The most commonly reported CT pattern is that of multiple abscesses with ring enhancement and edema after intravenous contrast, as seen in this patient. **B**, Repeat CT showing hemorrhage into the abscess and surrounding parenchyma.

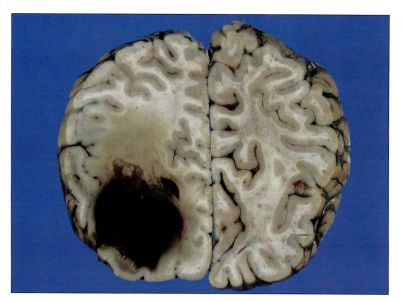

FIGURE 7-31. Postmortem findings in the patient shown in Fig. 7-31. The abscess cavity is seen with surrounding hemorrhage. (Photography *courtesy of* Dr. Marcia Cornford.)

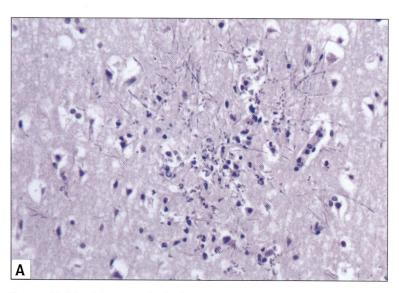
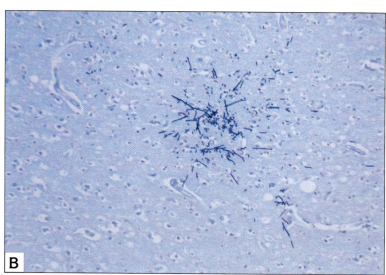

FIGURE 7-32. Microscopic findings in central nervous system candidiasis. **A**, Microabscess with fungal elements seen on hematoxylin-eosin stain. **B**, Microabscess with fungal elements seen on methanamine silver stain.

Candida Osteomyelitis

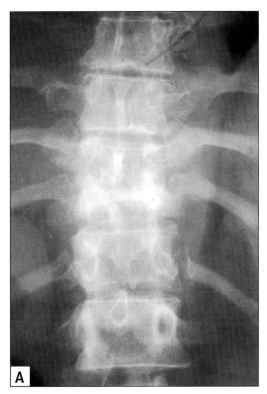
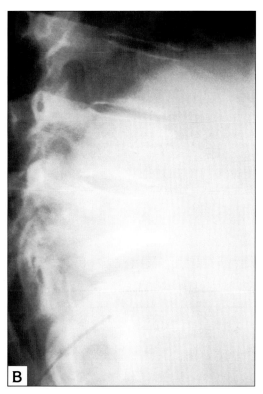
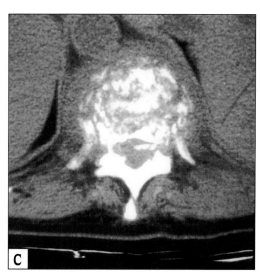

FIGURE 7-33. *Candida* spinal osteomyelitis. *Candida* osteomyelitis is usually a result of blood-borne infection. Osteomyelitis has been reported in the spine, wrist, femur, costochondral junction of ribs, scapula, and proximal humerus. Diagnosis typically is made via needle aspiration or open biopsy because blood cultures are frequently negative. **A,** Posteroanterior spine radiograph of a patient aged 50 years with a history of injection drug use. The patient presented with spinal osteomyelitis, which progressed to spinal cord compression despite broad-spectrum antibiotics. The patient underwent two fine-needle aspirations of her lesion, which were nondiagnostic. She ultimately required open decompression, at which time the diagnosis of *Candida* osteomyelitis was made. **B,** Lateral spine radiograph from the same patient. Note the involvement of T9, complete destruction of T10, and the marked compression of T11. **C,** Axial view of a computed tomogram from the same patient. Note the lytic destruction of the vertebral body.

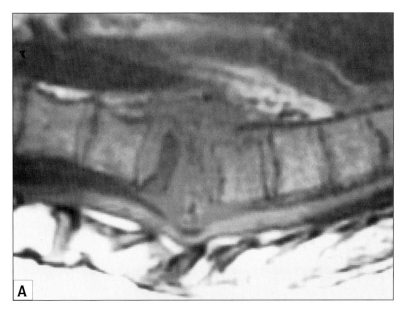
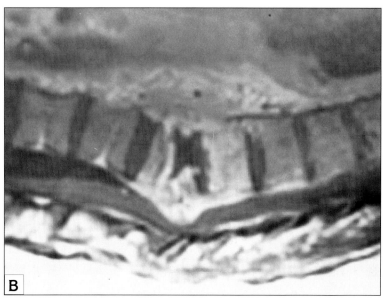

FIGURE 7-34. Magnetic resonance imaging findings in *Candida* spinal osteomyelitis. Magnetic resonance imaging scans were obtained in this patient prior to spinal cord decompression. **A,** Pregadolinium image showing marked destruction of the T9 to T11 vertebral bodies. **B,** Postgadolinium image showing compression of the spinal cord and increased signal intensity of the involved vertebral bodies, indicating hyperemia and inflammation.
(continued on next page)

Fungal Infections

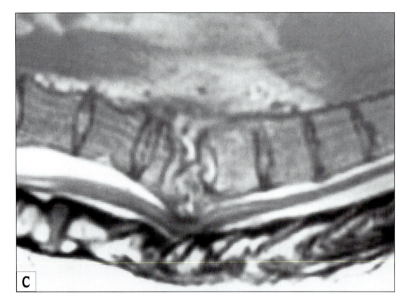

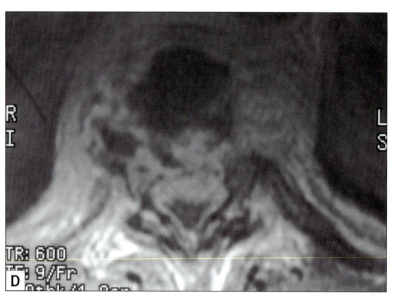

FIGURE 7-34. *(continued)* **C**, T2-weighted image showing subtle bright signal in the spinal cord, indicating edema due to compression. **D**, Axial reconstruction again showing spinal cord compression with surrounding paraspinous phlegmon.

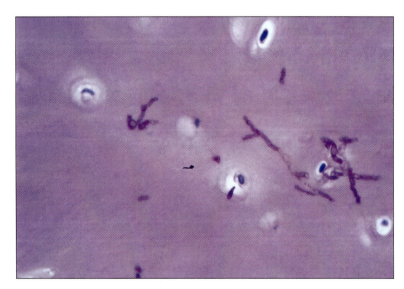

FIGURE 7-35. Microscopic findings in *Candida* spinal osteomyelitis. Periodic acid–Schiff stain of a surgical biopsy specimen was obtained during spinal cord decompression. Hyphal elements consistent with *Candida* species are seen invading the cartilage.

Candida Pneumonia

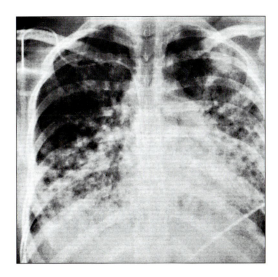

Figure 7-36. Chest radiograph from a patient with acute leukemia, neutropenia, and hematogenously disseminated candidiasis. Although *Candida albicans* is commonly isolated from sputum, it is rarely found invading the lung. Biopsy evidence of tissue invasion is required for definitive diagnosis. A diagnosis of *Candida* pneumonia cannot be made on the basis of sputum culture and radiographic findings alone. *Candida* pneumonia is usually seen in patients with neutropenia. Chest radiograph shows a finely nodular, diffuse interstitial infiltrate. Pathologic section revealed numerous foci of hematogenously seeded *Candida* species. (*From* Kwon-Chung and Bennett [16]; with permission.)

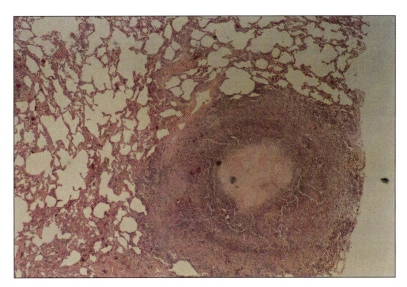

Figure 7-37. Microscopic section of lung from a patient with hematogenously disseminated candidiasis. Methanamine silver stain revealed organisms with evidence of alveolar hemorrhage and angioinvasion.

MANAGEMENT

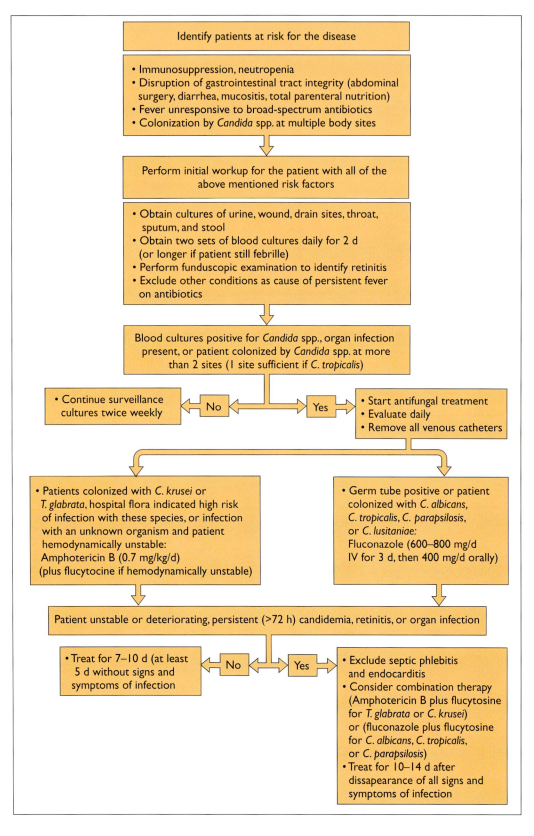

FIGURE 7-38. Algorithm for the management of disseminated candidiasis. It is well known that the rate of antemortem diagnosis of disseminated candidiasis is dismally low, thus a high level of suspicion is required on the part of the clinician. Definitive diagnosis occurs if there is histopathologic evidence of invasion in tissues. Single positive blood cultures also should be treated because there is no reliable way to distinguish "benign" candidemia from disseminated disease and the mortality rate associated with candidemia is at least 40%. An attempt should be made to rule out disseminated disease in patients with candidemia by evaluation for end-organ disease (*eg*, endophthalmitis, osteomyelitis, endocarditis, cutaneous lesions). (*Adapted from* Uzun and Anaissie [17]; with permission.)

Use of fluconazole versus amphotericin B	
Fluconazole	**Amphotericin B**
Isolation of *Candida* spp. routinely accepted as susceptible to fluconazole *C. albicans* *C. parapsilosis* *C. lusitanaie* *C. tropicalis*	Isolation of *C. krusei* and in some instances *C. glabrata*
No previous treatment with fluconazole	Previous treatment with fluconazole
Hemodynamically stable	Hemodynamically unstable

FIGURE 7-39. Use of fluconazole versus amphotericin B. The recommendations listed in the figure are based on the International Conference for the Development of a Consensus on the Management and Prevention of Severe Candidal Infections. In some instances, the recommendations are based on data from clinical trials. However, in some cases, not enough data are available, and the recommendations are based on the expert opinion of the attendees [18].

Acknowledgment

The authors would like to thank Dr. Louis Novoa-Takara for his help obtaining slides of pathologic sections.

References

1. Wenzell RP: Nosocomial candidemia: risk factors and attributable motrality. *Clin Infect Dis* 1995, 20:1531–1534.
2. Bodey GP: *Candidiasis: Pathogenesis, Diagnosis, and Treatment*, 2nd Ed. New York: Raven Press; 1993.
3. Pfaller MA: Nosocomial candidiasis: emerging species, reservoirs and modes of transmission. *Clin Infect Dis* 1996, 22(suppl 2):S89–S94.
4. Rex JH, Pfaller MA, Barry AL, *et al.*: Antifungal suceptibility testing of isolates from a randomized multicenter trial of fluconazole vs. amphotericin B as therapy of nonneutropenic patients with candidemia. *Antimicrob Agents Chemother* 1995, 39:40–44.
5. Wingard JR: Importance of *Candida* species other than *C. albicans* as pathogens in oncology patients. *Clin Infect Dis* 1995, 20:115–125.
6. Edwards JE: *Candida* species. In *Mandell, Douglas and Bennett's Principles and Practice of Infectious Diseases*, 4th Ed. Edited by Mandell GL, Bennett JH, Dolin R. New York: Churchill Livingstone; 1995:2289–2306.
7. Crissey JT, Lang H, Parish LC: *Manual of Medical Mycology*. Woburn: Blackwell Science, 1995.
8. Odds FC, Bernaerts RIA: CHROMagar Candida, a new differential isolation medium for presumptive identification of clinically important *Candida* species. *J Clin Microbiol* 1994, 32:1923–1929.
9. Pfaller MA, Houston A, Coffman S: Application of CHROMagar Candida for rapid screening of clinical specimens for *Candida albicans, Canidida tropicalis, Candida krusei* and *Candida (Torulopsis) glabrata*. *J Clin Microbiol* 1996, 34:58–61.
10. Thaler M, Pastakia B, Shawker TH, *et al.*: Hepatic candidiasis in cancer patients: the evolving picture of the syndrome. *Ann Intern Med* 1988, 108:88–100.
11. Clemente CD, ed.: *Gray's Anatomy*, 30th ed. Philadelphia: Lea & Febiger; 1985.
12. Edwards JE Jr. Candida endophlhalmitis. In *Current Clinical Topics in Infectious Diseases*. Edited by Remington JS, Swartz MN. New York: McGraw-Hill;1982: 386.
13. Fishman LS, Griffin JR, Sapico FL, Hecht R: Hematogenous *Candida* endophthalmitis: a complication of candidemia. *N Engl J Med* 1972, 286:675–681.
14. Herzog CA, Carson P, Michaud L, Asinger RW: Two-dimensional echocardiographic imaging of left ventricular vegetations. *Am Heart J* 1988, 115:684–686.
15. Gallis HA, Sobel JD: Candiduria. In *Atlas of Infectious Diseases*, vol 9. Edited by Mandell GL, Sobel JD. Philadelphia: Current Medicine; 1997:5.1–5.15.
16. Kwon-Chung, KJ, Bennett JE: Candidiasis. In *Medical Mycology*. Philadelphia: Lea & Febiger; 1992:280–336.
17. Uzun O, Anaissie EJ: Problems and controversies in the management of hematogenous candidiasis. *Clin Infect Dis* 1996, 22(suppl 2):S95–S101.
18. Edwards JE: International Conference for the Development of a Consensus on the Management and Prevention of Severe Candidal Infections. *Clin Infect Dis* 1997, 25:43–59.

CHAPTER 8

Mucocutaneous Candidiasis

Jack D. Sobel

Fungal Infections

Infections due to Candida species are the most common fungal infections, producing a broad range of infections. Mucocutaneous candidiasis, although rarely life threatening, is extremely common, frequently troublesome, and a major problem in compromised hosts.

A significant problem with mucosal and superficial candidiasis is the propensity for a small proportion of patients to suffer repeated relapses. In some situations, the explanation for such a relapse is obvious (eg, relapsing oropharyngeal candidiasis in a patient with advanced and uncontrolled HIV infection), but in other patients the cause is unknown (eg, healthy HIV-negative women with recurrent Candida vaginitis). Accurate diagnosis is essential for successful resolution of mucocutaneous candidiasis, especially given the availability of the safe and highly efficacious azole agents that remain the drugs of first choice for treatment of superficial candidiasis.

VULVOVAGINAL CANDIDIASIS

Candida Virulence Factors

Candida virulence factors
Adherence to epithelial cells
Protease elaboration
Germination (hyphae, pseudohyphae)
Phospholipase production
Switching colonies/phenotype variation
Immunosuppression
Hemolysin production
Iron utilization
Complement-binding receptors
Mycotoxins

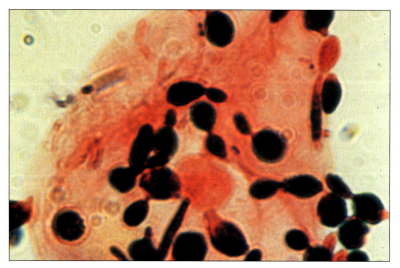

FIGURE 8-1. Microbial virulence factors expressed in *Candida*. To colonize, yeast blastospores adhere to epithelial cells and persist despite relatively antagonistic bacterial flora. Elaboration by *Candida* of phospholipase and proteases facilitates tissue invasion. Hemolysins lyse erythrocytes, releasing iron needed by *Candida* species. The ability of *Candida* blastospores to bind activated complement components interferes with complement binding to immunoglobulins and may prevent efficient phagocytosis of *Candida* in invasive candidiasis. The hyphal form of *Candida* is more virulent and invasive and is the morphotype associated with symptomatic mucositis. (*From* Sobel [1].)

FIGURE 8-2. Gram stain of vaginal squamous epithelial cell with adherent blastospores in budding phase. Yeasts are densely gram-positive. High-power view. (*From* Sobel [1].)

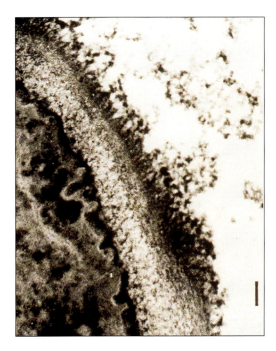

Figure 8-3. Transmission electron micrograph of *Candida albicans* cell wall. The micrograph shows the mannan surface layer containing mannoprotein (binding) ligands or adhesins. These mucopolysaccharide components adhere to fucose-containing receptors expressed on epithelial cells. (*From* Sobel [1].)

Epidemiology

Classification of vulvovaginal candidiasis	
Sporadic vaginitis	**Recurrent vaginitis (≥4 episodes/yr)**
Primary	Primary/idiopathic
Secondary	Secondary
Antibiotic therapy	Uncontrolled diabetes mellitus
Pregnancy	AIDS
	Estrogen replacement therapy
	Immunosuppressive therapy

Figure 8-4. Classification of vulvovaginal candidiasis. Most women suffer from sporadic, occasional attacks of vulvovaginal candidiasis, the most common precipitating factor being antibiotic use. Recurrent vulvovaginitis affects only a small percentage and, apart from in patients with uncontrolled diabetes and immunocompromised hosts, is usually idiopathic. (*From* Sobel [1].)

Epidemiology of vulvovaginal candidiasis
Second only on anaerobic bacterial vaginosis (*Gardnerella* spp.)
Approximately 75% of adults have at least one attack of vulvovaginal candidiasis
Three subpopulations:
No attacks
Infrequent episodes
Recurrent/chronic vulvovaginal candidiasis
45% have more than one episode

Figure 8-5. Epidemiology of vulvovaginal candidiasis. Vulvovaginal candidiasis is second only to bacterial vaginosis in prevalence, and because of its hormonal dependence, the infection is rare before puberty and after menopause. (*From* Sobel [1].)

Etiology

Microbiology of vulvovaginal candidiasis

>80% due to *Candida albicans*
3%–15% due to *Candida glabrata*
Incubation period: 24–96 hr
Inoculum: 10^2 microorganisms

FIGURE 8-6. Microbiology of vulvovaginal candidiasis. By far, the commonest pathogen in vulvovaginal candidiasis is *Candida albicans*; however, 5% to 15% of cases are due to non–*albicans* Candida species, the commonest of which is *Candida (Torulopsis) glabrata*. The minimal inoculum causing disease has been experimentally defined as 100 microorganisms. (*From* Sobel [1].)

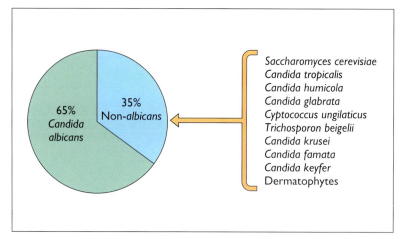

FIGURE 8-7. Subspeciation of yeast causing vulvovaginal candidiasis. Some authors have claimed a markedly increased prevalence of both *Candida glabrata* and *Candida tropicalis* in vulvovaginal candidiasis, although the data to support these recent claims have not been substantiated. Possibly women with HIV infection are more prone to infection with *C. glabrata* [2]. (*From* Sobel [1].)

Pathogenesis

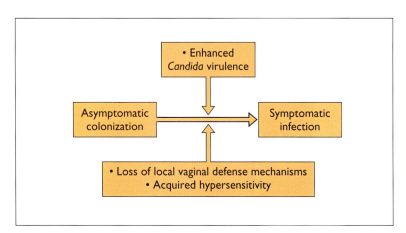

FIGURE 8-8. Transformation from asymptomatic colonization to symptomatic vaginitis. Low numbers of *Candida* species colonize the vagina as commensals but are capable of causing symptomatic vaginitis in the presence of local factors that enhance yeast virulence (*eg*, uncontrolled diabetes) or reduce local vaginal defense mechanisms (*eg*, antibiotics). (*From* Sobel [1].)

Natural anti-*Candida* vaginal defense mechanisms

Vaginal microbial flora dominated by *Lactobacillus* spp.
Intact vaginal (compartmentalized) cell-mediated immunity
Cervicovaginal immunoglobulins
  Candida-specific sIgA and IgG
Minor protective factors (?)
  Complement
  Phagocytic cells
Hormonal influence (anti-estrogen)

FIGURE 8-9. Natural anti-*Candida* defense mechanisms of the vagina. In contrast to oral thrush, vaginal candidiasis is not an opportunistic infection, because it occurs in otherwise healthy women. The normal *Lactobacillus*-dominant flora provides an essential defense mechanism, together with local vaginal cell-mediated immunity that involves *Candida*-specific T-lymphocyte clones expressing Th1 activity. Vaginal secretions contain antibodies that appear to have a minor protective role. (*From* Sobel [1].)

Risk factors for vulvovaginal candidiasis
Pregnancy
Uncontrolled diabetes mellitus
Corticosteroid therapy
Tight-fitting synthetic underclothing
Antimicrobial therapy (oral, parental, topical)
Estrogen therapy
Contraceptive use
Intrauterine device
Sponge
Nonoxynol-9 (?)
Diaphragm (?)
High-dose estrogen contraceptives
Increased frequency of coitus
"Candy binge"
Women frequenting sexually transmitted disease clinics
HIV infection

FIGURE 8-10. Risk factors for vulvovaginal candidiasis. The list of known exogenous and endogenous risk factors is large, but most episodes of vulvovaginal candidiasis occur in the absence of a recognizable precipitating factor. Although vulvovaginal candidiasis is not a sexually transmitted disease, sexual behavior, and possibly coital frequency, may contribute to symptomatic infection. (*From* Sobel [1].)

Pathogenesis of recurrent vulvovaginal candidiasis	
Source	Mechanism
1. More frequent vaginal inoculation/reinfection	1. Enhanced *Candida* virulence
Intestinal reservoir theory	2. Host
Sexual transmission	Depressed mucosal immunity (cell-mediated immunity)
2. Vaginal relapse	Immediate hypersensitivity reactivity (IgE)
	Loss of bacterial "colonization resistance"

FIGURE 8-11. Pathogenesis of idiopathic recurrent vulvovaginal candidiasis. For many years, recurrent vulvovaginal candidiasis was believed to be due to repeated reinfection from a gastrointestinal reservoir or possibly from sexual transmission. New evidence suggests that frequent reinfection is less likely to be responsible, and evidence instead points to frequent vaginal relapses resulting from subclinical persistence of yeasts in the vagina. Relapses occur because of the use of fungistatic antifungal agents and impaired local host defense mechanisms. Enhanced *Candida* virulence rarely may be due to antimycotic drug resistance. (*From* Sobel [3]; with permission.)

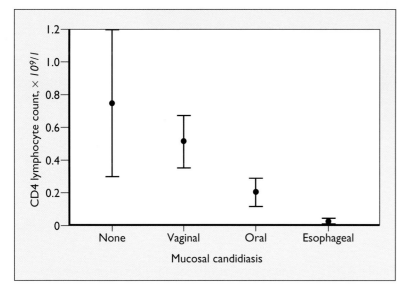

FIGURE 8-12. Occurrence of mucosal candidiasis correlating with CD4 cell counts in HIV-positive women. Esophageal candidiasis invariably occurs at CD4 counts less than 100/mm^3, whereas oral candidiasis frequently manifests at CD4 counts of 200 to 400/mm^3. Women reporting only vulvovaginal candidiasis (VVC) had CD4 counts within the normal range. The authors interpreted these findings as indicating that only a minimal immunosuppressive effect of HIV will result in chronic and recurrent VVC. This view has not been substantiated. (*From* Imam *et al.* [4]; with permission.)

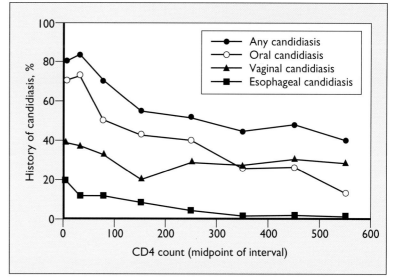

FIGURE 8-13. History of candidiasis by CD4 count. With a decline in CD4 cell counts in HIV-positive women, an increased susceptibility to oral and esophageal candidiasis is evident. However, no increased frequency of vulvovaginal candidiasis accompanies a decline in CD4 count. (*From* Sobel [1].)

Clinical Manifestations

Symptoms of acute vulvovaginal candidiasis
Pruritus
Discharge
Soreness, irritation, burning
Dysuria
Dyspareunia
Minimal nonoffensive color
Penile rash (men)

FIGURE 8-14. Symptoms of acute *Candida* vulvovaginitis. The symptoms of vulvovaginal candidiasis are nonspecific, not allowing diagnosis by history alone. Symptoms typically increase premenstrually and improve with onset of menstrual flow. A small portion of the male partners of women with vulvovaginal candidiasis will develop superficial genital candidiasis. (*From* Sobel [1].)

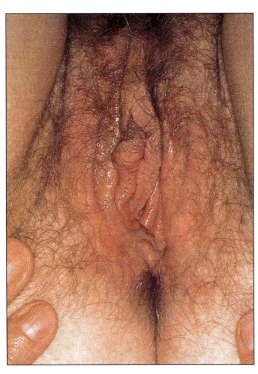

FIGURE 8-15. Vulvar erythema and pruritus extending into perianal area. Signs of vulvovaginal candidiasis are also nonspecific and preclude diagnosis without laboratory confirmation. (*From* Sobel [1].)

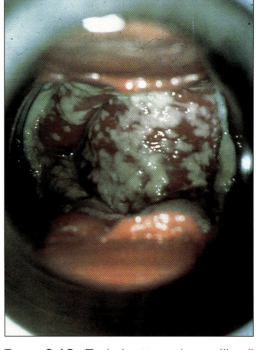

FIGURE 8-16. Typical cottage cheese–like discharges in vulvovaginitis candidiasis. The typical "cottage cheese," white discharge seen on speculum examination is found in only a minority of patients with *Candida* vaginitis. (*From* Sobel [1].)

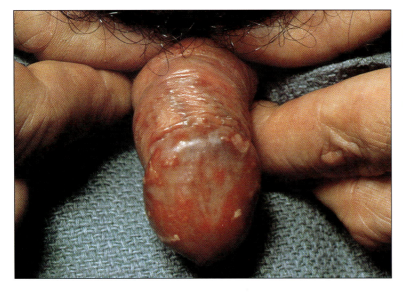

FIGURE 8-17. *Candida* balanoposthitis. *Candida* balanoposthitis presents with penile itching, irritation, and soreness, accompanied by edema, erythema, and excoriation. It is seen in the male partners of women with a vaginal culture positive for *Candida albicans*. Only a small fraction of the male partners of women with vulvovaginal candidiasis will develop superficial genital candidiasis. (*From* Sobel [1].)

Differential Diagnosis

Differential diagnosis of vulvovaginal candidiasis	
↑ pH	Normal pH
Bacterial vaginosis	Physiologic leukorrhea
Trichomoniasis	Allergic/hypersensitivity vaginitis
Atrophic vaginitis	Chemical/irritant (eg, nonoxynol-9)
Desquamative inflammatory vaginitis	Cytolytic vaginosis
Mixed (above + vulvovaginal candidiasis)	Vestibular adenitis/vulvovdynia
Erosive planus (vagina)	Erosive planus (vulva)
	Lichen simplex
	Lichen sclerosus
	Squamous papulomatosis
	Genital herpes

FIGURE 8-18. Differential diagnoses in vulvovaginal candidiasis. Considerations in the differential diagnosis of vulvovaginal candidiasis differ depending on measurement of the vaginal pH. (*From* Sobel [1].)

Diagnostic Procedures

Diagnostic tests in vulvovaginitis	
pH estimation	Nonspecific but extremely useful in suggesting bacterial and protozoal infection (*see* Fig. 8-13)
Amine test (whiff test, sniff test)	Low sensitivity and specificity; useful in suggestion bacterial vaginosis or trichomoniasis
Saline microscopy	Essential study in evaluating patients with vulvovaginitis; sensitivity in diagnosis of VVC only 30%–40%
10% potassium hydroxide microscopy	↑ sensitivity in diagnosing VVC (60%–80%)
Vaginal yeast culture	Gold standard for diagnosing presence of yeast, but a positive culture does not indicate vaginitis; culture uncommonly needed

VVC—vulvovaginal candidiasis.

FIGURE 8-19. Diagnostic tests in vulvovaginitis. Diagnosis of *Candida* vulvovaginitis typically includes measurement of vaginal pH, saline microscopy, and 10% potassium hydroxide microscopic examination. For each test, a swab is obtained from the middle third of the vagina. (*From* Sobel [1].)

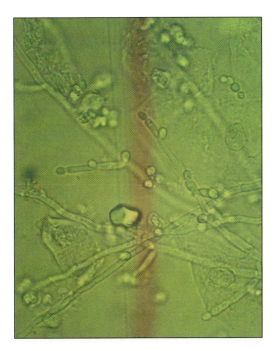

FIGURE 8-20. Saline microscopy. Although a number of techniques are used, most frequently a swab obtained from the middle third of the vagina is immediately placed in 0.5 mL of saline in a test tube. Then, a single drop of the resultant solution is placed on a clean, dry slide and a coverslip applied. Initially under low power, the presence of motile trichomonads, polymorphonuclear neutrophils (PMNs), and hyphae can be detected. Under high-power magnification, a search is made for clue cells, trichomonads, PMNs, yeast blastospores and pseudohyphae, and epithelial cell maturation (squamous versus basal and parabasal cells). Finally, the bacterial flora is assessed (rods versus cocci). (*From* Sobel [1].)

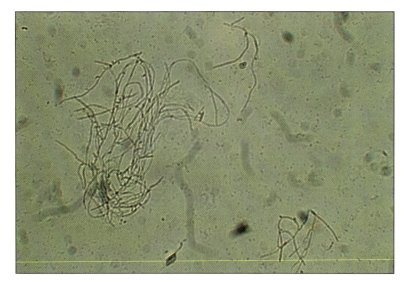

Figure 8-21. Potassium hydroxide (KOH) microscopy showing hyphae and blastospores. Ten percent KOH microscopy facilitates the diagnosis of *Candida* vulvovaginitis. KOH, by destroying epithelial cells, allows easier recognition of yeast and hyphae, improving on the sensitivity of the saline microscopy (30% to 40%) to reach levels of 60% to 80%. With the exception of *Candida glabrata* and *Saccharomyces cerevisiae*, KOH examination allows recognition of pseudohyphae and hyphae as well as blastospores. (*From* Sobel [1].)

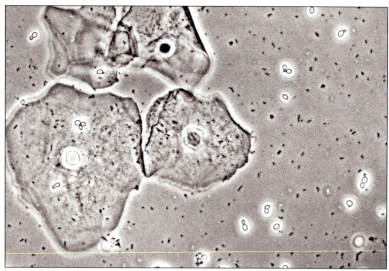

Figure 8-22. Phase contrast microscopy showing yeast cells without hyphae. Large numbers of yeast cells are seen as singlets or as budding yeast, but there is a complete absence of pseudohyphae and hyphae. This appearance is almost pathognomonic of *Candida glabrata* or *Saccharomyces cerevisiae*, two species of yeast that may resemble typical *Candida albicans* vaginitis but tend to be difficult to cure with conventional therapy. (*From* Sobel [1].)

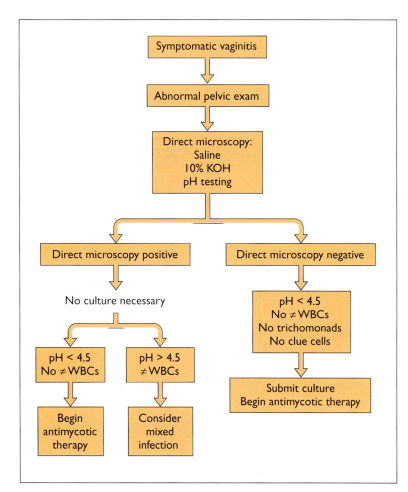

Figure 8-23. Diagnostic steps in vulvovaginitis candidiasis. All patients with symptomatic vaginitis require physical examination, pelvic examination, and vaginal swabs for laboratory diagnosis. If direct microscopy is positive for yeast, confirmatory culture for *Candida* species is unnecessary; however, if saline microscopy and potassium hydroxide (KOH) preparation are negative for yeast, culture is essential. A low pH in this situation would be a useful indication for a latex agglutination slide test. WBCs—white blood cells. (*From* Sobel [1].)

Treatment

Topical azole antimycotics for acute *Candida* vaginitis

Single day
  Clotrimazole (Mycelex)   500-mg vaginal tablets
  Tioconazole (Vagistat)   6.5% cream
3 days
  Butoconazole (Femstat)   2% cream (5 g)
  Clotrimazole (Mycelex, Gynelotrim)   200-mg vaginal tablet
  Miconazole (Monistat)   200-mg vaginal suppository
  Tioconazole   2% cream
  Terconazole (Terazol)   0.8% cream (5 g)
                                            80-mg vaginal suppository
7 days
  Clotrimazole   1% cream
                                            100-mg vaginal tablet
  Miconazole   2% cream
                                            100-mg vaginal suppository
  Terconazole   0.4% cream (5 g)

FIGURE 8-24. Topical azole preparations antimycotics for treatment of acute *Candida* vaginitis, stratified by duration of therapy. All the agents achieve 75% to 85% cure rates. The choice of formulation should be determined by patient preference and distribution of inflammation. Severity of inflammation also influences duration of therapy. (*From* Sobel [1].)

Nonazole topical agents for acute *Candida* vaginitis

14 days
  Nystatin (Mycostatin)   100,000-U vaginal tablet or suppository daily
  Boric acid   600-mg vaginal suppository daily
  Gentian violet   7–14 d

FIGURE 8-25. Nonazole topical agents for acute *Candida* vaginitis. Nonazole agents are also effective in treating *Candida* vulvovaginitis. Cure rates are slightly lower, 70% to 75%, and treatment requires more prolonged administration because of slower "killing rates" (*ie*, relatively more fungistatic). These agents may be particularly useful in therapy of non-*albicans* vaginitis and are also inexpensive despite protracted therapy. (*From* Sobel [1].)

Oral/systemic therapy for vulvovaginal candidiasis

Ketoconazole   400 mg/d × 5 d
Itraconazole   200 mg/d × 3 d
                   200 mg 2 times a day × 1 d
Fluconazole   150 mg/d × 1 d

FIGURE 8-26. Oral/systemic therapy for vulvovaginal candidiasis (VVC). Three agents—ketoconazole, itraconazole, and fluconazole—are all highly effective in achieving therapeutic cure in VVC. Ketoconazole is associated with significant toxicity, notably hepatotoxicity, and like the triazole itraconazole, is not approved for use for this indication in the United States. Single-dose fluconazole is approved and is now widely used for VVC. (*From* Sobel [1].)

Therapy for non-*albicans* *Candida* vaginitis

Trial of conventional azoles (not shortcourse)
Nystatin vaginal suppositories 100,000 U daily × 14 d
Boric acid 600 mg in gelatin capsule administered vaginally for 14 d
Topical flucytosine vaginally × 14 d
Combination systemic imidazole and vaginal nonazole

FIGURE 8-27. Therapy of non-*albicans Candida* vaginitis. Non-*albicans Candida* species (specifically *Candida glabrata*) are less susceptible to all azole antifungal agents and often respond clinically to older fungistatic nonazole agents when prescribed over protracted periods. Response of *C. glabrata* to azoles is less than 50%.

Fungal Infections

Therapy of recurrent vulvovaginal candidiasis

Confirm diagnosis (culture)
Eliminate predisposing factors
Treatment of sexual partner (?)
Reassure
Induction and maintenance regimen

FIGURE 8-28. Principles of therapy of recurrent vulvovaginal candidiasis. Because many women have been mislabeled as having chronic and recurrent vulvovaginal candidiasis, before any prolonged maintenance regimen is initiated, the role of *Candida* species as the cause of the chronic syndrome must be established by culture. Predisposing factors are usually absent, but when they are present (*eg*, uncontrolled diabetes), efforts to control precipitating factors should be attempted. Little evidence exists that treatment of male partners is beneficial. After a more intensive initial induction regimen, patients should be placed on a maintenance regimen for about 6 months. (*From* Sobel [1].)

FIGURE 8-29. Clinical and microbiologic patterns following antimycotic therapy. *Green bars* indicate the duration of signs and symptoms of vulvovaginal candidiasis, and *orange bars* reflect the patient's culture-positive status. Invariably following antimycotic therapy, symptoms disappear and a culture-negative status follows (*A*). In normal healthy women, vaginal recolonization with the same strain occurs in 20% to 25% of cases within 4 to 6 weeks, but is not associated with recurrence of symptoms (*B*). Women with recurrent vulvovaginal candidiasis do predictably develop recurrence of symptoms within 3 months of previous "successful" therapy (*C*). Because of these frequent recurrences following "successful" therapy, there is a need for maintenance therapy that can be prescribed on a weekly (*D*) or even daily basis (*E*). Infrequently, partial or incomplete symptomatic relief (*F*) or partial mycologic response only (*G*) follows appropriate intensive therapy. This is due to partial or complete resistance of yeast and requires that vaginal cultures and, rarely, fungal susceptibility tests be performed. *Asterisk* indicates maintenance regimen.

Maintenance regimens for recurrent vulvovaginal candidiasis (VVC). Two oral regimens (ketoconazole [100 mg daily] and fluconazole [100–200 mg weekly]) and one topical regimen (weekly clotrimazole [500 mg per vagina]) are highly effective in providing more than 90% protection against recurrence of vulvovaginal candidiasis (VVC) while prophylaxis is taken. Maintenance suppressive prophylaxis is prescribed for 6 months and then discontinued. Slightly more than half of women with recurrent VVC will remain in long-term remission. The remainder rapidly return to the same pattern of recurrent VVC and should be placed on maintenance suppressive therapy for 1 year and then reassessed. Other regimens include miconazole, 500 to 1200 mg, per vagina, and itraconazole, 200 mg three times per week, orally. (*From* Sobel [1].)

OROPHARYNGEAL CANDIDIASIS

Risk factors for oropharyngeal candidiasis

Antibiotic therapy (especially prolonged)
Neutropenia
Irradiation
Xerostomia
Diabetes mellitus (uncontrolled)
High-dosage corticosteroids
Chemotherapy
Newborns
AIDS
Debilitation
Prosthesis (dental)

FIGURE 8-30. Risk factors for oropharyngeal candidiasis. Most episodes of oropharyngeal candidiasis in patients without AIDS occur as nosocomial events in debilitated patients with single or multiple predisposing factors. In particular, patients with cancer frequently develop thrush owing to neutropenia, antibiotic therapy, irradication, direct tissue damage, and generalized debilitation. Patients at the extremes of age are also at high risk; in particular, elderly patients with dental prostheses frequently develop atrophic or erythematous glossitis and pharyngitis. Oropharyngeal candidiasis is a marker of depressed immunity. It develops in 80% to 95% of AIDS patients. It is also an indicator of the imminent arrival of opportunistic infections.

Pathogenesis of oropharyngeal candidiasis in AIDS
Xerostomia
Decreased sIgA (?)
Defective/absent protective mucosal cell-mediated immunity and T-cell function
Impaired polymorphonuclear cell and phagocyte function
Frequent antibiotic use for other opportunistic pathogens
Enhanced virulence of *Candida* spp. by HIV gene-products

Figure 8-31. Pathogenesis of oropharangeal candidiasis in patients with AIDS. Multiple contributory factors coexist to predispose to oropharyngeal candidiasis in HIV-seropositive patients. The dominant predisposing factor is the loss of protective mucosal superficial cell-mediated immunity with severe, recalcitrant, and recurrent disease accompanying advanced immunodeficiency. The use of highly active antiretroviral therapy often results in dramatic improvement of resistant candidiasis with only slight improvement in CD4 count. Recent studies suggest a role for HIV in directly enchancing the virulence of *Candida albicans*.

Microbiology of oropharyngeal and esophageal candidiasis
Usually single species
>90% *Candida albicans*
Mixed fungal infections (<10%)
C. albicans + *C. glabrata*
Role of non-*albicans Candida* spp. questionable
Rare infections caused by non-*albicans Candida* spp. only
Mixed infections with other pathogens (HSV, CMV)

HSV–herpes simplex virus; CMV–cytomegalovirus

Figure 8-32. Microbiology of oropharyngeal and esophageal candidiasis. The highly predictable presence of *Candida albicans* is a cause of oropharyngeal and esophageal candidiasis even in advanced immunodeficiency states. Whether a second concomitant potential pathogen such as *Candida glabrata* contributes to clinical disease and requires specific therapy is controversial. Non-*albicans Candida* species are selected for by azole therapy. In the 1980s, non-*albicans Candida* species accounted for 3.4% of oral isolates in HIV-infected patients, whereas in the 1990s, 16% to 18% of isolates recovered from symptomatic HIV-seropositive patients were non-*albicans Candida* species [5].

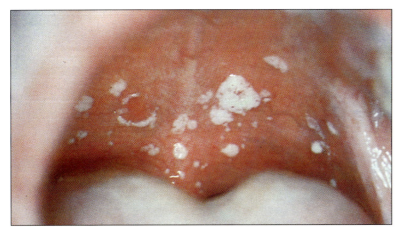

Figure 8-33. Pseudomembranous candidiasis (thrush). Thrush presents clinically as white patches on the oral mucosa, which wipe off to reveal a red or ulcerated area. Diagnosis is made by clinical appearance and demonstration of the organism on a stained smear from the lesion. It is a normal member of the oral flora that is low in virulence and is considered an opportunistic pathogen. Infection by *Candida* species usually indicates a lowering of the host's resistance or a change in the oral flora that permits *Candida* species to predominate. Its presence as a secondary infection in lesions such as angular cheilitis and erythema multiforme may mask the underlying disease process. Factors that may precipitate *Candida* infections include prolonged use of broad-spectrum antibiotics, chemotherapy, immunosuppressive drugs, irradiation, steroid therapy, and systemic or local disease that affects the patient's immune response. (*From* Gher and Quintero [6].)

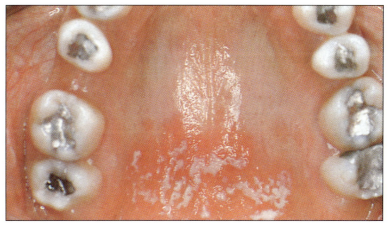

Figure 8-34. Chronic hyperplastic candidiasis. The condition presents clinically as a white, pebbly surfaced, slightly raised plaque or leukoplakia. Scattered erythematous areas may be noted. The plaque represents a hyperplastic response by the epithelium to the invading organism. The plaque will not wipe off as with pseudomembranous candidiasis. Biopsy and periodic acid–Schiff stain help make the diagnosis. (*From* Gher and Quintero [6].)

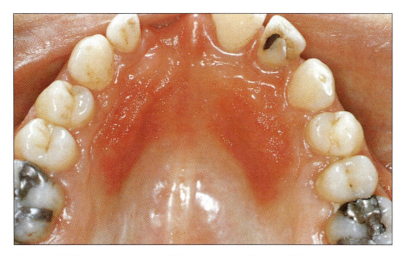

FIGURE 8-35. Atrophic candidiasis. Atrophic candidiasis presents clinically as an erythematous area under a denture base and is clinically diagnosed as denture stomatitis caused by an ill-fitting denture. Trauma from the denture is suspected as a precipitating or perpetuating factor for a candidial infection. (*From* Gher and Quintero [6].)

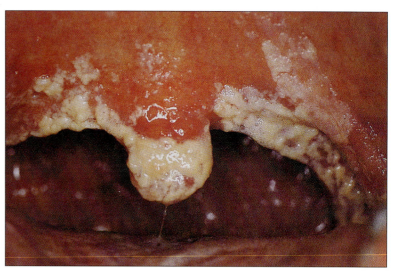

FIGURE 8-36. Extensive pharyngeal candidiasis involving the soft palette and uvula of a patient with AIDS. Oropharyngeal candidiasis can be a marker of T-cell immunosuppression. T cells are required to control *Candida* species growth on the mucosal surfaces. However, adequate neutrophil number and function are enough to prevent deep invasion, and there is surprisingly little tendency to develop disseminated candidiasis in patients who are T-cell deficient. (*From* Fitzpatrick *et al.* [7]; with permission.)

Therapy for oropharyngeal candidiasis

Clotrimazole troches 10 mg 5 times a day
Fluconazole 100–200 mg/d
Ketoconazole 200–600 mg/d
Itraconazole 200 mg/d (liquid or capsule)
Amphotericin B 0.6 mg/d IV or suspension

FIGURE 8-37. Therapy for oropharyngeal candidiasis. Clotrimazole is an effective treatment for mild cases of thrush. However, systemic therapy with oral imidazoles (ketoconazole) and triazoles (itraconazole and fluconazole) is preferred for achieving superior results. Triazole therapy is now the method of choice with the new cyclodextin itraconazole liquid/suspension, achieving cure rates equivalent to those of fluconazole. Clinical cure rates range from 75% to 95%, with mycologic cure rates of 65% to 85%, although most patients rapidly will become culture positive shortly after stopping therapy. Emerging resistance to fluconazole is a growing problem in patients with advanced AIDS.

ESOPHAGEAL CANDIDIASIS

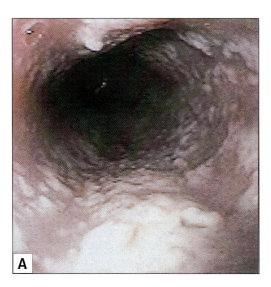

FIGURE 8-38. Invasive *Candida* esophagitis. *Candida* species is the most common opportunistic fungal pathogen affecting people with advancing HIV infection. Almost 100% of patients with AIDS will have had some clinical manifestation of mucosal candidial infection during the course of their illness. The upper gastrointestinal tract and anogenital areas are the most commonly involved. *Candida* esophagitis has been the most common initial AIDS-defining illness in at least two cohorts of HIV-infected women, which suggests that hormone differences may play a role in the risk of invasive disease. Involvement of the esophagus is the most common form of invasive candidal infection in patients with AIDS. **A**, The typical endoscopic appearance of *Candida* esophagitis is shown, presenting as superficial, often raised, white plaques on the mucosa. *(continued on next page)*

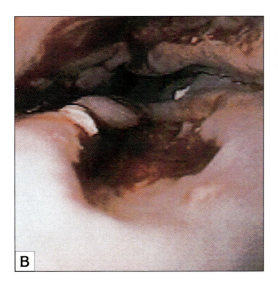

Figure 8-38. *(continued)* **B,** *Candida* species involvement of the esophageal mucosa in patients with advanced HIV infection can result in either superficially invasive disease or deep discrete ulcers. In this patient, who presented with fever and odynophagia, a large deep esophageal ulcer owing to *Candida* species was seen endoscopically. (*From* Kessler [8]; *courtesy of* Dr. J. Schaffner.)

Differential Diagnosis

Differential diagnosis of esophageal candidiasis

Herpes simplex virus
Cytomegalovirus
Other infections (rare)
  Bacterial infections (*Mycobacterium avium-intracellulare, Mycobacterium tuberculosis*)
  Cryptosporidium, histoplasmosis
Idiopathic apthous ulcer (giant single or multiple)
Reflux esophagitis
Neoplasia
  Primary cancer, lymphoma, Kaposi's sarcoma
Mixed

Figure 8-39. Differential diagnosis of esophageal candidiasis. Clinical symptoms of esophagitis are similar regardless of the etiology. Frequently, more than one pathogenic mechanism may occur simultaneously, and not infrequently two pathogens, such as cytomegalovirus and *Candida* species, may co-exist, hence the need to obtain multiple studies including tissue biopsy at the time of endoscopy. Cytomegalovirus esophagitis most frequently involves the distal esophagus and results in mucosal hemorrhage.

Treatment

Treatment of esophageal candidiasis

Fluconazole 100–200 mg/d (orally or IV)
Itraconazole 200–400 mg/d (liquid orally)
Amphotericin B 0.5–0.7 mg/kg/d (IV)

Figure 8-40. Treatment of esophageal candidiasis. Mild disease may respond to oral fluconazole or liquid itraconazole therapy. More severe disease is treated intravenously. Therapy is continued until resolution of symptoms and for several days, therapy switching from the IV to oral route to complete at least 2 weeks therapy. Ketoconazole 200 to 400 mg/d is also an option, with lower cure rates and no parenteral solution. Lower doses of amphotericin B are effective for mild disease in patients without AIDS, *eg*, 0.3 to 0.4 mg/kg/d. The role of highly active antiretroviral therapy should not be neglected in contributing to resolution of recalcitrant disease.

Cutaneous Candidiasis

Classification of cutaneous candidiasis

Primary (no candidemia)
  Mucocutaneous candidiasis
  Intertrigo
  Wound infection
  Diaper candidiasis
  Paronychium
  Onychomycosis
  Balanoposthitis
  Vulvitis
  Burns
Secondary (hematogenous)
  Receding or co-existent candidemia
  Granulocytopenia (usually severe and prolonged)
  IV catheter

FIGURE 8-41. Classification of cutaneous candidiasis. Primary cutaneous candidiasis is common, especially in neonates and women with vaginitis. Skin colonization by *Candida* species is infrequent but increases in patients with diabetes and when local factors provide a microenvironment, *eg*, maceration. Systemic and local antibiotic agents also enhance local yeast manifestations.

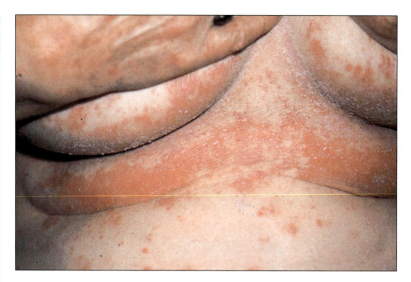

FIGURE 8-42. Intertriginous candidiasis. The typical appearance of candidiasis is with bright red erythema and satellite papules and pustules, occurring in the axillae, groin, or other skin folds, as beneath pendulous breasts in this woman. The vigorous neutrophilic response is believed to be due to release of complement-derived chemotactic factors by fungal polysaccharides. (*From* Raugi [9].)

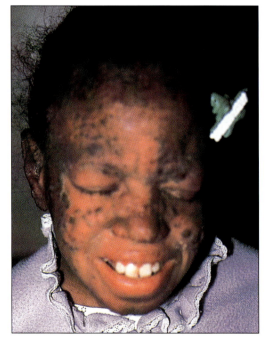

FIGURE 8-43. Chronic mucocutaneous candidiasis. This distinctive clinical syndrome occurs in patients with defective cellular immunity. Multiple acral and periorificial sites are involved with nonhealing, verrucous, hyperkeratotic plaques. Biopsy shows invasion of organisms into the dermis and subcutaneous fat, in contrast to the superficial invasion in other cutaneous forms of candidiasis. (*From* Raugi [9]; *courtesy of* Dr. J. Francis.)

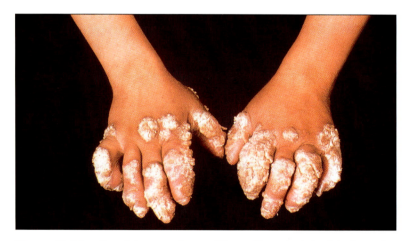

FIGURE 8-44. *Candida* granuloma. The solitary indolent lesion of *Candida* granuloma typically contains organisms only in the cornified cell layer of the epidermis, but the reactive inflammatory infiltrate may extend into the subcutaneous fat. An example on the hand demonstrates part of the clinical spectrum of this condition. (*From* Raugi [9]; *courtesy of* Dr. K. Abson.)

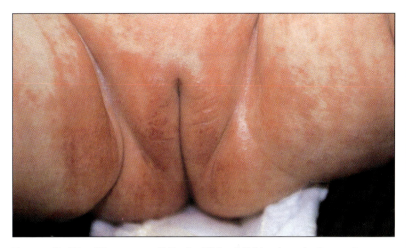

FIGURE 8-45. Diaper candidiasis. This child had an irritant diaper dermatitis (note the characteristic sparing of the depths of the creases) with secondary colonization and infection with *Candida* species. (*From* Raugi [9]; *courtesy of* Dr. J. Francis.)

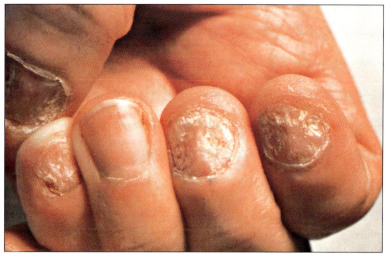

FIGURE 8-46. Candidal infection of the periungual tissue. Candidal infection of the periungual tissue, known as paronychia, is characterized by swelling, erythema, and tenderness, sometimes with a purulent around the nails. When the nails are involved, they become brittle, thickened, and opaque. (*From* Friedman-Kien [10].)

CANDIDA ONYCHOMYCOSIS

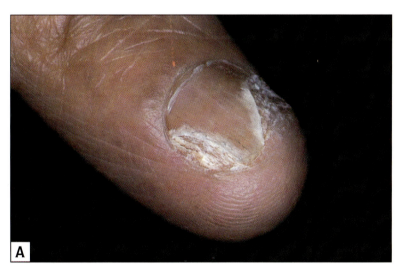
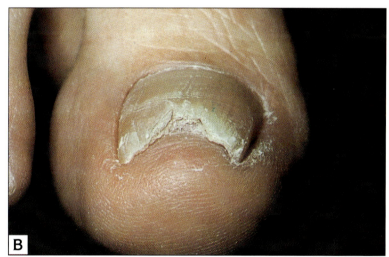

FIGURE 8-47. Candidal infection of the nail plate. **A,** Onychomycosis is a prominent feature of candidal infection of the nail plate with especially exuberant subungual debris. Culture is required to definitively establish *Candida* species as the etiologic agent. **B,** The nail may become hyperconvex with the piled-up subungual debris. (*From* Raugi [9]; *courtesy of* Dr. P. Fleckman.)

Hematogenous Candidiasis

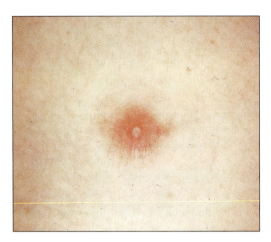

FIGURE 8-48. Skin lesion in disseminated candidiasis. Fungi may produce a variety of skin lesions, but they are usually papular with or without a necrotic or pustular center. This lesion was due to *Candida albicans*; the source was probably the gastrointestinal tract, with the skin being infected by hematogenous spread. The patient also had hematogenous spread of infection to the lungs. Another route of entry for *Candida* species is an indwelling intravenous catheter. (*From* Armstrong [11].)

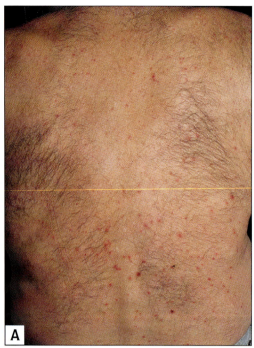 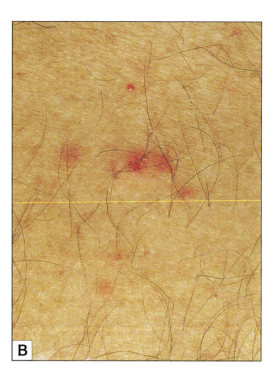

FIGURE 8-49. Pustular cutaneous lesions of disseminated candidiasis. **A**, Diffuse erythematous pustular lesions arose over the course of 24 hours on the trunk of a man aged 67 years with chronic lymphocytic leukemia and neutropenia. He had been febrile and on broad-spectrum antibiotics for 8 days when these lesions occurred. **B**, Close-up view of the lesions shows small pustules on an erythematous base. The lesions were nontender. (*From* Kauffman [12].)

Drug-resistant Candidiasis

Azole-resistant mucocutaneous candidiasis	
Intrinsic resistance to non-*albicans Candida* spp.	
Candida glabrata (all azoles)	++
Candida krusei (fluconazole)	+++
Candida tropicalis (all azoles)	+
Candida parapsilosis (all azoles)	+
Increasing frequency in vaginitis	
Controversial role in oropharyngeal and esophageal candidiasis in patients with AIDS	

FIGURE 8-50. Azole-resistant mucocutaneous candidiasis. Intrinsic resistance of non-*albicans Candida* species to azoles, especially fluconazole, is emerging as a growing problem in superficial and invasive candidiasis. Widespread use of topical and systemic azoles especially in low-dosage as well as abbreviated courses may be responsible for selecting for non-*albicans Candida* species. *Candida krusei* is usually susceptible to other imidazoles and triazoles. For vaginal candidiasis, topical boric acid or flucytosine is effective.

Fluconazole-resistant *Candida albicans* infection
Growing problem in oropharyngeal and esophageal candidiasis in patients with AIDS
Rare in vaginitis (even in patients with AIDS)
Clinical failure
Inadequate dosing
Decreased absorption
Lack of adherence
Drug interaction
Acquired resistance (↑ MIC)
Cross-resistance to other azoles

FIGURE 8-51. Fluconazole-resistant *Candida albicans* infection. Although extremely rare in vaginitis and cutaneous candidiasis, approximately 5% to 10% of patients with AIDS, advanced immunodeficiency, and high viral loads develop recalcitrant oropharyngeal and esophageal candidiasis. Achlorhydria noted in many patients with advanced HIV reduces ketoconazole but not fluconazole absorption. Approximately 30% to 40% of fluconazole-resistant strains retain sensitivity of itraconazole and ketoconazole, but resistance to these agents predictably and rapidly occurs. Amphotericin B IV may be required to achieve clinical improvement, which is often short lived.

Azole resistance in *Candida albicans*

Risk factors	Mechanisms
Previous oropharyngeal candidiasis (repeated)	Altered cytochrome P450 lanosterol demethylase enzyme
Lower median CD4 counts	Changes in Δ^{5-6}-sterol desaturase
Longer duration of previous azole therapy [16]	↓ Permeability of fungal cell wall
	Energy-dependent drug efflux mechanism

FIGURE 8-52. Azole resistance in *Candida albicans*. The dominant mechanism for acquired resistance appears to the energy-dependent drug efflux mechanism, responsible for pumping active drug from the fungal intracellular compartment into the exterior of the yeast cell. A similar resistance mechanism has been reported in non-*albicans Candida* species.

REFERENCES

1. Sobel JD: Vulvovaginal candidiasis. In *Atlas of Infectious Diseases*, vol 5. Edited by Mandell GL, Rein MF. Philadelphia: Current Medicine; 1996:7.1–7.17.

2. Horowitz BJ, Giaqunta D, Ito S: Evolving pathogens in vulvovaginal candidiasis: implications for patient care. *J Clin Pharmacol* 1992, 32:248–255.

3. Sobel JD: Genital candidiasis. In *Candidiasis: Pathogenesis, Diagnosis, and Treatment*, 2nd ed. Edited by Bodey GP. New York: Raven Press; 1953:232.

4. Imam N, Carpenter CC, Mayer KH, *et al.*: Hierarchical pattern of mucosal candida infections in HIV-seropositive women. *Am J Med* 1990, 89:142–146.

5. Barchiesi F, Morbiducci V, Ancarani F, Scalise G: Emergence of oropharyngeal candidiasis caused by non-*albicans* species of *Candida* in HIV-infected patients. *Eur J Epidemiol* 1993, 9:455–456.

6. Gher ME Jr, Quintero G: Infectious diseases of the oral cavity. In *Atlas of Infectious Diseases*, vol 4. Edited by Mandell GL, Brook I. Philadelphia: Current Medicine; 1995:5.1–5.27.

7. Fitzpatrick TB, Johnson RA, Polano MR, *et al.* (eds): *Color Atlas and Synopsis of Clinical Dermatology*, 2nd ed. New York: McGraw-Hill; 1992.

8. Kessler HA: Clinical manifestations in opportunistic infections. In *Atlas of Infectious Diseases*, vol 1, 2nd ed. Edited by Mandell GL, Mildvan D. Philadelphia: Current Medicine; 1997:14.1–14.14.

9. Raugi GJ: Fungal and yeast infections of the skin, appendages, and subcutaneous tissue. In *Atlas of Infectious Diseases*, vol 2. Edited by Mandell GL, Stevens DL. Philadelphia: Current Medicine; 1995:6.1–6.28.

10. Friedman-Kien AE: Cutaneous manifestations. In *Atlas of Infectious Diseases*, vol 1, 2nd ed. Edited by Mandell GL, Mildvan D. Philadelphia: Current Medicine; 1997:5.1–5.18.

11. Armstrong D: Cutaneous manifestations of infection in the immunocompromised host. In *Atlas of Infectious Diseases*, vol 8. Edited by Mandell GL, Fekety R. Philadelphia: Current Medicine; 1997:13.1–13.12.

12. Kauffman CA: Systemic fungal infections. In *Atlas of Infectious Diseases*, vol 8. Edited by Mandell GL, Fekety R. Philadelphia: Current Medicine; 1997:11.1–11.18.

CHAPTER 9

Aspergillosis

Andreas H. Groll
Thomas J. Walsh

Moulds of the genus *Aspergillus* are among the most common fungi of all environments. They grow well in soil and decaying vegetation and can be found on all types of organic debris. In hospitals, ventilation systems and dust associated with construction activity have been implicated as the main habitats of the organism.

The term *aspergillosis* refers to a group of human diseases owing to *Aspergillus* species. The usual portal of entry of the airborne conidia (spores) is the respiratory tract, but any laceration of the integument can serve as a nidus for infection in the appropriate setting. Despite the existence of many hundreds of species, only a few have been regularly and consistently involved in human disease; and among these, *Aspergillus fumigatus*, *Aspergillus flavus*, and *Aspergillus niger* most commonly are encountered. The spectrum of possible pathologic processes is broad and includes hypersensitivity conditions, saprophytic disease, and, in patients with impaired host defenses, chronic granulomatous or life-threatening invasive infections. Notably, in all of these conditions, the most important determinant of disease is the individual predisposition of the patient, not the intensity of exposure or virulence factors of the infecting organism.

The first descriptions of human disease due to *Aspergillus* species were published in the middle of the 18th century. Over the ensuing 100 years, almost all forms of aspergillosis in humans had been delineated, and allergic and saprophytic manifestations of aspergillosis had been recognized as not uncommon causes of human disease [1]. However, aspergillosis probably would have remained something of marginal clinical interest had it not been for the dramatic increase of severely immunocompromised patients that has occurred over the past three decades in conjunction with advances in anticancer treatment, organ transplantation, therapeutic immunosuppression, and the advent of the AIDS epidemic [2]. Along with these developments, invasive aspergillosis has emerged as an important cause of morbidity and mortality in the hospital, and in some centers, *Aspergillus* species has replaced *Candida* species as the leading pathogen of invasive opportunistic fungal disease over time found at postmortem [3].

The major and quantitatively most important risk factors for invasive disease owing to *Aspergillus* species are profound and protracted granulocytopenia and functional phagocytic defects such as those that occur after systemic treatment with high dosages of corticosteroids. Accordingly, invasive aspergillosis has become a leading cause of attributable mortality in patients undergoing bone marrow transplantations [4,5]; it is the most significant fungal infection in patients with hematologic malignancies [6] and aplastic anemia [7] and in patients after solid organ transplantation [8]. It also has been increasingly observed in patients with advanced stages of HIV infection [3,9,10].

Various forms of invasive aspergillosis exist. The lungs are by far the most common focus of infection, and dissemination to virtually any body site is quite frequent. Except for the integument, all forms of invasive aspergillosis are both difficult to diagnose and difficult to treat, and mortality is close to 100% in patients with persistent granulocytopenia independent of all therapeutic interventions. However, early presumptive diagnosis is now facilitated in the appropriate clinical setting by high-resolution computed tomography. Prompt institution of aggressive medical and surgical treatment in conjunction with the concept of empirical antifungal therapy may improve the outcomes in patients who ultimately recover from neutropenia or other life-threatening complications of their underlying conditions. Molecular and immunologic diagnostics, novel and potent antifungal compounds, and approaches to augmenting host defenses are under intensive preclinical and early clinical investigation and hopefully will provide avenues for better diagnosis and treatment for invasive aspergillosis.

Description of the Organism and Spectrum of Diseases

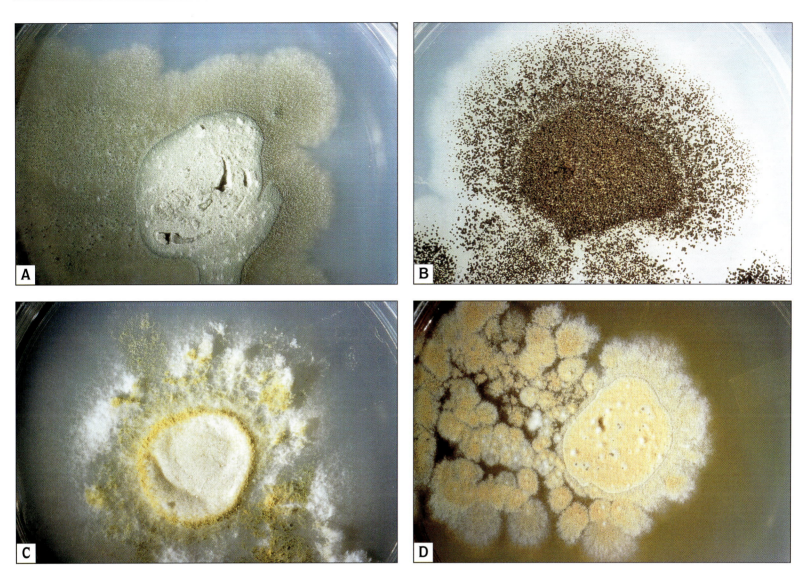

FIGURE 9-1. Colonial morphology of *Aspergillus* species. Four clinically relevant organisms are shown 7 days after inoculation on Czapek-Dox agar. **A**, With the production of conidia, *Aspergillus fumigatus* produces a flat, velvety gray-green colony. **B**, *Aspergillus niger* has a white to yellow basal mycelium, which bears abundant black conidial structures. **C**, *Aspergillus flavus* develops a white mycelium and produces intense yellow to yellow-green conidial heads. **D**, *Aspergillus terreus* produces a whitish mycelium and has cinnamon-buff to wood-brown conidial structures.

Fungal Infections

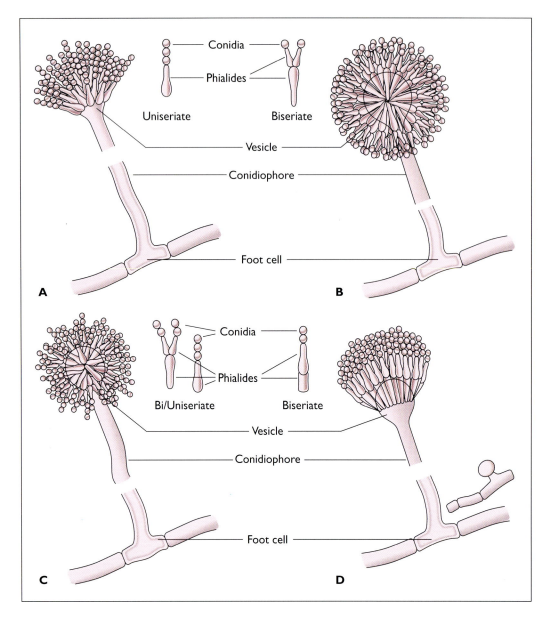

FIGURE 9-2. Microscopic morphology of *Aspergillus* species. The figure depicts the characteristic fine structure of the fruiting organ of four *Aspergillus* species. Each fruiting organ consists of a foot cell, the conidiophore, and the vesicle. Arising from the vesicle are the conidia-bearing phialides, which may be uniseriate or biseriate. **A**, *Aspergillus fumigatus* possesses uniseriate phialides, which usually arise from the upper two thirds of the vesicle and are parallel to the axis of the conidiophore. **B**, The phialides of *Aspergillus niger* are biseriate and cover the entire vesicle to form a radiate head. **C**, *Aspergillus flavus* exhibits uniseriate and biseriate phialides, which cover the entire vesicle and point in all directions. **D**, *Aspergillus terreus* typically possesses biseriate and compactly columnar phialides. (*Adapted from* Larone [11].)

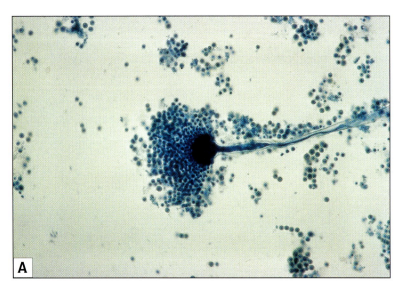
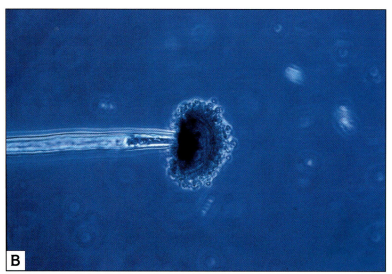

FIGURE 9-3. Microscopic morphology of *Aspergillus* species. (Lactophenol cotton blue, x500.) **A**, *Aspergillus fumigatus*. **B**, *Aspergillus niger*. *(continued on next page)*

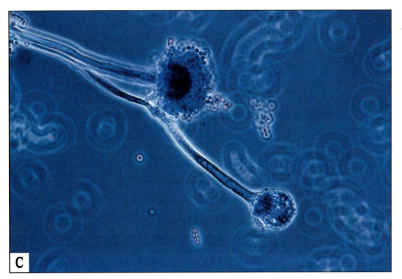
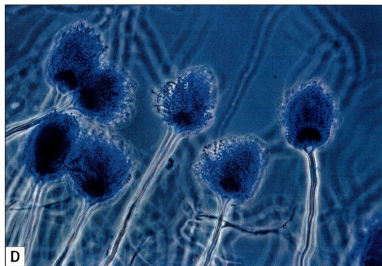

FIGURE 9-3. *(continued)* **C**, *Aspergillus flavus*. **D**, *Aspergillus terreus*.

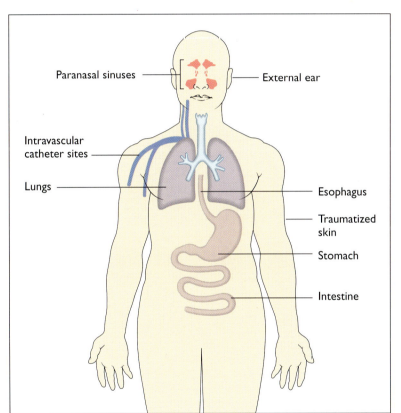

FIGURE 9-4. Portals of entry for *Aspergillus* species. Owing to the airborne route of infection, the respiratory tract, including the paranasal sinuses, is the major portal of entry. The small (2.5 to 3.5 µm) diameter of *Aspergillus* conidia from most pathogenic species permits them to reach the pulmonary alveolar spaces where they may germinate to form hyphae. However, in patients with neutropenia, the main route of tissue invasion probably is through the lacerated bronchial mucosa into lung parenchyma and anatomically adjacent pulmonary arteries, leading to arterial thrombosis and hemorrhagic infarction. (*Adapted from* Walsh and Dixon [12].)

Disease manifestations of aspergillosis in humans

Noninvasive forms of aspergillosis
  Allergic manifestations
  Saprophytic disease
  Superficial infection
Invasive aspergillosis
  Pulmonary aspergillosis
  Paranasal sinus aspergillosis
  Primary cutaneous aspergillosis
  Alimentary tract aspergillosis
  Disseminated aspergillosis

FIGURE 9-5. Disease manifestations of aspergillosis in humans. The spectrum of possible disease processes is broad and includes hypersensitivity conditions, saprophytic disease, and life-threatening invasive infections in patients with impaired host defenses.

NONINVASIVE DISEASE MANIFESTATIONS OF ASPERGILLOSIS

Noninvasive manifestations of aspergillosis

Allergic disease
  Extrinsic asthma
  Allergic bronchopulmonary aspergillosis
  Extrinsic allergic alveolitis
Saprophytic disease
  Aspergilloma
  Saprophytic bronchopulmonary and sinus aspergillosis
Superficial infection
  Onychomycosis
  Otomycosis

FIGURE 9-6. Noninvasive manifestations of aspergillosis. Noninvasive disease manifestations associated with *Aspergillus* species include allergic diseases, saprophytic diseases, and, rarely, superficial infections of the skin and its appendages.

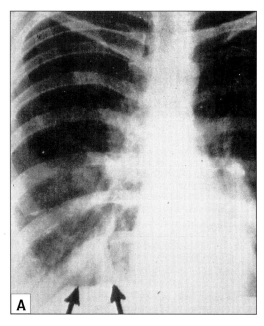
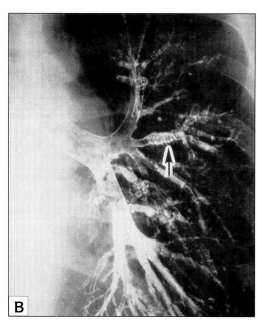
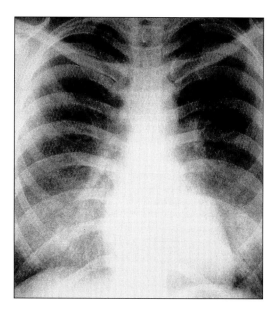

FIGURE 9-7. Allergic bronchopulmonary aspergillosis. Allergic bronchopulmonary aspergillosis is a type I hypersensitivity reaction and occurs in patients with asthma who become sensitized to *Aspergillus* species. It is characterized by pulmonary infiltrates, peripheral eosinophilia, and increased levels of total and *Aspergillus*-specific IgE, and, in advanced stages, by central bronchiectases. Clinical symptoms include worsening bronchial obstruction, productive cough, fever, weight loss, and hemoptysis. **A,** Posterioranterior chest radiograph shows "gloved finger" shadows (*arrows*). These and more homogenous parenchymal consolidations are the most frequent radiologic findings during acute episodes. **B,** Bronchogram demonstrates the classic picture of proximal bronchiectasis with normal peripheral filling (*arrow*) during a disease-free interval. (Panel A *from* Bayer [13]; with permission; panel B *from* Malo [14]; with permission.)

FIGURE 9-8. Early subacute allergic alveolitis. Pathophysiologically, allergic alveolitis is believed to be a type III or IV hypersensitivity reaction. In general, patients have an elevated IgG against the specific allergen, and no elevated IgE. Of note, *Aspergillus* species is only one of many organic agents that can lead to allergic alveolitis. The chest radiograph shows a marked small nodular infiltrate in the lower parts of both lungs. These infiltrates may resolve completely with the resolution of clinical illness that resembles a restrictive lung disease with fever and malaise. In chronic late stages, however, the radiographic findings consist of fibrosis and cystic changes and become indistinguishable from other forms of end-stage lung disease. (*From* Kryda *et al.* [15]; with permission.)

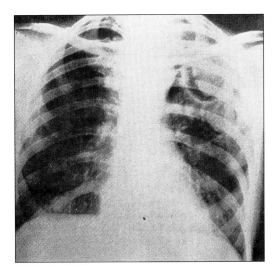

FIGURE 9-9. Aspergillomata of the left upper lung lobe. The posterioranterior chest radiograph shows two cavities in which a central opacity is partially surrounded by a crescent patch of air (Monod's sign). An aspergilloma (mycetoma, "fungus ball") typically develops in a preformed and poorly drained, mostly tuberculous lung cavity, and consists of a ball of saprophytically growing fungus. In most instances, the mycetomal lesion is caused by *Aspergillus* species, but mycetomas owing to other filamentous fungi also have been described. Aspergillomata must not be confused with cavitating lesions in patients with invasive pulmonary aspergillosis who are recovering from neutropenia. Although these lesions look quite similar, they are pathophysiologically different and represent sequestration of necrotic lung tissue after hemorrhagic infarction during neutropenia. (*From* Bardana [16]; with permission.)

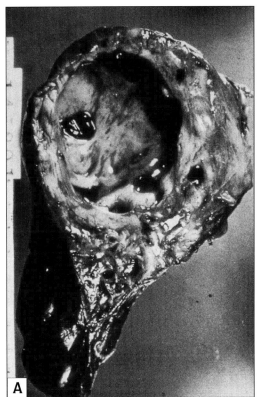
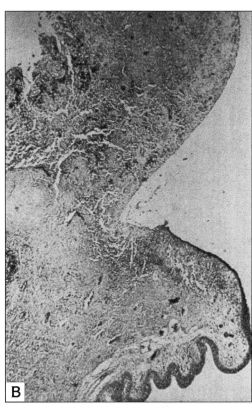

FIGURE 9-10. Surgical resectate of aspergilloma. **A**, Cavity after removal of the mycetoma and blood clots is shown. Note the thick, fibrous wall and the ectatic bronchi leading from the cavity. **B**, Microscopic section of the cavity wall is shown (x100). In one area, the epithelial lining is eroded, giving rise to a potential source for hemorrhage from the underlying granulation tissue. (*From* Rippon [1]; with permission.)

Treatment for allergic and saprophytic aspergillosis
Allergic manifestations
Extrinsic asthma
Avoidance of allergen exposure
Anti-inflammatory agents/bronchodilators
Allergic bronchopulmonary aspergillosis
Corticosteroids (prednisone)
Antifungal chemotherapy (itraconazole)
Extrinsic allergic alveolitis
Avoidance of allergen exposure
Corticosteroids (prednisone)
Saprophytic aspergillosis
Aspergilloma
Conservative
In the case of major hemoptysis: surgery (intralesional instillations of amphotericin B/sclerosing agents; itraconazole)
Saprophytic bronchopulmonary and sinus aspergillosis
Itraconazole
Drainage

FIGURE 9-11. Treatment for allergic and saprophytic aspergillosis. The mainstay of treatment for conditions associated with hypersensitivity to *Aspergillus* species is the administration of anti-inflammatory corticosteroids. Medical treatment with itraconazole may be a reasonable adjunct in the management of allergic bronchopulmonary aspergillosis. The treatment of aspergilloma is controversial and includes observation, medical therapy, and surgical resection. There is agreement that systemic antifungal agents in general are not effective, mainly due to their poor intralesional penetration. Percutaneous instillations of amphotericin B and adstringent agents have been applied with varying success and cannot be generally supported. Surgical resection of an aspergilloma is the only certain method of cure and has been advocated by a number of investigators. However, most patients with aspergilloma have preexisting lung disease and therefore are poor surgical candidates [17]. Management of patients with aspergilloma thus must be individualized. Surgery should be performed in cases of severe hemoptysis under perioperative amphotericin B coverage. If this approach is not feasible, bronchial artery embolization and intracavitary instillations can be useful to control hemorrhage. Itraconazole may be useful for symptomatic aspergilloma when surgery is not indicated [18]. In saprophytic bronchopulmonary or sinus aspergillosis in patients with preexisting chronic destructive airway disease, adjunctive medical therapy with a systemic antifungal agent may reduce suppuration and improve clinical symptoms.

Invasive Aspergillosis

Classification and Epidemiology

Manifestations of invasive aspergillosis

Invasive pulmonary aspergillosis
  Airway
    Necrotizing *Aspergillus* tracheobronchitis
    Obstructing bronchial aspergillosis
  Parenchymal
    Chronic necrotizing pulmonary aspergillosis
    Acute invasive pulmonary aspergillosis
Invasive aspergillosis of the paranasal sinus and the mastoid air cells
Primary cutaneous and soft-tissue aspergillosis
Primary alimentary tract aspergillosis
Disseminated aspergillosis

FIGURE 9-12. Manifestations of invasive aspergillosis. Invasive aspergillosis usually is further classified according to the affected site or, in the case of more than one major site of infection, referred to as disseminated aspergillosis.

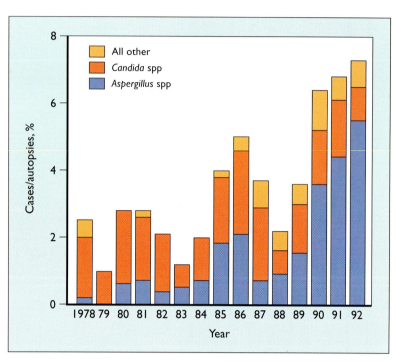

FIGURE 9-13. Epidemiology of invasive aspergillosis at postmortem. The analysis is based on data from 8124 autopsies performed between 1978 and 1992 on patients who died at the University Hospital of Frankfurt/Main, Germany. During that period, a total of 278 cases of invasive fungal infections were diagnosed, and among these, 119 cases of invasive aspergillosis. Although the prevalence of invasive *Candida* infections was stable and even showed a declining trend within the past years, there was a significant, steady increase of invasive *Aspergillus* infections from 0.4% and 1.2% in 1978 to 1982 and 1983 to 1987, respectively, to 3.1% during 1988 to 1992 ($P<0.001$ by 3x2 chi-squared test). In 1992, the last year of the survey, invasive aspergillosis was found in 5.5% of all patients who died at the hospital and underwent postmortem examination. (*Adapted from* Groll *et al.* [3]; with permission.)

Approximate frequency of invasive aspergillosis in immunocompromised hosts

Condition	Range, %
Acute leukemia	5–24
Allogeneic BMT	4–9
Autologous BMT	0.5–6
AIDS	0–12
Liver transplantation	1.5–10
Heart and renal transplantation	0.5–10
Heart and lung or lung transplantation	19–26*
Chronic granulomatous disease	25–40†

*Both colonization and disease.
†Lifetime frequency.
BMT—bone marrow transplantation.

FIGURE 9-14. Approximate frequency of invasive aspergillosis in immunocompromised hosts. Data represent approximate frequencies at different centers. (*Adapted from* Denning [19]; with permission.)

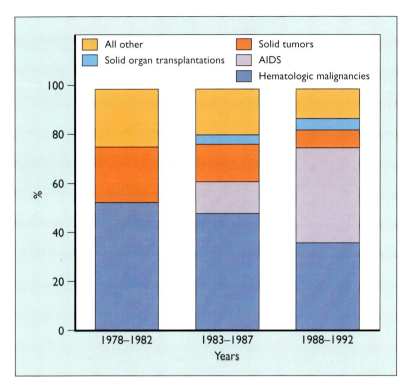

Figure 9-15. Emergence of AIDS as the underlying condition in invasive aspergillosis. The data are from the same postmortem study cited in Fig. 9-13. In this analysis, AIDS has evolved into the most common primary condition in patients who had a postmortem diagnosis of invasive aspergillosis. During 1988 to 1992, 13% of patients with AIDS who died at the hospital and underwent autopsy were diagnosed with invasive aspergillosis, as compared with 12% of patients with hematologic malignancies. (*Adapted from* Groll *et al.* [3]; with permission.)

Experimental Pathogenesis and Clinical Risk Factors

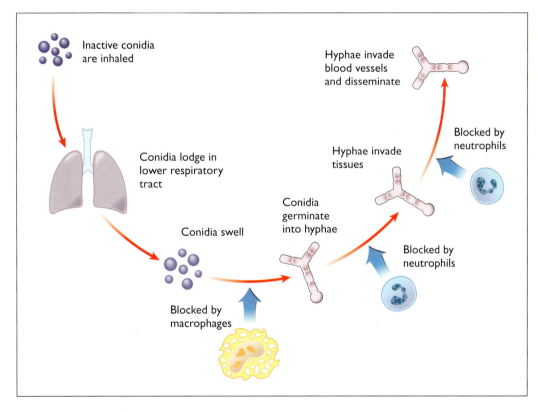

Figure 9-16. Summary of host defenses against *Aspergillus* species. Phagocytosis and intracellular killing by phagocytes is the main line of host defense against *Aspergillus* species [20]. Normal macrophages ingest and kill inhaled *Aspergillus* conidia, thus preventing germination and invasive hyphal growth. Normal neutrophils stop hyphal growth and dissemination and eradicate mycelia through oxidative and nonoxidative microbicidal mechanisms. Granulocytopenia permits the growth of hyphae, whereas administration of corticosteroids rapidly impairs the accumulation and fungicidal activity of mononuclear and polymorphonuclear phagocytes, thus allowing germination and invasive hyphal growth. (*Courtesy of* Dr. Richard Diamond.)

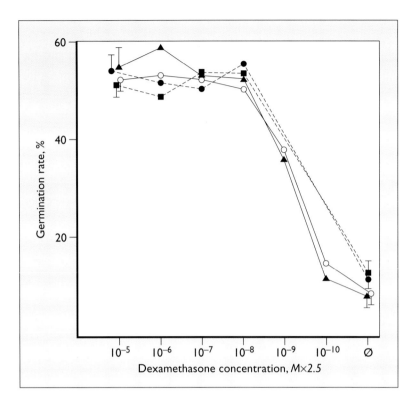

Figure 9-17. Suppressive effects of dexamethasone on the activity of macrophages against *Aspergillus* conidia. Macrophages were preincubated with dexamethasone for 36 hours before challenge. Germination rates of conidia were measured 24 hours after phagocytosis by blood-derived (*solid line*) and alveolar (*dotted line*) macrophages. (*Adapted from* Schaffner *et al.* [21]; with permission.)

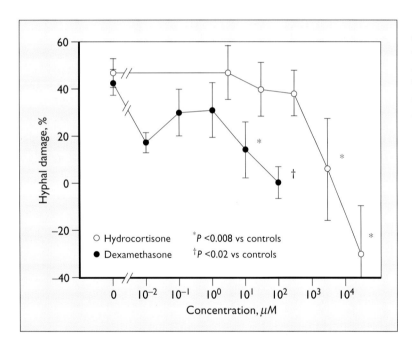

Figure 9-18. Suppressive effects of corticosteroids on the antifungal activity of neutrophils against *Aspergillus* hyphae. Hyphae were incubated with either hydrocortisone or dexamethasone. The effector-to-target cell ratio was 10:1. Neutrophils were added to wells containing 10^5 hyphae per well without serum with the indicated concentrations of corticosteroids and incubated at 37°C for 2 hours. (*Adapted from* Roilides *et al.* [22]; with permission.)

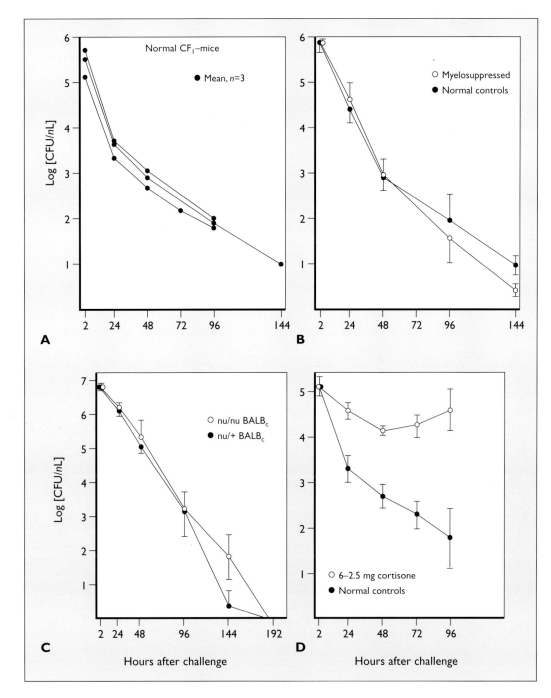

FIGURE 9-19. A–D, Clearance of inhaled conidia from lung tissue after exposure of normal (*panel A*), myelosuppressed (*panel B*), athymic (*panel C*), and cortisone-treated (*panel D*) mice to aerosolized spores of *Aspergillus fumigatus*. Normal as well as severely neutropenic and athymic mice cleared inhaled conidia efficiently. Cortisone-treated mice exhibited significantly impaired clearance with histologic sections showing progressive transition to mycelial growth, providing indirect evidence for the critical role of pulmonary macrophages in preventing germination and establishment of invasive infection. (*Adapted from* Schaffner *et al.* [21]; with permission.)

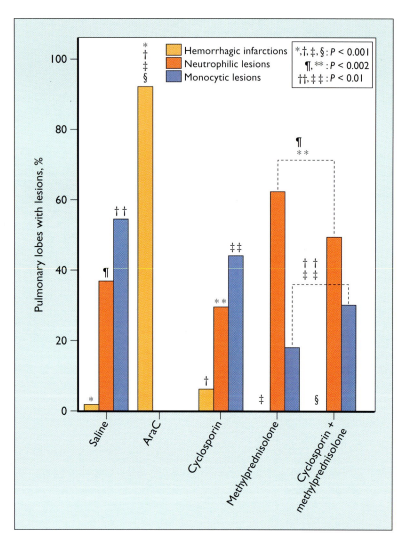

FIGURE 9-20. Experimental pathogenesis of pulmonary aspergillosis in granulocytopenic vs cyclosporine- and methylprednisolone-induced immunosuppression. To compare the pathogenesis of aspergillosis in two distinct patient populations at high risk, patterns of infection and inflammation were studied in two rabbit models of pulmonary aspergillosis, which closely resemble the situation encountered in patients treated for cancer or in patients treated for graft/transplant rejection. There were substantial differences according to the type of immunosuppression. Although pulmonary lesions in cytarabine-treated, granulocytopenic rabbits were predominantly hemorrhagic infarcts with a conspicuous absence of inflammatory infiltrates, rabbits immunosuppressed with methylprednisolone or cyclosporine plus methylprednisolone (CSA/MP) had mainly neutrophilic and monocytic infiltrates and inflammatory necrosis. Extensive infiltration by hyphae with angioinvasion was seen in granulocytopenic rabbits. In animals treated with CSA/MP, conidia in various stages of germination dominated. Mortality was 100% in profoundly granulocytopenic rabbits in comparison with 100% survival in all other regimens. Methylprednisolone was the major immunosuppressive drug in animals treated with CSA/MP. Cyclosporine alone did not increase the progression of pulmonary aspergillosis and did so only when used in conjunction with methylprednisolone. (*From* Berenguer *et al.* [23]; with permission.)

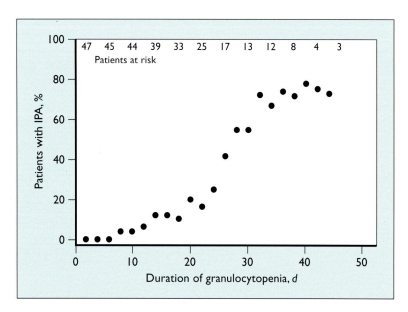

FIGURE 9-21. Granulocytopenia and incidence of invasive pulmonary aspergillosis. The figure, based on a case control study in adult patients with acute leukemia, shows the percentage of all patients with granulocytopenia who developed invasive pulmonary aspergillosis (IPA) as a function of duration of granulocytopenia. Only a few patients developed evidence of IPA early in the course of granulocytopenia. However, with increasing duration of granulocytopenia, the percentage of patients with granulocytopenia and radiographic signs of IPA increased and exceeded 50% in the 13 patients remaining granulocytopenic on day 28. Seven patients had developed signs of IPA. In this study, only granulocytopenia was associated with development of IPA, whereas cytotoxic regimens and exposure to antibacterial agents or corticosteroids were not significantly different between the 15 patients and 45 control subjects. (*From* Gerson *et al.* [24]; with permission.)

Major clinical risk factors for invasive aspergillosis
Profound and prolonged granulocytopenia (<500/µL for >10 d)
Qualitative defects of neutrophil and macrophage function
Corticosteroid therapy
Advanced HIV infection
Chronic granulomatous disease
Graft-vs-host disease after allogenic marrow transplantation*
Acute rejection after solid organ transplantation*
Tissue damage†
Concomitant invasive infections‡

*Both conditions are treated with high dosages of corticosteroids.

†Such as disrupted mucosal barriers after cytotoxic chemotherapy, cutaneous lacerations, burns, surgical trauma.

‡Such as by causing tissue injury (cytomegalovirus lung infection, other lung infections) or by obscuring the early clinical diagnosis (bacterial pneumonias).

FIGURE 9-22. Major clinical risk factors for invasive aspergillosis. Consistent with the experimental data, quantitative and qualitative deficiencies of phagocytosis and intracellular killing have been found to be the major underlying clinical risk factors for invasive *Aspergillus* infections.

Invasive Pulmonary Aspergillosis

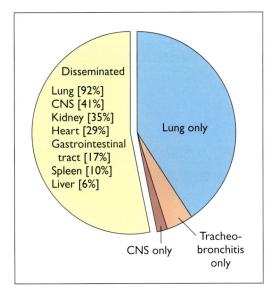

FIGURE 9-23. Organ involvement in 119 autopsy cases of invasive aspergillosis. Similar to other large case series [25,26], the lung was the most frequently affected organ site in this more recent survey. Forty-one percent of all cases were confined to the lung, and disseminated disease was found in 53% of all cases, of which almost all had lung involvement. Of note, the central nervous system was the second most common site, and 41% of patients with disseminated diseases had central nervous system lesions. (*Adapted from* Groll *et al.* [3]; with permission.)

Patterns of lung involvement in invasive aspergillosis in the setting of anticancer treatment	
Type of involvement	Cases, *n* (%)
Necrotizing bronchopneumonia	34 (38)
Hemorrhagic infarction	32 (36)
Focal necrosis	5 (6)
Aspergilloma (cavitating)	5 (6)
Bronchitis	5 (6)
Microabscesses	4 (4)
Interstitial disease	2 (2)
Lobular pneumonia	2 (2)
Lobar pneumonia	1 (1)

FIGURE 9-24. Patterns of lung involvement in invasive pulmonary aspergillosis in the setting of anticancer treatment. The data are from a large autopsy series reported from the Memorial Sloan Kettering Cancer Center in the early 1970s and thus may represent the natural course of lung disease. Necrotizing bronchopneumonia and hemorrhagic infarction were the predominant patterns of invasive aspergillosis of the lung. (*From* Meyer *et al.* [26]; with permission.)

Fungal Infections

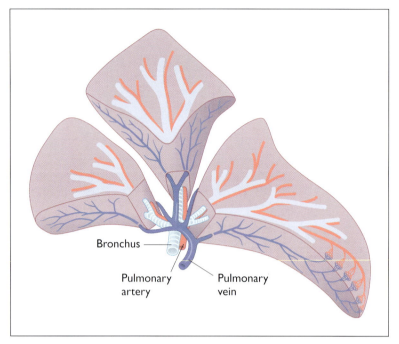

FIGURE 9-25. Anatomic relation of airways and major vessels in the lung. In patients with neutropenia, hyphae may penetrate through the walls of bronchi and bronchioles into anatomically adjacent arteries. Subsequent thrombomycotic occlusion may lead to mostly multiple nodular or wedge-shaped hemorrhagic infarctions, which may progress to minor hemoptysis or hematogenous dissemination [23]. In patients who survive the phase of neutropenia, the influx of neutrophilic granulocytes may lead to cavitation and sequestration of the infarcted parenchyma but also to massive and often lethal pulmonary hemorrhage by the erosion of adjacent arterial vessels. Thus, the time during recovery of granulocytes is a danger period with respect to massive pulmonary hemorrhage [27]. Computed tomography can be helpful in identifying lesions with close proximity to major vessels that may be amenable to surgery [28].

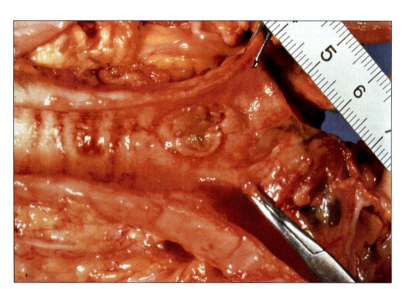

FIGURE 9-26. Necrotizing tracheitis caused by *Aspergillus* species. Note the two circumscript lacerations in the distal part of the trachea.

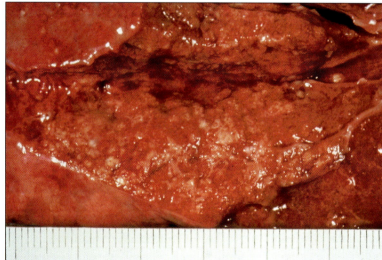

FIGURE 9-27. Cut section from a nodular lung lesion. The infectious lesion originates from a segmental bronchus and extends into the parenchyma in a radial fashion. (*Courtesy of* Prof. Markward Schneider.)

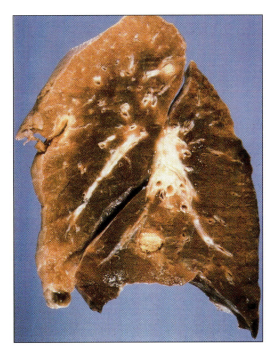

FIGURE 9-28. Necrotic lung nodule in a patient with leukemia and invasive pulmonary aspergillosis who died from pulmonary hemorrhage during recovery from neutropenia. The figure shows the left, formalinized lung, whose dark color is a result of massive blood aspiration. A necrotic lung nodule can be appreciated in the upper and lower lung lobe each. Note the presence of an air crescent in both lesions. Necrotic lung nodules are not to be confused with an aspergilloma. In patients who can be treated successfully, these lesions regress over time to form small cavities or cysts or, alternatively, to longitudinal scars, which often extend to the pleura. (*From* Groll *et al.* [27]; with permission.)

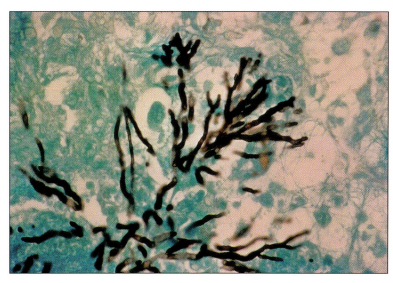

FIGURE 9-29. Microscopic morphology of *Aspergillus* species in tissue sections. This section from infarcted lung tissue shows tissue invasion by dichotomously branching, septate hyphae, suggestive of *Aspergillus* species. However, because *Fusarium* species and some of the dematiaceous moulds have a similar microscopic appearance, definite diagnosis relies on cultures obtained from the same material. (Gomori methenamine silver stain, x400.)

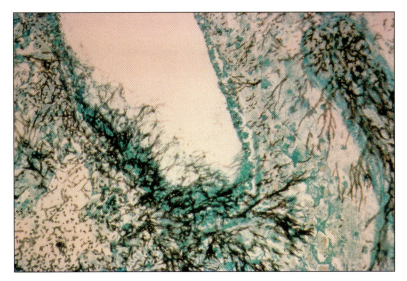

FIGURE 9-30. Invasion of a small blood vessel by *Aspergillus* species. Angioinvasion is a hallmark of invasive aspergillosis. Invasion of an arterial blood vessel may result in occlusion and infarction of downstream parenchyma or in dissemination of the organism to distant sites. Although this process is characteristic for *Aspergillus* species, blood cultures from patients with invasive infections are only rarely positive. (Gomori methenamine silver stain, x250.)

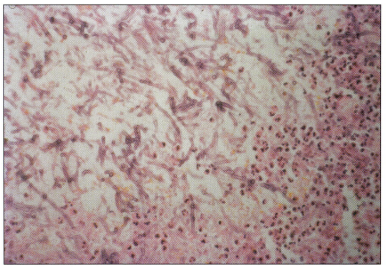

FIGURE 9-31. Invasive pulmonary aspergillosis in a patient with acute leukemia recovering from neutropenia after intensive chemotherapy. The figure shows necrotic tissue with an abundance of dichotomously branching hyphae. At the left upper corner, freshly recruited neutrophilic granulocytes have begun to invade the lesion. (Hematoxylin-eosin stain, x400.)

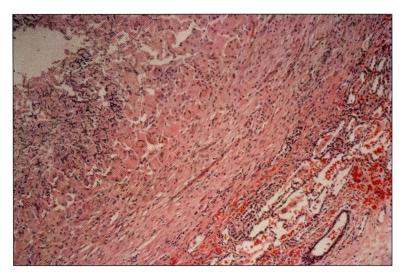

Figure 9-32. Chronic invasive pulmonary aspergillosis in a patient without neutropenia who has advanced HIV infection. The figure shows a lung lesion with central necrosis and dichotomously branching hyphae invading necrotic tissue with relatively few granulocytes, walled off from normal lung parenchyma by an incomplete granulomatous reaction consisting of mostly multinucleated histiocytes and fibrous tissue. (Hematoxylin-eosin stain, x250.)

Options for the recovery of *Aspergillus* species from the respiratory tract

Procedure	Comment
Expectorated sputum, bronchial washings	Low sensitivity but high positive predictive value in immunocompromised patients
Bronchoscopy BAL	Low sensitivity but high positive predictive value in immunocompromised patients
Transbronchial biopsy	Recommended in conjunction with BAL whenever feasible due to additive diagnostic yield
Percutaneous needle biopsy	Useful for obtaining diagnostic specimens from peripheral lesions
Thoracoscopy	Alternative to open lung biopsy in patients without thromboytopenia
Open lung biopsy	Gold standard for diagnosis of invasive aspergillosis

BAL—bronchoalveolar lavage.

Figure 9-33. Options for the recovery of *Aspergillus* species from the respiratory tract. If an invasive procedure is contemplated, a chest computed tomogram should be performed to define the area of interest and to delineate the most appropriate procedure. Central lesions are the domain of bronchoscopic procedures, whereas peripheral lesions may be amenable to computed tomography- or fluoroscopy-guided fine-needle aspiration or thoracoscopy. In either circumstance, risk, diagnostic yield, and the impact of a positive or negative finding on the individual patient's management must be thoroughly evaluated. Although fiberoptic bronchoscopy with bronchoalveolar lavage is feasible in almost any clinical situation, biopsy procedures carry a considerable risk of pulmonary air leakage or hemorrhage.

Diagnostic yield of bronchoalveolar lavage in invasive pulmonary aspergillosis

Bronchoalveolar lavage analysis	Aspergillosis present Positive specimens, n (%) $n=17$	No aspergillosis present Positive specimens, n (%) $n=65$	Specificity, %
Stain	9 (53)	3 (5)	95
Culture	4 (23)	3 (5)	95
Stain and/or culture	10 (59)	5 (8)	92

Figure 9-34. Diagnostic yield of bronchoalveolar lavage (BAL) in invasive pulmonary aspergillosis. Cultures and histochemical stains for fungi were performed on concentrated, cytocentrifuged BAL samples from 82 immunocompromised, mostly oncologic patients undergoing bronchoscopic evaluation of new pulmonary infiltrates. *Aspergillus* hyphae were identified by microscopy in nine of 17 BAL samples from patients with tissue proven invasive pulmonary aspergillosis and from three of the remaining 65 study patients without this diagnosis. BAL fungal cultures were positive only in four of the 17 cases. The combination of fungal stains and cultures yielded a diagnostic sensitivity of 58% and a specificity of 92% [29]. Other studies in mostly neutropenic cancer patients reported diagnostic yields between 50% and 69% [28,30,31], but notably, a sensitivity of close to 100% when *Aspergillus* species was detected in respiratory specimen [32]. (*Adapted from* Khan *et al.* [29]; with permission.)

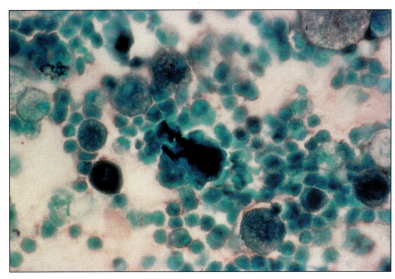

Figure 9-35. Bronchoalveolar lavage material obtained from a patient with invasive pulmonary aspergillosis. A small bundle of apparently damaged hyphal structures is seen in the center of the photomicrograph. The diagnosis of chronic necrotizing pulmonary aspergillosis was later confirmed by microscopy and culture of material obtained at the surgical resection of the lesion. Of note, the culture from the lavage material remained sterile. (Gomori methenamine silver stain, x450.)

Radiographic and computed tomographic patterns of invasive pulmonary aspergillosis

Radiography
  Normal parenchyma
  Peribronchitis/bronchopneumonia
  Segmental/subsegmental consolidation
  Diffuse consolidation
  Pleura-based, wedge-shaped infiltrates
  Ill-defined nodular lesions
  Air crescent (Monod's) sign/cavitation
  Pneumothorax (infrequent)
  Pleural effusion (rare)
CT
  Nodules, masslike infiltrates, and segmental/subsegmental consolidation
  ±Incomplete halo of ground-glass attenuation ("CT halo sign")
  ±Air crescent between lesion and adjacent parenchyma

CT—computed tomography.

Figure 9-36. Radiographic and computed tomographic (CT) patterns of invasive pulmonary aspergillosis. There is a wide spectrum of radiographic appearances including normal radiographic findings in the presence of yet abnormal CT films [33,34]. Relatively characteristic CT findings are found in angioinvasive pulmonary aspergillosis. They include the CT halo sign, which typically is seen in patients with neutropenia and represents hemorrhagic necrosis, and the air crescent sign, a late finding representing air between retracted, infarcted lung and the adjacent lung parenchyma.

Radiographic differential diagnosis of invasive pulmonary aspergillosis

Infectious
  Bacterial processes (*eg*, *Pseudomonas* spp)
  Infection by other filamentous fungi (*eg*, *Fusarium* spp, *Zygomycetes* spp, dematiaceous fungi)
  Nocardiosis
  Tuberculosis
  Parasitic diseases (strongyloidiasis, echinococcosis, cysticercosis, paragonimiasis, amebiasis)
Noninfectious
  Thromboembolic infarction
  Cancer infiltrate/metastases
  Obstruction/atelectasis

Figure 9-37. Radiographic differential diagnosis of invasive pulmonary aspergillosis. The most important differential diagnoses are pulmonary lesions caused by bacteria of the patient's endogenous flora, in particular *Pseudomonas aeruginosa*; pulmonary emboli from a coexisting deep-vein thrombosis or thrombotic material associated with indwelling central venous catheters; pulmonary atelectasis of various causes; and tuberculosis.

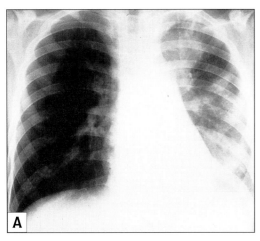
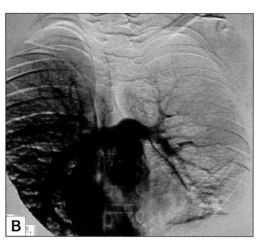
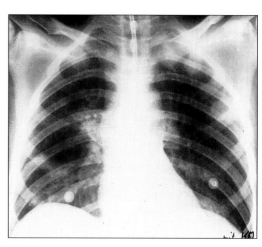

FIGURE 9-38. Invasive pulmonary aspergillosis. **A,** Posteroanterior chest radiograph demonstrates inhomogenous opacification of the left lung in a patient with neutropenia. **B,** Digital subtraction angiography reveals severely impaired perfusion of the left lung and several occluded arteries, consistent with multiple pulmonary infarctions. (*Courtesy of* Prof. Fritz Ball.)

FIGURE 9-39. Posteroanterior chest radiograph showing invasive pulmonary aspergillosis. Several rounded lesions can be seen in a patient with acute leukemia recovering from neutropenia. (*Courtesy of* Dr. Christina Engelcke.)

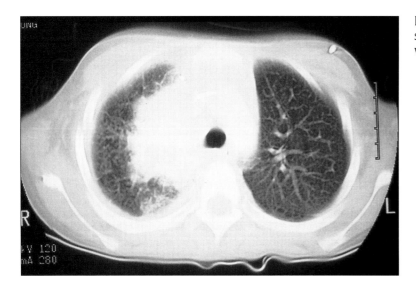

FIGURE 9-40. High-resolution computed tomogram showing invasive pulmonary aspergillosis. Masslike lesion is shown in a patient with advanced HIV infection and marrow aplasia.

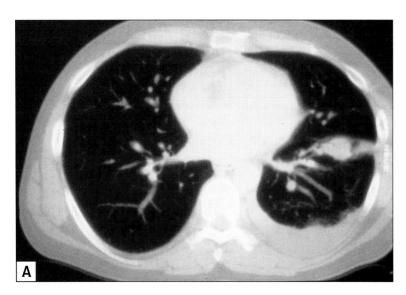
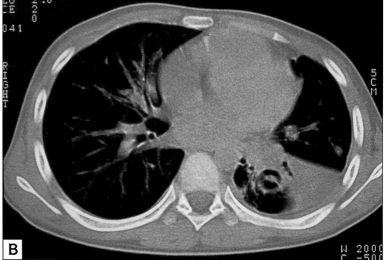

FIGURE 9-41. High-resolution computed tomogram showing invasive pulmonary aspergillosis. **A,** Nodular lesion and pleural effusion (an uncommon, and in this case, unrelated finding) are shown. **B,** A cavitating lesion can be seen. Note the small rim of ground-glass opacification, which is consistent with the "halo sign."

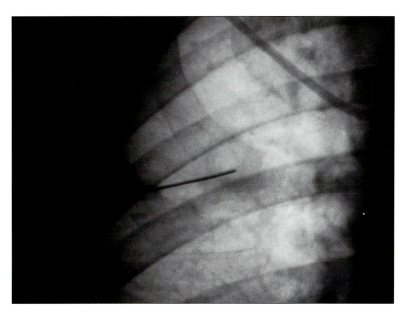

FIGURE 9-42. Fluoroscopy of invasive pulmonary aspergillosis. Diagnostic percutaneous needle aspiration from a peripheral nodular lesion is shown.

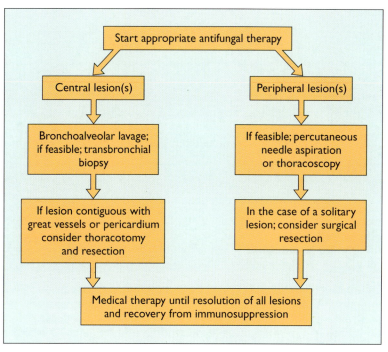

FIGURE 9-43. Algorithm for the management of presumed invasive pulmonary aspergillosis.

Extrapulmonary Manifestations of Invasive Aspergillosis

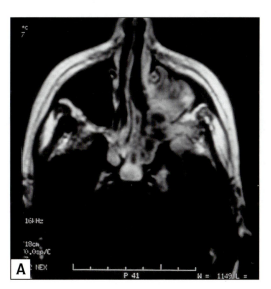
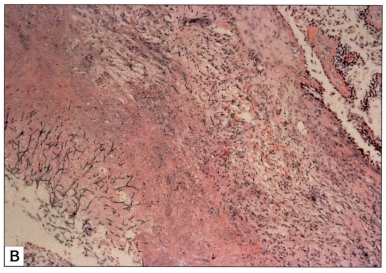

FIGURE 9-44. *Aspergillus* sinusitis in a patient with advanced HIV infection. **A**, The gadolinium-enhanced magnetic resonance imaging scan shows pansinusitis sparing the right maxillary sinus. **B**, Histologic section from material obtained from the sinuses during surgical debridement shows tissue invasion by dichotomously branching septate hyphae, extensive necrosis, and a wall of highly vascularized granulation tissue. (Hematoxylin-eosin stain, x125.)

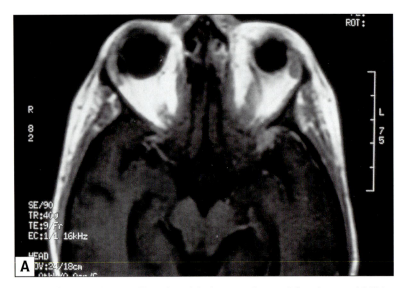
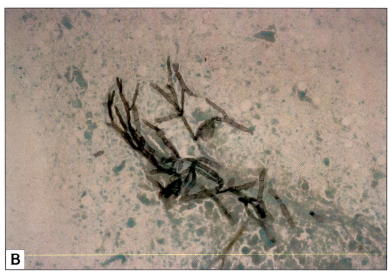

FIGURE 9-45. *Aspergillus* sinusitis in a patient with advanced HIV infection. **A**, Additional rostral cuts reveal enhanced uptake of contrast material near the anterior horn of the temporal lobe. **B**, Scrapings from that area at postmortem examination 1 month later reveal an abundance of hyphae morphologically consistent with *Aspergillus* species, suggesting extension of the infectious process from the sphenoidal sinus to the base of the medial cranial fossa. (Gomori methenamine silver stain, x300.)

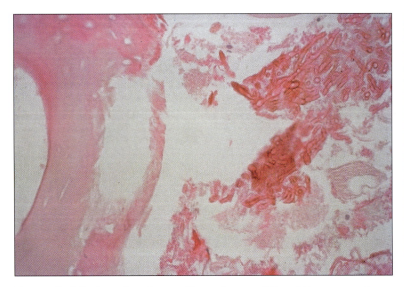
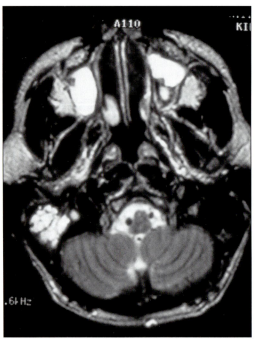

FIGURE 9-46. Invasive *Aspergillus* osteomyelitis of the vomer in a patient with acute leukemia and clinically inapparent sinusitis maxillaris invading the hard palate. The patient presented with a perforation of the hard palate during morning rounds. (Hematoxylin-eosin stain, x500.)

FIGURE 9-47. *Aspergillus* otomycosis and mastoiditis in a patient with advanced HIV infection. The T2-weighted magnetic resonance imaging scan shows complete opacification of the right middle ear cavity and the mastoid air cells. Invasive aspergillosis subsequently was confirmed by culture and histology from material obtained during surgical debridement. The image also reveals pansinusitis (nonfungal in this case).

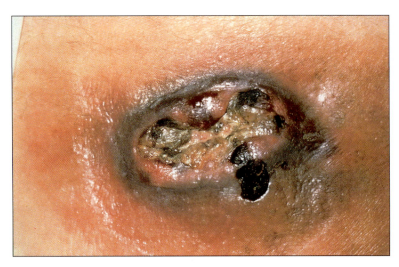

FIGURE 9-48. Primary cutaneous aspergillosis in a patient with neutropenia. Preceeding trauma is almost always a prerequisite when invasive aspergillosis originates in the skin. Primary cutaneous aspergillosis has been described in immunocompromised patients at the insertion sites of central venous catheters, at peripheral intravenous sites, and in association with lacerations by armboards or tape. It also has been described in patients with burn wounds and soft-tissue trauma and, in recent years, in very immature neonates of 3 weeks of age or younger [35,36].

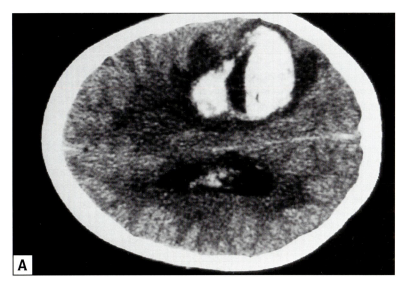
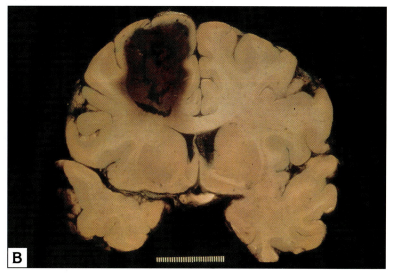

Figure 9-49. **A** and **B**, Aspergillosis of the central nervous system presenting as intracerebral hemorrhage in a patient with acute leukemia and invasive pulmonary aspergillosis recovering from neutropenia. Aspergillosis of the central nervous system is a devastating event, and mortality in immunocompromised patients is close to 100% [37–39]. Apart from the typical setting of hematologic malignancies, aplastic anemia, and transplantation, it also may occur in patients with AIDS or in individuals receiving high dosages of corticosteroids. The principal neuropathologic event is *Aspergillus* invasion of blood vessels causing hemorrhagic infarction or hemorrhage. Accordingly, the most common clinical presentation is a strokelike syndrome in an immunocompromised patient with pulmonary aspergillosis. Meningeal signs are rare, and the cerebrospinal fluid is usually nondiagnostic.

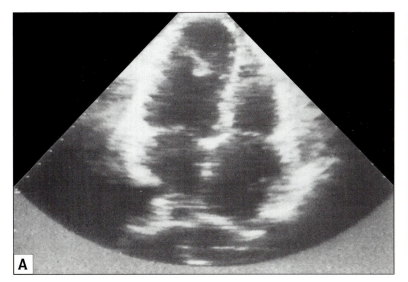
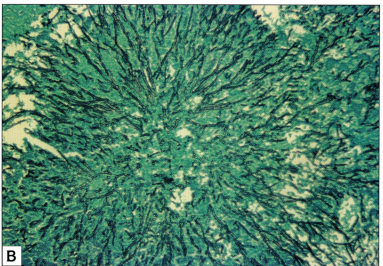
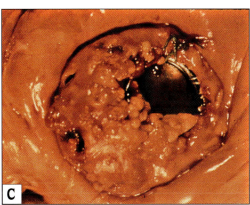
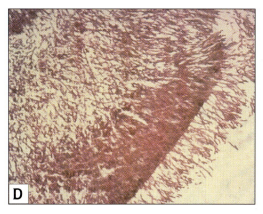

Figure 9-50. Infectious endocarditis due to *Aspergillus* species. **A**, Two-dimensional echocardiogram shows a pedunculated mural mass in the left ventricle involving the posterior papillary muscle. **B**, The surgically resected mass reveals dichotomously angular branching septate hyphae consistent with *Aspergillus* thrombus material. (Gomori methenamine silver stain, ×100.) **C**, Prosthetic valve endocarditis is shown. **D**, Microscopic aspect of the vegetation is shown. Large, friable vegetations are characteristic, but not diagnostic, for *Aspergillus* species. *Aspergillus* endocarditis is rare and mostly associated with central venous catheters or prosthetic valve surgery [40]. (*From* Mullen *et al.* [41]; with permission.)

Treatment

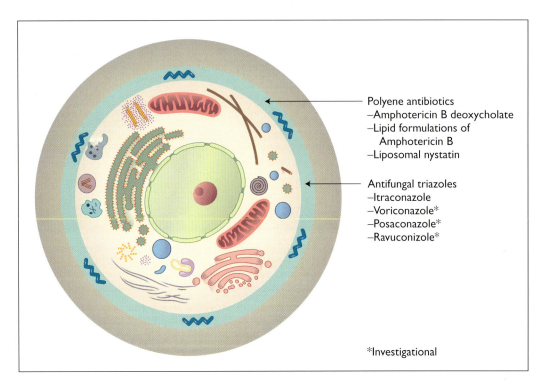

Figure 9-51. Currently available antifungal agents used for systemic treatment of invasive aspergillosis and their target site at the cellular level. The polyene antibiotics interact with ergosterol, the main sterol of the fungal membrane, which leads to the formation of aqueous channels and, ultimately, cell death. The antifungal azoles act by inhibiting the cytochrome P-450–dependent C-14 demethylation of lanosterol, thereby causing ergosterol depletion and accumulation of toxic sterols in the cell membrane. (*Adapted from* Groll and Walsh [42]; with permission.)

Treatment for invasive aspergillosis

Antimicrobial chemotherapy
  Amphotericin B deoxycholate (1–1.5 mg/kg/d)
  Lipid formulations of amphotericin B (5 mg/kg/d)*
  Itraconazole (5–12 [max] mg/kg/d)†‡
  Voriconazole (investigational)*
  Posaconazole (investigational)*
  Ravuconazole (investigational)*
Surgery (as appropriate)
  Infections of skin and soft tissues; invasive sinusitis; hemoptysis from a single lung lesion; progressive focal lung lesions; lung lesions extending into pericardium, great vessels, bone, and soft tissue; endocarditis; endophthalmitis; and other focal lesions amenable to surgery
Restoration of host defenses
  Discontinuation of immunosuppressive therapy, if feasible
  Use of colony-stimulating factors in patients with neutropenia
Removal/exchange of infected foreign material

*In patients intolerant or refractory to amphotericin B deoxycholate.

†For maintenance in stable patients.

‡Monitoring of serum levels recommended (>0.5 µg/mL [high-pressure liquid chromatography] or >2.0 µg/mL [bioassay] before next dose; loading dose: 4 mg/kg 3 times per day for 3 d).

Figure 9-52. Treatment for invasive aspergillosis.

Response to therapy with amphotericin B deoxycholate among patients with invasive aspergillosis treated for ≥14 days

Site/patient group	Responders, n (%)
Pulmonary aspergillosis	
Bone marrow transplantation	5/15 (33)
Leukemia, neutropenia, aplastic anemia	44/81 (54)
Renal transplantation	10/12* (83)
Heart transplantation[†]	10/12 (83)
Liver transplantation	1/5 (20)
AIDS	20/54 (37)
Aspergillus rhinosinusitis	17/35 (49)
Cerebral aspergillosis	
Immunocompromised	0/7 (0)
Nonimmunocompromised	3/9 (33)

*Four of the 10 survivors experienced graft failure because of reduced immunosuppression and/or amphotericin B therapy.

[†]All seven patients of another series died despite therapy with amphotericin B, but the exact amount given was not stated.

FIGURE 9-53. Response to therapy with amphotericin B deoxycholate among patients with invasive aspergillosis treated for 14 days or longer. Only amphotericin B deoxycholate was given, except to patients with AIDS, most of whom received both amphotericin B and itraconazole. The data stem from a review of a series of 4 or more cases of invasive aspergillosis (total, 1223 cases), which aimed at establishing crude mortality and response rates to amphotericin B deoxycholate in the major risk groups. There were no survivors among the 151 untreated patients, and only one of 84 patients treated for 13 days or less responded. (*Adapted from* Denning [19]; with permission.)

Response to therapy in patients with suspected or documented invasive aspergillosis*

Study	Agent	Overall response rate, %
Denning *et al.* [43]	Itraconazole	39
White *et al.* [44]	Amphotericin B colloidal dispersion	49
Walsh *et al.* [45]	ABLC	47
Wingard [46]	ABLC	38
Hiemenz *et al.* [47]	ABLC	40
	Amphotericin B deoxycholate[†]	23
Ringden *et al.* [48]	Amphotericin B encapsulated in liposome	66

*Only studies with >20 reported patients were included. Please note that due to differences in patient populations, study design, and efficacy criteria, these trials are not comparable.

[†]Retrospective, matched control group.

ABLC—amphotericin B lipid complex.

FIGURE 9-54. Response to therapy in patients with suspected or documented invasive aspergillosis in recent prospective studies.

Cause of death in patients with invasive aspergillosis

Necrotizing pneumonia/diffuse pulmonary hemorrhage
Massive pulmonary infarction
Erosion of a major vessel and hemorrhage
Cerebral hemorrhagic infarction
Brain lesions with mass effect
Brain lesions with rupture into ventricles
Erosion of intestinal wall and perforation
Asphyxia by occlusion of lower airways by debris
Intestinal infarction
Cardiac insufficiency after valve destruction
Cardiac tamponade owing to *Aspergillus* pericarditis

FIGURE 9-55. Cause of death in patients with invasive aspergillosis.

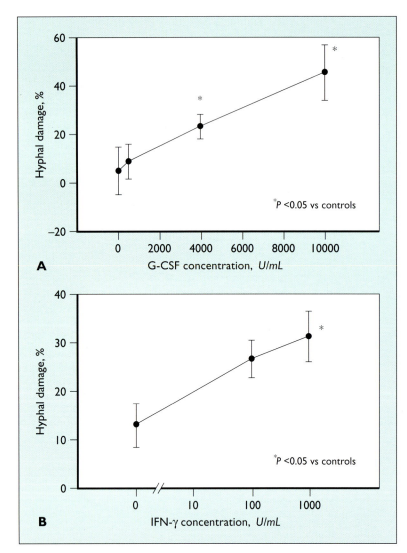

FIGURE 9-56. Enhancement of neutrophil-induced hyphal damage by granulocyte colony-stimulating factor (G-CSF) or interferon-γ (IFN-γ) in vitro. Neutrophils were preincubated with the indicated concentrations of G-CSF or IFN-γ for 90 minutes, and the antihyphal activites were assessed after a 2-hour incubation of the cells with 10^5 nonopsonized hyphae at 37°C. The effector-to-target cell ratio was 5:1. (Adapted from Roilides et al. [49]; with permission.)

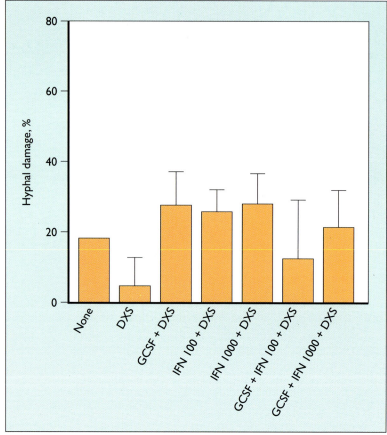

FIGURE 9-57. Reversal of corticosteroid-induced suppression of neutrophil-induced damage of *Aspergillus fumigatus* hyphae by granulocyte colony-stimulating factor (G-CSF) and interferon-γ (IFN-γ). The figure shows the effects of G-CSF (4000 U/L), IFN-γ (100 and 1000 U/mL), or their combination on the hyphal damage induced by dexamethsone (10 μM)-treated neutrophils at an effector-to-target cell ratio of 5:1. Nonopsonized hyphae were used. All treatments resulted in hyphal damage significantly greater than that of dexamethsone-only treated control neutrophils ($P<0.05$). (Adapted from Roilides et al. [49]; with permission.)

Antimicrobial prophylaxis for invasive aspergillosis

Empirical antifungal therapy
  Patients with fever and neutropenia unresponsive to broad-spectrum antibiotics
  Patients with neutropenia receiving broad-spectrum antibiotics and with new fever
  Patients with neutropenia and new pulmonary infiltrates or respiratory symptoms
Secondary chemoprophylaxis
  Patients with successfully treated invasive aspergillosis undergoing repeat cycles of chemotherapy or scheduled for marrow transplantation

FIGURE 9-58. Antimicrobial prophylaxis for invasive aspergillosis. Although a variety of different approaches has been investigated, including intranasal amphotericin B, aerosolized amphotericin B, intravenous amphotericin B, and itraconazole, none of these measures has been proved to be effective in reducing the incidence of invasive aspergillosis in a prospective, randomized study. Thus, the concept of empirical antifungal chemotherapy remains the mainstay for prevention or early treatment of invasive aspergillosis in the high-risk groups of patients with neutropenia and cancer or undergoing bone marrow transplantation. Although data are limited, secondary chemoprophylaxis is recommended at the indications delineated in the figure.

Infection control measures for the prevention of invasive aspergillosis in high-risk patients
Routinely review air supply by hospital engineering and infection control
Regularly supervise and review new cases of aspergillosis by infection control
Relocate immunocompromised patients from floors adjacent to construction
Seal off areas of patient care by floor-to-ceiling plastic or drywall barriers
Direct staff and visitor traffic to prevent dust from being tracked into patient areas
Prevent penetration of unfiltered air through elevators, windows, or doors in hospital air supplying system
Ensure proper function of ventilation system, including status of filters, air exchange rate, and pressure relationships
Ensure air is not circulated from construction areas into other hospital areas; provide negative air pressure at construction sites, if feasible
Install High Efficiency Particulate Air (HEPA) filters in rooms housing patients with profound and prolonged neutropenia
Vacuum areas above false ceilings and air supplying ducts
Clean construction areas and new wards; decontaminate with Copper-8-quinolinolate

FIGURE 9-59. Infection control measures for the prevention of invasive aspergillosis in high-risk patients. (*Adapted from* Walsh and Dixon [50].)

REFERENCES

1. Rippon JW: Aspergillosis. In *Medical Mycology: The Pathogenic Fungi and the Pathogenic Actinomycetes*. Edited by Rippon JW. Philadelphia: WB Saunders; 1988:618–650.

2. Cohen J: Clinical manifestations and management of aspergillosis in the compromised patient. In *Fungal Infections in the Compromised Patient*. Edited by Warnock DW, Richardson MD. Chichester: John Wiley & Sons; 1991:117–152.

3. Groll AH, Shah PM, Mentzel C, *et al.*: Trends in the postmortem epidemiology of invasive fungal infections at a university hospital. *J Infect* 1996, 33:23–32.

4. Pannuti CS, Gingrich RD, Pfaller MA, Wenzel RP: Nosocomial pneumonia in adult patients undergoing bone marrow transplantation: a 9-year study. *J Clin Oncol* 1991, 9:77–84.

5. Wald A, Leisenring W, vanBurik JA, Bowden RA: Epidemiology of *Aspergillus* infections in a large cohort of patients undergoing bone marrow transplantation. *J Infect Dis* 1997, 175:1459–1466.

6. Anaissie E: Opportunistic mycoses in the immunocompromised host: experience at a cancer center and review. *Clin Infect Dis* 1992, 14 (suppl 1):S43–S53.

7. Weinberger M, Elattor I, Marshall D, *et al.*: Patterns of infection in patients with aplastic anemia and the emergence of *Aspergillus* as major cause of death. *Medicine* 1992, 71:24–43.

8. Hibberd PL, Rubin RH: Clinical aspects of fungal infection in organ transplant recipients. *Clin Infect Dis* 1994, 19 (suppl 1):33–40.

9. Khoo SH, Denning DW: Invasive aspergillosis in patients with AIDS. *Clin Infect Dis* 1994, 19 (suppl 1):41–48.

10. Shetty D, Giri N, Gonzalez CE, *et al.*: Invasive aspergillosis in human immunodeficiency virus infected children. *Pediatr Infect Dis J* 1997, 16:216–221.

11. Larone DH: *Medically Important Fungi: A Guide to Identification*, 2nd ed. Edited by Larone DH. Amsterdam: Elsevier Science Publishing; 1991:90–91.

12. Walsh TJ, Dixon DM: Spectrum of mycoses. In *Medical Microbiology*, 4th ed. Edited by Baron S. New York: Churchill Livingstone; 1996:919–925.

13. Bayer AS: Diagnosis of aspergillosis. In *Aspergillosis*. Edited by Al-Doory Y, Wagner GE. Springfield: Charles Thomas Publisher; 1985:129–146.

14. Malo JL: Allergic bronchopulmonary aspergillosis. In *Aspergillosis*. Edited by Al-Doory Y, Wagner GE. Springfield: Charles Thomas Publisher; 1985:79–95.

15. Kryda MJ, Marx JJ, Emanuel DA: Farmer's lung disease and other hypersensitivity pneumonitides. In *Fungal Diseases of the Lung*, 2nd ed. Edited by Sarosi GA, Davies SF. New York: Raven Press; 1993:215–227.

16. Bardana EJ: Pulmonary aspergillosis. In *Aspergillosis*. Edited by Al-Doory Y, Wagner GE. Springfield: Charles Thomas Publisher; 1985:43–78.

17. Daly RC: Pulmonary aspergilloma: results of surgical treatment. *J Thorac Cardiovasc Surg* 1986, 92:981–998.

18. Patterson TF: Commentary: management of *Aspergillus* fungus ball—role of antifungal therapy. *Infect Dis Clin Pract* 1998, 7:127–128.

19. Denning DW: Diagnosis and management of invasive aspergillosis. *Curr Clin Top Infect Dis* 1996, 16:277–299.

20. Diamond RD: Invasive aspergillosis: host defenses. *Recent Results Cancer Res* 1993, 132:109–115.

21. Schaffner A, Douglas H, Braude A: Selective protection against conidia by mononuclear and against mycelia by polymorphonuclear phagocytes in resistance to *Aspergillus*. *J Clin Invest* 1982, 69:617–631.

22. Roilides E, Uhlig K, Venzon D, *et al.*: Enhancement of oxidative response and damage caused by human neutrophils to *Aspergillus fumigatus* hyphae by granulocyte colony-stimulating factor and gamma interferon. *Infect Immun* 1993, 61:1185–1193.

23. Berenguer J, Allende MC, Lee JW, *et al.*: Pathogenesis of pulmonary aspergillosis: granulocytopenia vs. cyclosporine and methylprednisolone-induced immunosuppression. *Am J Respir Crit Care Med* 1995, 152:1079–1086.

24. Gerson SL, Talbot GH, Hurwitz S, *et al.*: Prolonged granulocytopenia: the major risk factor for invasive pulmonary aspergillosis in patients with acute leukemia. *Ann Intern Med* 1984, 100:345–351.

25. Young RC, Bennet JE, Vogel CL, *et al.*: Aspergillosis: the spectrum of the disease in 98 patients. *Medicine* 1970, 49:147–173.

26. Meyer RD, Young LS, Armstrong D, Yu B: Aspergillosis complicating neoplastic disease. *Am J Med* 1983, 54:6–15.

27. Groll AH, Renz S, Gerein V, et al.: Fatal haemoptysis associated with invasive pulmonary aspergillosis treated with high-dose amphotericin B and granulocyte macrophage colony-stimulating factor (GM-CSF). *Mycoses* 1992, 35:67–75.

28. Caillot D, Casasnovas O, Bernard A, et al.: Improved management of invasive pulmonary aspergillosis in neutropenic patients using early thoracic computed tomography scan and surgery. *J Clin Oncol* 1997, 15:139–147.

29. Khan FW, Jones JM, England DM: The role of bronchoalveolar lavage in the diagnosis of invasive pulmonary aspergillosis. *Am J Clin Pathol* 1986, 86:518–523.

30. Albelda SM, Talbot GH, Gerson SL, et al.: Role of fiberoptic bronchoscopy in the diagnosis of invasive pulmonary aspergillosis in patients with acute leukemia. *Am J Med* 1984, 76:1027–1034.

31. McWhinney PHM, Kibbler CC, Hamon MD, et al.: Progress in the diagnosis and management of aspergillosis in bone marrow transplantation: 13 years experience. *Clin Infect Dis* 1993, 17:397–404.

32. Yu VL, Muder RR, Poorsattar A: Significance of isolation of *Aspergillus* from the respiratory tract in diagnosis of invasive pulmonary aspergillosis: results from a three year prospective study. *Am J Med* 1986, 81:249–254.

33. Pagani JJ, Libshitz HI: Opportunistic fungal pneumonias in cancer patients. *Am J Radiol* 1981, 137:1033–1039.

34. Kuhlman JE, Fishman EK, Siegelman SS: Invasive pulmonary aspergillosis in acute leukemia: characteristic findings on CT, the CT halo sign, and the role of CT in early diagnosis. *Radiology* 1985, 157:611–614.

35. Walmsley S, Devi S, King S, et al.: Invasive *Aspergillus* infections in a pediatric hospital: a ten-year review. *Pediatr Infect Dis J* 1993, 12:673–682.

36. Groll AH, Jaeger G, Allendorf A, et al.: Invasive pulmonary aspergillosis in a critically ill neonate: case report and review of invasive aspergillosis in the first three months of life. *Clin Infect Dis* 1998, 27:437–452.

37. Walsh TJ, Hier DB, Caplan LR: Aspergillosis of the central nervous system: clinicopathological analysis of 17 patients. *Ann Neurol* 1985, 18:574–582.

38. Denning DW, Stevens D: Antifungal and surgical treatment of invasive aspergillosis: review of 2121 published cases. *Rev Infect Dis* 1990, 12:1147–1201.

39. Boes B, Hahn F, Bashir R, et al.: Central nervous system aspergillosis: analysis of 26 patients. *J Neuroimag* 1994, 4:123–129.

40. Walsh TJ, Hutchins GM, Bulkley BH, Mendelsohn G: Fungal infections of the heart: analysis of 51 autopsy cases. *Am J Cardiol* 1980, 45:357–366.

41. Mullen P, Jude C, Borkon M, et al.: *Aspergillus* mural endocarditis: clinical and echocardiographic diagnosis. *Chest* 1986, 90:451–452.

42. Groll AH, Walsh TJ: Potential new antifungal agents. *Curr Opin Infect Dis* 1997, 10:449–458.

43. Denning DW, Lee JY, Hostetler JS, et al.: NIAID Mycoses Study Group multicenter trial of oral itraconazole therapy for invasive aspergillosis. *Am J Med* 1994, 97:135–144.

44. White MH, Anaissie EJ, Kusne S, et al.: Amphotericin B colloidal dispersion vs. amphotericin B as therapy for invasive aspergillosis. *Clin Infect Dis* 1997, 24:635–642.

45. Walsh TJ, Hiemenz JW, Seibel N, et al.: Amphotericin B lipid complex in invasive fungal infections: analysis of safety and efficacy in 556 cases [Abstr P-571]. *Abstracts of the 13th Congress of the International Society for Human and Animal Mycology*. Parma, Italy: International Society for Human and Animal Mycology, 1997.

46. Wingard JR: Efficacy of amphotericin B lipid complex injection (ABLC) in bone marrow transplant recipients with life-threatening systemic mycoses. *Bone Marrow Transplant* 1997, 19:343–347.

47. Hiemenz JW, Lister EJ, Anaissie E, et al.: Emergency use of amphotericin B lipid complex (ABLC) in the treatment of patients with aspergillosis: historical control comparison with amphotericin B. *Blood* 1995, 86 (suppl 1):849a.

48. Ringden O, Meunier F, Tollemar J, et al.: Efficacy of amphotericin B encapsulated in liposome (AmBisome™) in the treatment of invasive fungal infections in immunocompromised patients. *J Antimicrob Chemother* 1991, 28 (suppl B):73–82.

49. Roilides E, Uhlig K, Venzon D, et al.: Prevention of corticosteroid-induced suppression of human polymorphonuclear leukocyte-induced damage of *Aspergillus fumigatus* hyphae by granulocyte colony-stimulating factor and gamma interferon. *Infect Immun* 1993, 61:4870–4877.

50. Walsh TJ, Dixon DM: Nosocomial aspergillosis: environmental microbiology, hospital epidemiology, diagnosis and treatment. *Eur J Epidemiol* 1989, 5:131–142.

Chapter 10

Mucormycosis and Entomophthoromycosis

Alan M. Sugar

Fungal Infections

Mucormycosis is an uncommon fungal infection that requires rapid diagnosis in order to minimize morbidity and mortality. The fungi of the order Mucorales are responsible for causing this infection. The more commonly isolated representatives include Rhizopus, Rhizomucor, and Mucor. Absidia, Cunninghamella, and Apophysomyces are also being increasingly recovered from clinical specimens. Details of the class of fungi that cause human illness can be found below and in the references to Figure 1.

Classically, patients with diabetes mellitus and diabetic ketoacidosis present with evidence of a progressive sinusitis, with extension of the process to the periorbital region, face, and brain. Other manifestations of the infection have been described in recent years and these are presented in the figures that follow. Treatment with amphotericin B and aggressive surgical debridement of the involved areas usually represent the best chance for cure of the infection. The role of newer antifungal drugs to replace or to supplement amphotericin B is not yet known.

Once suspected by the physician as a possible explanation for a patient's presentation, appropriate diagnostic procedures and therapeutic interventions can be done. The characteristic appearance of these fungi under the microscope help to make a presumptive diagnosis easier than for other mycoses. The figures that follow provide a sampling of the different clinical presentations of mucormycosis and illustrate the remarkable pathologic changes that occur during the course of this infection.

Classification of the Mucorales

Zygomycetes
  Mucorales
    Mucoraceae
      Absidia
        A. corymbifera
        A. ramosa
      Mucor
        M. circinelloides
      Rhizomucor
        R. pusillus
      Rhizopus
        R. oryzae
        R. arrhizus
        R. rhizopodiformis
    Cunninghamellacaeae
      Cunninghamella
        C. bertholletiae
    Mortierellaceae
      Mortierella
        M. wolfii
    Saksenaeaceae
      Saksenaea
        S. vasiformis
    Syncephalastraceae
      Syncephalastrum
    Apophysomyceae
      Apophysomyces
        A. elegans
    Thamnidiaceae
      Cokeromyces
        C. recurvatus
  Entomophthorales
    Conidiobolus
      C. coronatus (Entomophthora coronata)*
      C. incongruans
    Basidiobolus
      B. haptosporus (B. meristosporus, B. ranarum)*

*Obsolete synonyms.

FIGURE 10-1. Classification of the Mucorales. The fungi grouped together in the class Zygomycetes have been known by many different names over the years. Many of these names are obsolete owing to advances in taxonomy and the application of rules of nomenclature. Most cases of mucormycosis are due to one of the Mucoraceae (*Absidia*, *Mucor*, *Rhizomucor*, or *Rhizopus* species). Representatives from the genera *Cunninghamella*, *Saksenaea*, and *Apophymyces*, however, increasingly are being recovered. Entomophthoramycosis is the designation given to disease caused by the other large group of Zygomycetes, the Entomophthorales. These infections primarily are caused by *Conidiobolus* or *Basidiobolus* species. Although mucormycosis and entomophthoromycosis were distinct infections in the past, recent cases of infection by the Entomophthorales involving tissue invasion similar to that seen in mucormycosis have been described. This discovery has blurred the lines of demarcation that had separated the two clinical and pathologic syndromes caused by these fungi. (*From* Sugar [1].)

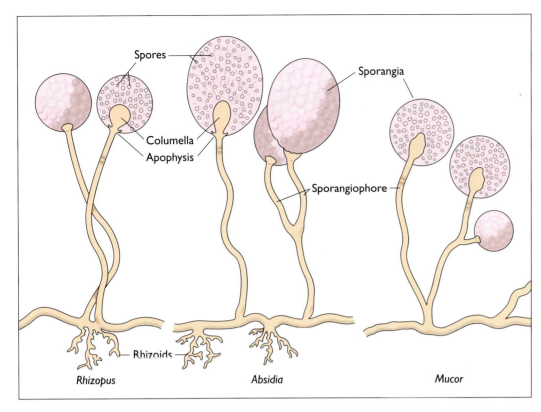

FIGURE 10-2. Distinguishing morphologic features of three of the more common Mucorales. Assignment of genus is based on the presence or absence of rhizoids and their location with respect to the sporangiophore, characteristics of the columella, and the shape of the sporangia. Zygomycetes are widely distributed in nature and grow in the environment and tissue as hyphae. The anatomic features of the fungi in the laboratory are not found in tissue; thus, definitive identification of genus and species is dependent on growing the fungus in the laboratory so that the fungus can be examined. All Zygomycetes share similar morphology in tissue (see Fig. 10-4). (Adapted from Sugar [1].)

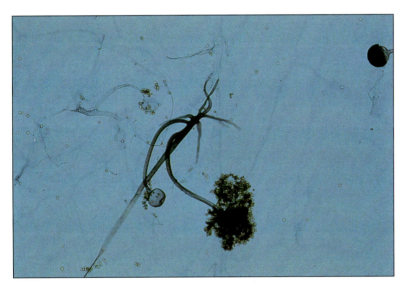

FIGURE 10-3. Lactophenol cotton blue preparation of *Rhizopus* species. The figure demonstrates the morphology of *Rhizopus* species as seen under the microscope in the laboratory. Note that the sporangiophore arises directly from the rhizoids ("roots"). (*Courtesy of* Dr. K. Abson; *from* Raugi [2].)

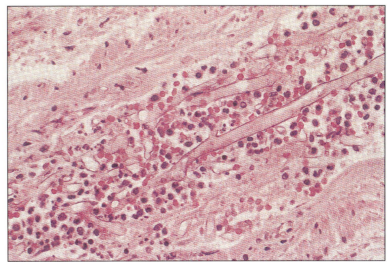

FIGURE 10-4. Histopathologic appearance of mucormycosis. This section of lung stained with hematoxylin-eosin clearly shows the presence of the characteristic broad, nonseptate hyphae present in the pulmonary artery. The culture grew *Rhizopus* species. (*From* Kauffman [3].)

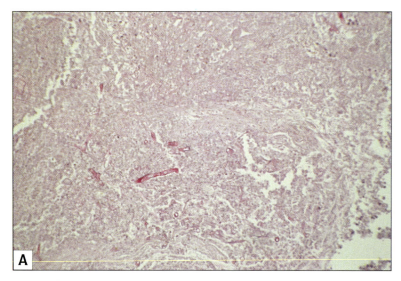
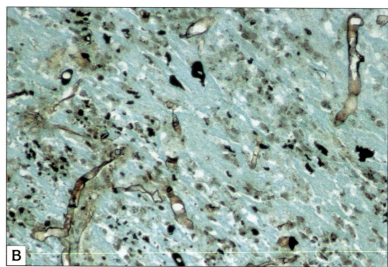

Figure 10-5. Histopathology of the lung obtained from a patient with pulmonary mucormycosis. **A,** Hematoxylin-eosin stain clearly shows the characteristic broad, nonseptate hyphae. An inflammatory vasculitis with extensive tissue necrosis with thrombosis of the small arteries and pulmonary veins also is present. **B,** Methenamine silver stain also shows the hyphae with characteristic right angle branching consistent with one of the Mucorales. (*From* Fishman and Rubin [4].)

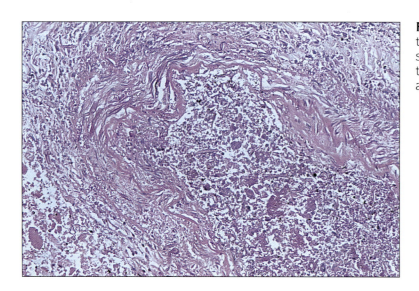

Figure 10-6. Blood vessel invasion in mucormycosis. As seen in the figure, the characteristic hyphae of the Mucorales easily are seen on sections stained with hematoxylin-eosin. Involvement of the blood vessels results in thrombosis, hemorrhage, infarction, and tissue necrosis. (*From* Buckley [5].)

Clinical syndromes of mucormycosis

Rhinocerebral
Pulmonary
Gastrointestinal
Cutaneous
Central nervous system
Disseminated infection
Miscellaneous (myocardium, endocardium, bones, kidneys, allergic sinusitis)

Figure 10-7. Clinical syndromes of mucormycosis. Mucormycosis usually presents in several characteristic ways as detailed in this table. Symptoms depend on extent and location of the infection.

Predisposing factors for the development of mucormycosis
Diabetes mellitus
Neutropenia
Iron overload and deferoxamine administration
Trauma (wound contamination with soil; colonized adhesive tape)
Protein calorie malnutrition
Corticosteroids

FIGURE 10-8. Predisposing factors for the development of mucormycosis. Mucormycosis is not commonly seen in patients without a predisposing condition. Patients with diabetes mellitus, especially ketoacidosis, are at increased risk for the development of rhinocerebral mucormycosis. Some patients present with mucormycosis as the first indication of diabetes. It is not clear what the exact mechanism is for the increased risk of this infection, but it is probably a combination of metabolic abnormalities present in the patient with diabetes. In patients with neutropenia, usually secondary to chemotherapy, pulmonary mucormycosis is the most common presentation. Because the fungus has a predilection for blood vessel invasion, radiographic abnormalities are secondary to thrombosis, necrosis, and hemorrhage into the lungs. Rarely, patients can present with a subacute syndrome of pulmonary nodule or pulmonary cavity in the setting of minimal or no underlying immunosuppressive condition. Iron overload and treatment with the chelator deferoxamine also have been implicated as predisposing factors for the development of mucormycosis. Once diagnosed, mucormycosis in this setting is very aggressive and mortality is high. Most patients present with the rhinocerebral form of the infection. Deferoxamine may have been prescribed for iron overload syndromes or more commonly for aluminum overload in patients receiving hemodialysis for chronic renal failure. Contaminated adhesive bandages were once a major cause of cutaneous mucormycosis in hospitalized patients. Once this association was recognized, appropriate steps to sterilize these products were taken, and this form of the infection is now rare. However, patients who are involved in traumatic accidents resulting in wounds contaminated with soil may develop an aggressive infection of the subcutaneous and cutaneous tissues. This infection may result in extensive tissue destruction requiring amputation and dramatic surgical debridement and may result in death.

RHINOCEREBRAL MUCORMYCOSIS

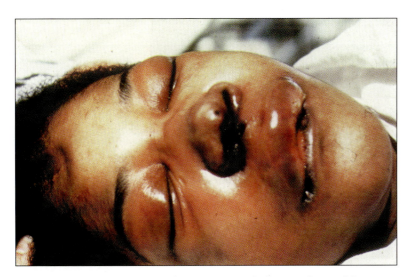

FIGURE 10-9. Rhinocerebral mucormycosis in a patient with diabetes. Swelling of the eyelids and nose is indicative of extensive sinus and periorbital involvement. (*Courtesy of* Drs. J.J. Herdegen and R. Bone; *from* Buckley [5].)

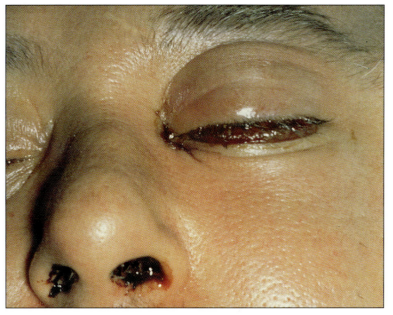

FIGURE 10-10. Rhinocerebral mucormycosis involving the left nose and orbit. Note the proptosis, chemosis, and edema resulting in the eye being closed. Black discharge in the left nare is indicative of hemorrhage and tissue necrosis. (*From* Davies and Sarosi [6].)

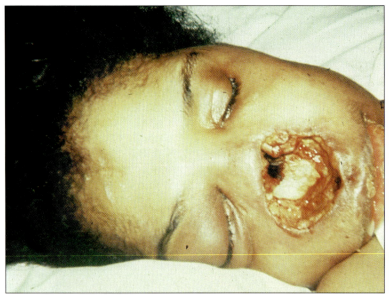
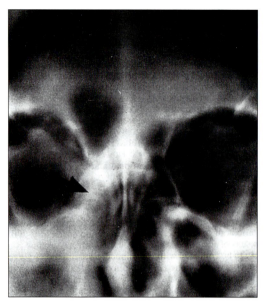

FIGURE 10-11. Residual sinus infection after surgical debridement of rhinocerebral mucormycosis. Following debridement, many patients are left with significant defects, which can be later corrected with plastic surgical procedures. (*From* Herdegen and Bone [7].)

FIGURE 10-12. Radiograph of the sinuses of a patient with mucormycosis, showing involvement of both ethmoid and maxillary sinuses.

PULMONARY MUCORMYCOSIS

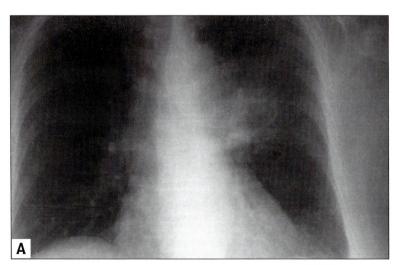
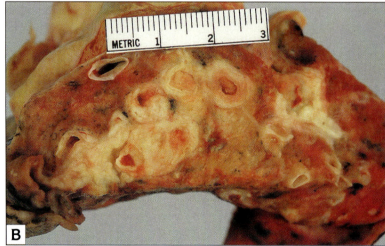

FIGURE 10-13. Pulmonary mucormycosis. **A**, Chest radiograph is shown from a 60-year-old woman who had myelodysplastic syndrome and who was treated with deferoxamine for iron overload. She presented to the hospital with fever and confusion, became hypotensive, and died 4 days later. A left hilar infiltrate is present. **B**, Lung specimen obtained at autopsy showed multiple thrombi in major pulmonary arteries. (*From* Kauffman [3].)

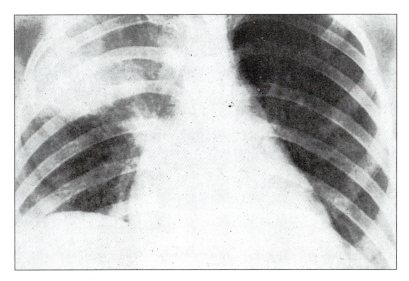

Figure 10-14. Chest radiograph from an 18-year-old woman who presented with neutropenia, persistent fever, cough, and generalized weakness. She died from the infection, which was histopathologically documented as mucormycosis on the basis of widespread pulmonary involvement with broad, nonseptate hyphae throughout the lungs. (*From* Dartrum *et al.* [8]; with permission.)

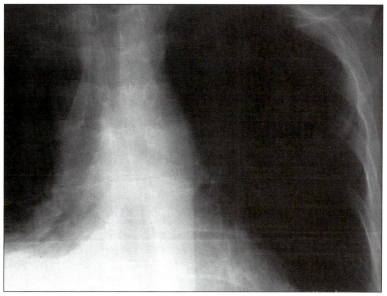

Figure 10-15. Chest radiograph from a 48-year-old woman taken 4 years after liver transplantation. A right middle lobe cavity is present, which was diagnosed as a result of mucormycosis. The radiographic appearance is indistinguishable from other causes of pulmonary cavitation, including aspergillosis and other fungi, pyogenic bacterial infections, and tuberculosis. (*From* Fishman and Rubin [4].)

INVOLVEMENT OF THE STOMACH IN DISSEMINATED MUCORMYCOSIS

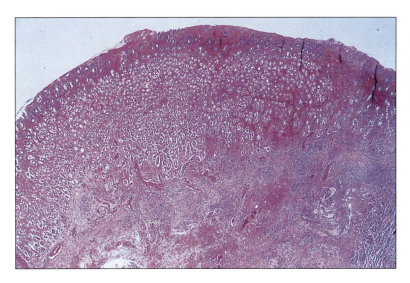

Figure 10-16. Hemorrhagic necrosis of gastric mucosa in a patient with a fatal case of disseminated *Rhizopus* infection. Virtually any organ can be involved in disseminated infection. Similar lesions characterized by hemorrhage and necrosis can be found throughout the gastrointestinal tract in patients with disseminated infection. In patients with protein calorie malnutrition, localized gastrointestinal infection occurs, with the same histopathologic features as the lesions that develop as a result of disseminated infection. (*From* Buckley [5].)

TREATMENT OF MUCORMYCOSIS

Treatment of mucormycosis

- Aggressive surgical debridement
- Reversal of underlying predisposing factors to the greatest extent possible
- Amphotericin B, 1.0–1.5 mg/kg/d, as tolerated
- Lipid formulations of amphotericin B doses up to 15–20 mg/kg/d depending on formulation

Figure 10-17. Aggressive surgical debridement. Because blood vessel invasion is a prominent component of mucormycosis, tissue necrosis is a common occurrence. Such necrotic tissue requires removal because it serves as a nidus for continued infection and possible superinfection of the area. Thus, surgical debridement should be considered in every case of mucormycosis. The temptation for small daily, "piecemeal"-type bedside debridement should be resisted, if clinically possible, because the end result of this approach is usually further morbidity and possibly increased mortality.

Cutaneous Mucormycosis

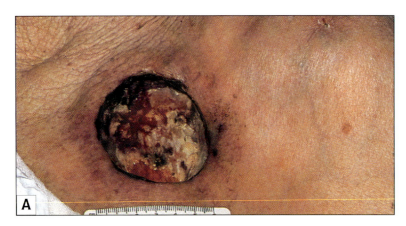
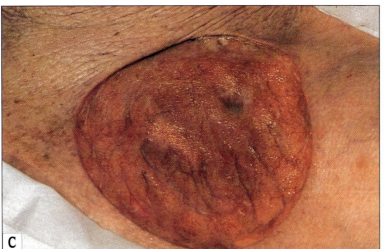
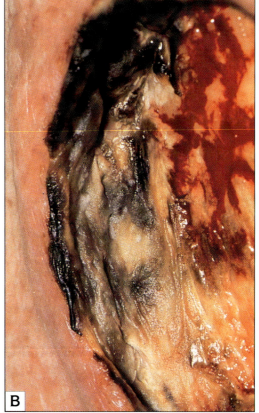

FIGURE 10-18. *Rhizopus* infection at the site of an intravenous catheter. Typically, this infection begins as a cellulitis, and a necrotic area soon develops secondary to vascular invasion and thrombosis. A similar appearance can develop in infection with *Aspergillus* species and with bacterial infections owing to, for example, *Pseudomonas* and *Aeromonas* species and other gram-negative bacilli. **A,** The infected area is shown 48 hours after debridement. **B,** Close-up view of the lesion in *panel A* shows fungus growing on subcutaneous tissue and muscle. **C,** After additional debridement, the size of the wound greatly increased. Following additional antifungal therapy, the area is ready for skin grafting. (*From* Raugi [2].)

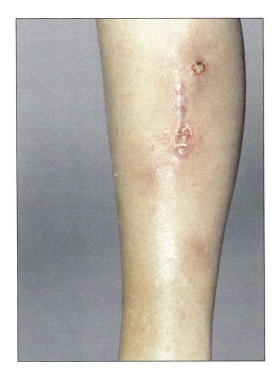

FIGURE 10-19. Mucormycosis affecting the lower leg. This infection developed on the calf of a 72-year-old man who had myelodysplastic syndrome and received deferoxamine for the treatment of iron overload secondary to repeated blood transfusions. The cellulitis did not respond to antistaphylococcal antibiotics. The lesions became painful and necrotic, and purulent material drained from the calf lesion. Two weeks later, nodules appeared on the patient's heel. These nodules also became painful and progressed to necrosis. Biopsy of the calf lesion revealed broad, nonseptate hyphae, and the culture grew *Rhizopus* species.

CONIDIOBOLUS INFECTION

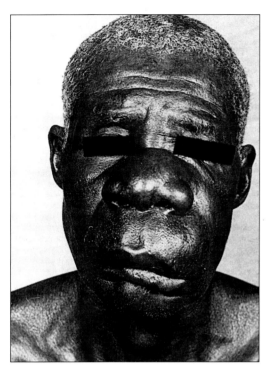

FIGURE 10-20. Infection of the nose and paranasal sinuses with *Conidiobolus* species. In contrast to mucormycosis, most infections with the Entomophthorales do not invade tissue and blood vessels. Rather, they produce swelling and symptoms secondary to mass effect. Thus, nasal congestion, sinus pain, and nasal discharge commonly are seen. Nodular masses can be seen and palpated in the affected areas of the face. In contrast to *Conidiobolus* infections that primarily involve the face, infections due to *Basidiobolus* species typically involve the trunk, arms, legs, or buttocks. Nodular subcutaneous masses are characteristic of this infection, but invasion into underlying muscle also may be found. Other diagnoses to be considered include malignancy, including lymphoma; bacterial abscesses; tuberculosis and other mycobacterial infections; sporotrichosis; elephantiasis; onchocerciasis; and pythiosis. Most patients suffer from a slowly progressive infection until therapy can be administered. Data concerning the most appropriate therapy are lacking, but success with potassium iodide, trimethoprim-sulfamethoxazole, and amphotericin B has been noted. Azoles such as ketoconazole and fluconazole also have been reported to have some beneficial effects in the treatment of these infections. Surgery remains an important part of the management of patients with entomophthoromycosis and removal of the subcutaneous masses is palliative and sometimes curative.

REFERENCES

1. Sugar AM: Agents of mucormycosis and related species. In *Principles and Practice of Infectious Diseases*, 4th ed. Edited by Mandell GL, Bennett JE, Dolin R. New York: Churchill Livingstone; 1995:2311–2321.
2. Raugi GJ: Fungal and yeast infections of the skin, appendages, and subcutaneous tissues. In *Atlas of Infectious Diseases*, vol 2. Edited by Mandell GL, Stevens DL. Philadelphia: Current Medicine; 1995:6.1–6.28.
3. Kauffman CA: Systemic fungal infections. In *Atlas of Infectious Diseases*, vol 8. Edited by Mandell GL, Fekety R. Philadelphia: Current Medicine; 1997:11.1–11.18.
4. Fishman JA, Rubin RH: Respiratory infections in transplant recipients. In *Atlas of Infectious Diseases*, vol 6. Edited by Mandell GL, Simberkoff MS. Philadelphia: Current Medicine; 1996:11.1–11.26.
5. Buckley H: Fungal enteritis. In *Atlas of Infectious Diseases*, vol 7. Edited by Mandell GL, Lorber B. Philadelphia: Current Medicine; 1996:7.1–7.9.
6. Davies SF, Sarosi GA: Fungal infections. In *Atlas of Infectious Diseases*, vol 6. Edited by Mandell GL, Simberkoff MS. Philadelphia: Current Medicine; 1996:5.1–5.32.
7. Herdegen JJ, Bone RC: Pulmonary manifestations of extrapulmonary infection. In *Atlas of Infectious Diseases*, vol 6. Edited by Mandell GL, Simberkoff MS. Philadelphia: Current Medicine; 1996:12.1–12.20.
8. Bartrum RJ Jr, Watnick M, Herman PG: Roentgenographic findings in pulmonary mucormycosis. *Am J Roentgenol* 1973, 117:810–815.

SELECTED BIBLIOGRAPHY

Kwon-Chung KJ, Bennett JE: *Medical Mycology*. Philadelphia: Lea & Febiger; 1992.

Harloff KJ, Stoehr A, Wasmuth R, *et al.*: Pulmonary mucormycosis in an HIV-infected patient. *Dtsch Med Wochenschr* 1995, 120:94–98.

Gaziev D, Baronciani D, Galimberti M, *et al.*: Mucormycosis after bone marrow transplantation: report of four cases in thalassemia and review of the literature. *Bone Marrow Transplant* 1996, 17:409–414.

Leong KW, Crowley B, White B, *et al.*: Cutaneous mucormycosis due to *Absidia corymbifera* occurring after bone marrow transplantation. *Bone Marrow Transplant* 1997, 19:513–515.

McAdams HP, deChristenson MR, Strollo DC, Patz EF: Pulmonary mucormycosis: radiologic findings in 32 cases. *Am J Roentgenol* 1997, 168:1541–1548.

PastorPons E, MartinezLeon MI, AlvarezBustos G, *et al.*: Isolated renal mucormycosis in two patients with AIDS: case report. *Am J Roentgenol* 1996, 166:1282–1284.

Jantunen E, Kolho E, Ruutu P, *et al.*: Invasive cutaneous mucormycosis caused by *Absidia corymbifera* after allogeneic bone marrow transplantation. *Bone Marrow Transplant* 1996, 18:229–230.

Jamadar DA, Kazerooni EA, Daly BD, *et al.*: Pulmonary zygomycosis: CT appearance. *J Comput Assist Tomogr* 1995, 19:733–738.

Perolada Valmana JM, Morera Perez C, Blanes Julia M, *et al.*: Mucormycosis of the paranasal sinuses. *Rev Laryngol Otol Rhinol* 1996, 117:51–52.

Peterson KL, Wang M, Canalis RF, Abemayor E: Rhinocerebral mucormycosis: evolution of the disease and treatment options. *Laryngoscope* 1997, 107:855–862.

Rangel-Guerra RA, Martinez HR, Saenz C, *et al.*: Rhinocerebral and systemic mucormycosis: clinical experience with 36 cases. *J Neurol Sci* 1996, 143:19–30.

Shpitzer T, Stern Y, Anavi Y, *et al.*: Mucormycosis: experience with 10 patients. *Clin Otolaryngol* 1995, 20:374–379.

CHAPTER 11

Penicillium marneffei Infections

Khuanchai Supparatpinyo
Thira Sirisanthana

Fungal Infections

Penicillium marneffei is a dimorphic fungal pathogen, which can cause disseminated disease both in immunocompetent and immunocompromised patients. The prevalence of disseminated *P. marneffei* infection has increased markedly over the past few years. This increase is due exclusively to infection among patients infected with HIV. Less than 40 cases of *P. marneffei* infection were reported prior to the HIV epidemic in southeast Asia, whereas more than 1000 patients have been diagnosed at Chiang Mai University Hospital alone since the beginning of the HIV/AIDS epidemic in northern Thailand. In addition, cases of disseminated *P. marneffei* infection have been reported in individuals with HIV infection from the United States, the United Kingdom, the Netherlands, Italy, France, Germany, Switzerland, and Australia following visits to the endemic region.

INCIDENCE AND DISTRIBUTION

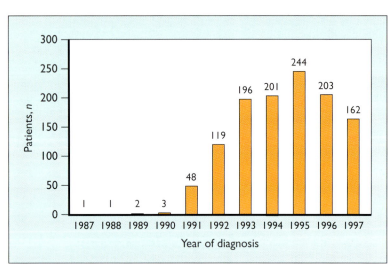

FIGURE 11-1. Number of patients diagnosed with *Penicillium marneffei* infection at Chiang Mai University Hospital from 1987 to 1997. A total of 1180 patients were found to have *P. marneffei* infection between January 1991 and December 1997. Ninety-nine percent of these patients also were infected with HIV. In northern Thailand, infection with *P. marneffei* is the third most common opportunistic infection in patients with AIDS after tuberculosis and cryptococcal meningitis.

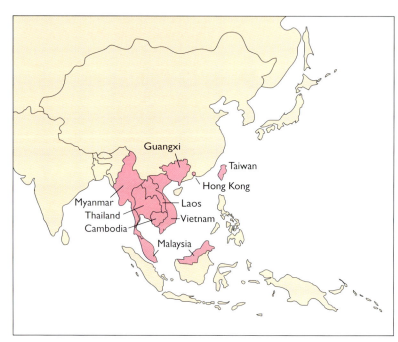

FIGURE 11-2. Geographic regions of *Penicillium marneffei* infection. The endemic area of *P. marneffei* infection includes southeast Asia, the Guangxi province of China, Taiwan, and Hong Kong.

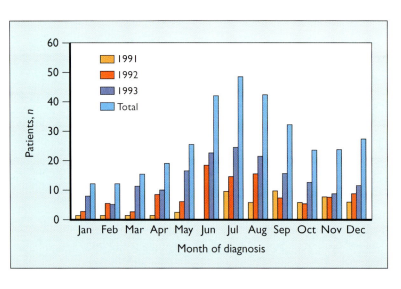

FIGURE 11-3. Distribution of cases with *Penicillium marneffei* infection at Chiang Mai University Hospital by month of diagnosis. Patients with *P. marneffei* infection were more likely to be seen during the rainy season (May through November) in each year of the study. (*Adapted from* Chariyalertsak, *et al.* [1].)

CLINICAL APPEARANCE

Clinical manifestations in 80 patients infected with HIV and *Penicillium marneffei* in Chiang Mai, Thailand

Patient characteristics	
Male-to-female ratio	74 : 6
Age, *mean* (*range*)	32.4 y (18–63 y)
Acquisition of HIV infection	Patients, *n*
Blood transfusion	2
IV drug use	2
Heterosexual transmission	76
Symptoms	Patients, *n* (%)
Fever	74 (92.5)
Skin lesions	54 (67.5)
Cough	39 (48.7)
Diarrhea	25 (31.2)
Signs	
Elevated body temperature (≥38.3°C)	79 (95.0)
Marked weight loss	61 (76.2)
Anemia	62 (77.5)
Jaundice	6 (7.5)
Oral candidiasis	59 (73.7)
Hairy leukoplakia	6 (7.5)
Palatal papules	3 (3.7)
Generalized lymphadenopathy	46 (57.5)
Hepatomegaly	41 (51.2)
Splenomegaly	13 (16.2)
Skin lesions	57 (71.2)
Genital ulcer	5 (6.2)
Laboratory findings, *mean* (*range*)	
Hemoglobin	96 (54–167) g/L
Leukocyte count	6.2 (1.6–17.2) x 10^9/L
Lymphocyte count	1.3 (0.2–4.0) x 10^9/L
Blood urea nitrogen	6.8 (2.5–16.4) mmol/L
Serum creatinine	97 (53–530) µmol/L
Serum aspartate aminotransferase	122 (4–650) U/L*
Serum alanine aminotransferase	43 (5–194) U/L†
Serum alkaline phosphatase	226 (38–755) U/L‡
Serum bilirubin	26.0 (3.2–138.2) µmol/L

*Normal range, 3–35 U/L.
†Normal range, 7–33 U/L.
‡Normal range, 23–98 U/L.

FIGURE 11-4. Signs and symptoms of *Penicillium marneffei* infection. The clinical manifestations of 80 patients infected with HIV and *P. marneffei* in Chiang Mai, Thailand, are shown. (*From* Supparatpinyo *et al.* [2]; with permission.)

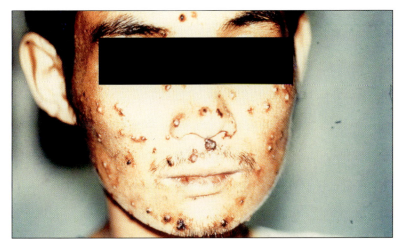

FIGURE 11-5. Multiple papulonecrotic lesions on the face of a patient with HIV and disseminated *Penicillium marneffei* infection. The skin lesions typically distribute over the face, head, neck, and upper extremities.

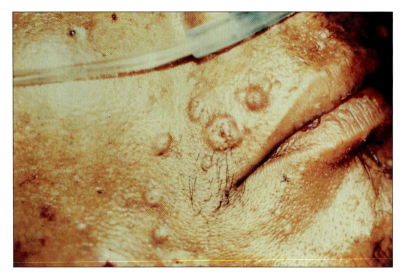

FIGURE 11-6. Close-up view of skin lesions in a patient infected with HIV and *Penicillium marneffei*. The findings of discrete skin-colored papules, 5 to 10 mm in diameter, with central umbilication are characteristic. These typical lesions are observed in about 70% of patients with disseminated *P. marneffei* infection. The lesions are sometimes described as molluscum contagiosum–like lesions. (*From* Supparatpinyo *et al.* [2]; with permission.)

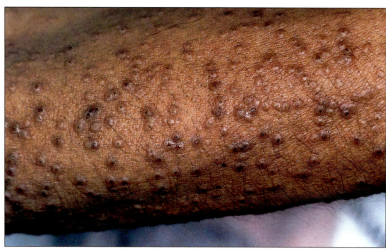

FIGURE 11-7. Numerous skin lesions on the forearm of a patient with HIV and disseminated *Penicillium marneffei* infection. Several papules show the characteristic molluscum contagiosum–like lesions.

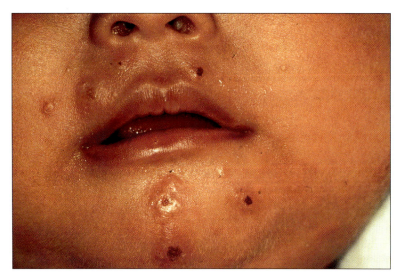

FIGURE 11-8. Skin lesions on the face of an infant with HIV and disseminated *Penicillium marneffei* infection. The lesions are papulonecrotic in appearance, similar to those found in adult patients. More than 40 pediatric patients with disseminated *P. marneffei* infection were diagnosed at Chiang Mai University Hospital in Thailand. All of these patients acquired HIV infection via vertical transmission. (*From* Sirisanthana and Sirisanthana [3]; with permission.)

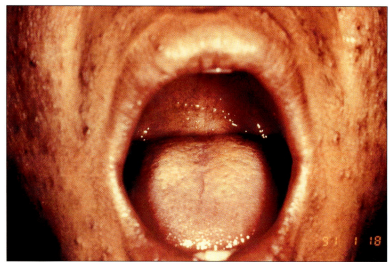

FIGURE 11-9. Papules on the hard palate of a patient with HIV and *Penicillium marneffei* infection. The patient also had skin lesions on his face. Findings from the microscopic examination and culture of the scraping from the palatal papule confirmed the diagnosis of *P. marneffei* infection.

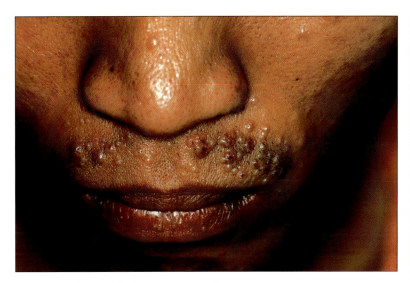

FIGURE 11-10. Skin lesions above the upper lip in a patient with HIV and disseminated cryptococcosis. Some lesions are papulonecrotic in appearance, giving a molluscum contagiosum–like feature. In Thailand, the differential diagnoses of febrile patients with HIV and molluscum contagiosum–like lesions include disseminated cryptococcosis and disseminated histoplasmosis.

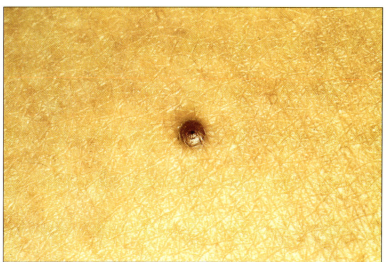

FIGURE 11-11. Skin lesions in a patient with AIDS and disseminated histoplasmosis. This erythematous papule–type of skin lesion is not specific and could be found in patients with penicilliosis, cryptococcosis, or histoplasmosis.

MICROSCOPIC APPEARANCE

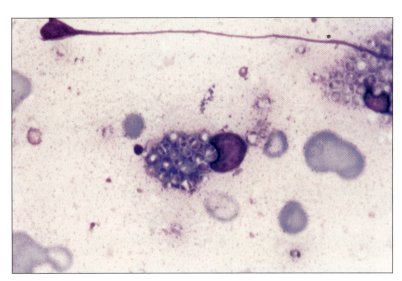

FIGURE 11-12. Photomicrograph from a Wright's-stained skin biopsy touch smear showing numerous yeastlike organisms in a macrophage. Some of these cells have clear central septation, which is the characteristic feature of *Penicillium marneffei*. Microscopic examination of Wright's-stained touch smears of skin biopsy specimens, lymph node biopsy specimens, and bone marrow aspirate is the useful bedside procedure for differential diagnosis of skin lesions in patients with AIDS. Presumptive diagnosis of *P. marneffei* infection could be made in 63% of patients several days before the results of fungal culture were available. (×1000.) (*From* Supparatpinyo *et al.* [2]; with permission.)

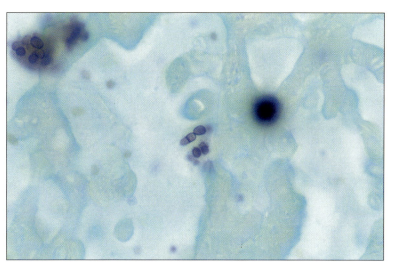

FIGURE 11-13. Photomicrograph of the Gomori methenamine silver–stained skin biopsy touch smear confirming the presence of a septate yeastlike organism. This characteristic of *Penicillium marneffei* is the result of the organism dividing itself by binary fission and not by budding. (×1000.)

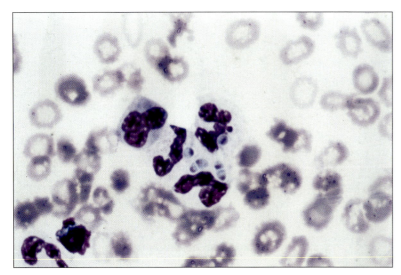

FIGURE 11-14. Photomicrograph of a Wright's-stained peripheral blood smear from a patient with AIDS and severe disseminated *Penicillium marneffei* infection. The blood smear shows typical features, including intracellular spherical, oval, and elliptical yeast-like organisms with clear central septation. Through examination of peripheral blood smear, presumptive diagnosis of penicilliosis could be made on the first day of admission in this patient. Patients with *P. marneffei* observed in the peripheral blood smear usually had severe disease and died soon after admission. (x1000.)

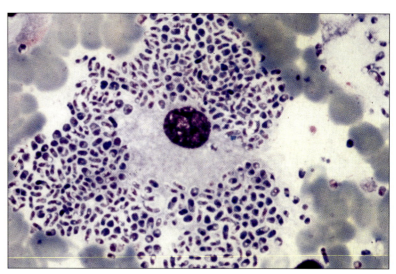

FIGURE 11-15. Photomicrograph of a Wright's-stained smear of bone marrow aspirate from a patient with HIV and *Penicillium marneffei* infection. The smear shows numerous yeastlike organisms in a histiocyte. In addition to the septate yeastlike form, *P. marneffei* is frequently elongated in a smear of bone marrow aspirate, giving a sausagelike appearance. (x1000.)

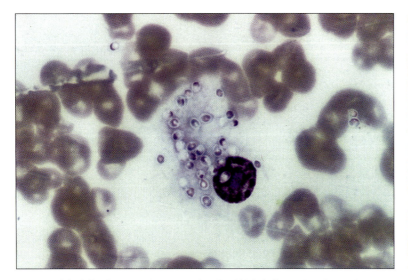

FIGURE 11-16. Photomicrograph of a Wright's-stained touch smear of the skin biopsy specimen from the patient in Fig. 11-11 who had disseminated histoplasmosis showing many yeastlike organisms in a macrophage. It is usually difficult to differentiate between *Penicillium marneffei* and *Histoplasma capsulatum* by the microscopic examination. However, *H. capsulatum* is typically round or oval in shape and more uniform. The presence of budding yeast forms suggests the diagnosis of histoplasmosis, whereas the presence of septate yeast forms suggests the diagnosis of penicilliosis. (x1000.)

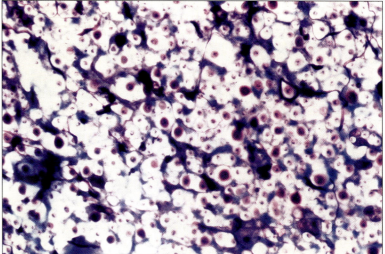

FIGURE 11-17. Photomicrograph of a Wright's-stained touch smear of the skin biopsy specimen from the patient in Fig. 11-10 who had disseminated cryptococcosis. The figure shows many yeastlike organisms with surrounding haloes. Differential diagnosis between cryptococcosis and penicilliosis by microscopic examination of specimens obtained from skin biopsy is usually easier than that of penicilliosis and histoplasmosis. Yeastlike organisms with surrounding haloes is the typical feature of *Cryptococcus neoformans*. Definite diagnosis could be made by special staining with mucicarmine or fungal culture. (x100.)

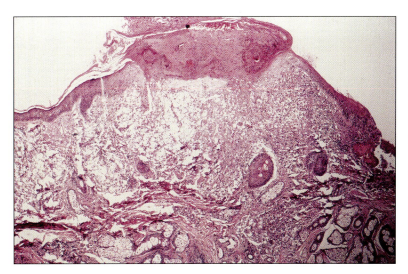

FIGURE 11-18. Photomicrograph of a skin biopsy tissue section stained with hematoxylin-eosin from a papulonecrotic skin lesion of a patient with HIV and *Penicillium marneffei* infection. The figure shows a volcano-like appearance. The upper part of the skin lesion contains necrotic tissue abundant with intra- and extracellular fungi. (x40.)

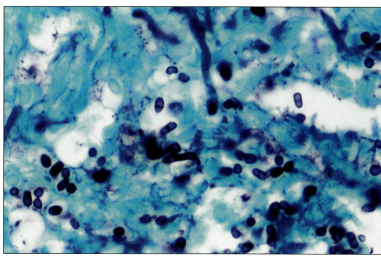

FIGURE 11-19. Photomicrograph of the same specimen in Fig. 11-18 specially stained with Gomori methenamine silver. The figure shows the black fungal elements in subcutaneous tissue underneath the skin lesion. Some of these cells show a typical yeastlike organism with central septation. (x1000.)

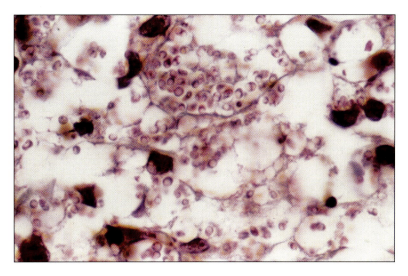

FIGURE 11-20. Photomicrograph of the same specimen in Fig. 11-18 specially stained with periodic acid–Schiff. The figure shows the red yeastlike organisms in subcutaneous tissue underneath the skin lesion. A careful examination usually reveals the characteristic septate yeastlike organisms. (x1000.)

CULTURE

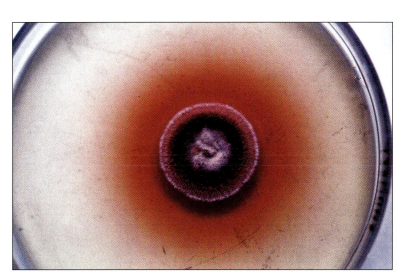

FIGURE 11-21. Colony of mycelium phase. *Penicillium marneffei* is the only dimorphic fungus of the genus *Penicillium*. The figure shows the colony of *Penicillium marneffei* growing as mold at 25°C on Sabouraud's dextrose agar. The colony of mycelial phase is grayish white and downy. During differentiation, the color of the colony turns grayish pink. The reverse side becomes brownish red, as a soluble red pigment diffuses into the surrounding agar.

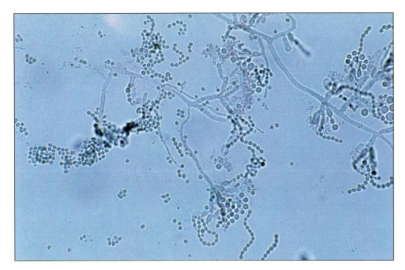

FIGURE 11-22. Mycelium culture. Photomicrograph of a fresh smear of the mycelial colony in Fig. 11-21 shows the hyaline, septate branching hyphae with lateral and terminal conidiophores. The conidiophores consist of basal stripes with terminal verticils of three to five metulae, with each metula bearing three to seven phialides. The conidia are oval and smooth-walled, measuring approximately 2 by 3 μm. They are formed basipetally in chains from each phialide. (×400.)

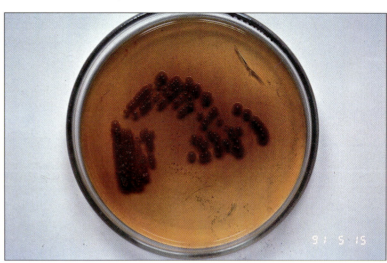

FIGURE 11-23. Colony yeast phase. Yeast colonies of *Penicillium marneffei* are shown after incubation at 37°C on brain–heart infusion agar for a few days. The colony is rough, glabrous, and tan in color. No soluble pigment could be seen in the agar.

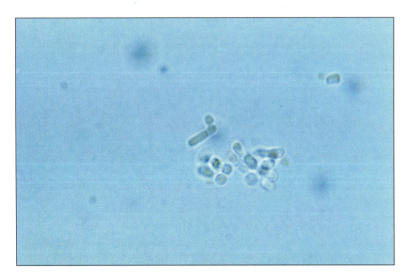

FIGURE 11-24. Yeast culture. Photomicrograph of a fresh smear of the yeast colony in Fig. 11-23 showing unicellular, pleomorphic, ellipsoidal-to-rectangular yeastlike cells with septation. Short segments of hyphae occasionally could be seen. (×400.)

Route of Infection

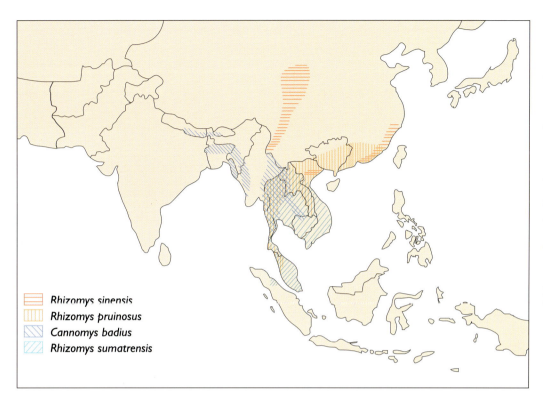

Figure 11-25. Geographic distribution of population of bamboo rats (*Rhizomys sinensis*, *Rhizomys sumatrensis*, *Rhizomys pruinosus*, and *Cannomys badius*). *Penicillium marneffei* was first isolated from bamboo rats (*R. sinensis*) in Vietnam in 1956. In the Guangxi province of China, the fungus has been isolated from the internal organs of more than 90% of another species of bamboo rats, *R. pruinosus*. In Thailand, *P. marneffei* was isolated from *R. pruinosus* and two other species of bamboo rats, *C. badius* and *R. sumatrensis*. Because the bamboo rats usually live near the forest and have limited contact with people, it is believed that both humans and bamboo rats are infected with *P. marneffei* from a common source, rather than the patients being infected from the rats.

- *Rhizomys sinensis*
- *Rhizomys pruinosus*
- *Cannomys badius*
- *Rhizomys sumatrensis*

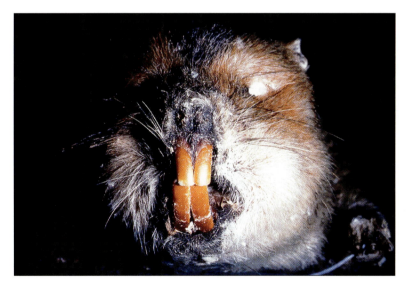

Figure 11-26. Bamboo rat. *Rhizomys sumatrensis*, a species of bamboo rat, captured from a village in Chiang Mai, Thailand, has a triangular shape of darker hairs on the forehead. From the 14 captured animals in a study in Chiang Mai, the average mean weight of the rat was approximately 2 kg. The average measurement of the head and body was 382 mm. The tail was naked and long (average length, 150 mm). The posterior footpads were granular and joined. *Penicillium marneffei* could be isolated from the internal organs of 13 of 14 (92.8%) bamboo rats of this species. (*From* Chariyalertsak *et al.* [4]; with permission.)

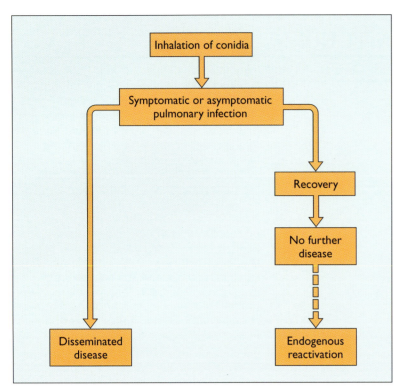

FIGURE 11-27. Natural history of *Penicillium marneffei*. The route of infection of *P. marneffei* is unknown. By analogy with other endemic systemic mycoses, it is likely that *P. marneffei* conidia may be inhaled from a contaminated reservoir in the environment and subsequently disseminate from the lungs when the infected hosts experience immunosuppression. Because the disease is significantly more likely to occur in the rainy season (*see* Fig. 11-3), there may be an expansion of the environmental reservoirs with favorable conditions for growth in the rainy months. In endemic areas, it is likely that a certain proportion of the general population is infected but remains asymptomatic. Patients have been reported with long periods of asymptomatic infection prior to presentation with disseminated disease. In other instances, the clinical appearance of disseminated disease occurs shortly after exposure to the organism. Appearance of *P. marneffei* infection in infants with HIV also suggests that the duration between infection and clinical manifestation sometimes may be brief (*see* Fig. 11-8).

TREATMENT

In vitro susceptibility of *Penicillium marneffei*

Antifungal agent	Isolates, n	MIC, µg/mL	
		Median	Range
Fluconazole	30	10.0	0.313–20.0
Itraconazole	28	0.009	<0.002–0.19
Ketoconazole	29	0.078	<0.002–0.078
Miconazole	29	<0.002	<0.002–0.156
Amphotericin B	29	1.0	0.25–4.0
5-Flucytosine	29	0.23	<0.015–0.46

FIGURE 11-28. In vitro susceptibility of *Penicillium marneffei*. The mortality rate of patients with disseminated *P. marneffei* infection had been very high, most likely owing to failure to make a timely diagnosis. When treatment was started early, the response to therapy was much better. The fungus was sensitive to amphotericin B, itraconazole, and ketoconazole. Our current treatment regimen is to give amphotericin B 0.6 mg/kg/d for 2 weeks, followed by itraconazole 400 mg/d orally for the next 10 weeks. At Chiang Mai University Hospital, all 73 patients treated with this regimen responded well. After the initial therapy, patients with HIV should be given itraconazole 200 mg/d orally as secondary prophylaxis for life. (*From* Supparatpinyo *et al.* [5]; with permission.)

REFERENCES

1. Chariyalertsak S, Sirisanthana T, Supparatpinyo K, Nelson KE. Seasonal variation of disseminated Penicillium marneffei infections in northern Thailand: a clue to the reservoir? J Infect Dis 1996, 173:1490–1493.

2. Supparatpinyo K, Khamwan C, Baosoung V, *et al.*: Disseminated *Penicillium marneffei* infection in Southeast Asia. *Lancet* 1994, 344:110–113.

3. Sirisanthana V, Sirisanthana T: *Penicillium marneffei* infection in children infected with human immunodeficiency virus. *Pediatr Infect Dis J* 1993, 12:1021–1025.

4. Chariyalertsak S, Vanittanakom P, Nelson KE, *et al.*: *Rhizomys sumatrensis* and *Cannomys badius*, new natural animal hosts of *Penicillium marneffei*. *J Med Vet Mycol* 1996, 34:105–110.

5. Supparatpinyo K, Nelson KE, Merz WG, *et al.*: Response to antifungal therapy by human immunodeficiency virus infected patients with disseminated *Penicillium marneffei* infections and in vitro susceptibilities of isolates from clinical specimens. *Antimicrob Agents Chemother* 1993, 37:2407–2411.

Chapter 12

Mycetoma

El Sheikh Mahgoub

Mycetoma (Madura Foot) is a localized destructive infection of the skin and subcutaneous tissues which slowly progresses to involve contiguous muscle, fascia, and bone. Lesions are usually painless. Infections are initiated where organisms present in soil or plant debris are inoculated into skin and may involve any area subject to local trauma by contaminated objects. Feet or hands are most commonly affected, but carriage of contaminated sacks or other objects may lead to infections involving, the shoulders, back, chest wall, head, or neck, and the buttocks may be inoculated during sitting. A localized papular or nodular swelling containing suppurative granulomas develops, with progressive extension and formation of multiple sinus tracts which exude characteristic grains or granules representing colonies of causative organisms. Grains are 0.2 to 30 mm in diameter and may be colored black, white, yellow, pink, or red depending on the causative organism. Extensive tissue swelling, induration, and destruction develop. Extensive chronic lesions typically contain healed, scarred, sometimes closed sinus tracts with new open suppurative tracts in other adjacent areas. Over a period of months to years, invasion of bone cortex results in replacement of osseous tissues and marrow by masses of grains, manifested on x-rays by cavitary osteolytic lesions and periosteal new bone formation. There may be some regional lymphadenopathy but hematogenous spread does not occur. Systemic signs or symptoms such as fever typically do not develop unless there is secondary bacterial infection.

Infections occur worldwide between the tropics of Cancer and Capricorn but are most common in areas of Africa (eg, Niger, Senegal, Somalia, Sudan, Zaire), India, the Middle East (eg, Saudi Arabia, Yemen), and the Americas (eg, Mexico, Venezuela). Young adult male farmers, outdoor laborers, or bedouins are most often exposed and infected. Mycetomas are divided into two groups. Those caused by true fungi are termed eumycetomas, in contrast to actinomycetomas, caused by aerobic bacterial actinomycetes. Fungi causing eumycetoma include *Pseudallescheria boydii*, the most common cause in the United States, *Madurella mycetomatis*, *Madurella grisea*, *Phialophora jeanselmei*, *Pyrenochaeta romeroi*, *Leptosphaeria senegaliensis*, *Curvularia lunata*, *Neotestudina rosatii*, *Aspergillus nidulans*, *Aspergillus flavus*, and species of *Fusarium*, *Cylindrocarpon*, and *Acremonium*. The causative bacterial agents of actinomycetoma include *Actinomadura madurae* and *A. pelletieri*, *Streptomyces somaliensis* (predominant in tropical African areas and India), and several species and varieties of *Nocardia*, particularly *N. brasiliensis*. Some dermatophyte species cause mycetoma-like scalp or neck infections but do not invade bone and are not considered mycetomas. Differential diagnosis includes botriomycosis due to gram-positive (*Staphylococcus*, *Streptococcus*) or gram-negative (*Escherichia coli*, species of *Proteus* or *Pseudomonas*) bacteria.

The clinical appearance of established lesions can be characteristic. Differences in the morphology and color of grains offer important presumptive diagnostic information for experienced observers. Tissue gram stain distinguishes the narrow bacterial filaments of actinomycetoma. Silver and PAS stains for true fungi hyphae of eumycetoma. Culture provides definitive etiologic diagnosis. Grains may contain nonviable organisms or surface contaminants, so are not ideal sources of diagnostic material. Ideally, wedge biopsies of involved tissues are obtained, then washed in 70% alcohol and several times in saline prior to culturing.

Not all mycetomas are responsive to antimicrobial agents. Many actinomycetomas can be cured by prolonged treatment with two drugs, dapsone or trimethoprim-sulfamethoxazole plus streptomycin or amikacin for 10 months or longer. Some eumycetomas caused by *Madurella mycetomatis* have responded to ketoconazole. Itraconazole has been effective in rare cases caused by *Aspergillus*. Lipid formulations of amphotericin B have reportedly effected improvement but only temporary remissions in infections caused by *Madurella grisea* or species of *Fusarium*. Surgical debridement of affected tissues helps speed up the treatment, although amputation may be necessary at times. Although mycetoma is a localized process, secondary bacterial superinfections and septicemia may cause life-threatening systemic illness.

Definition and Clinical Appearance

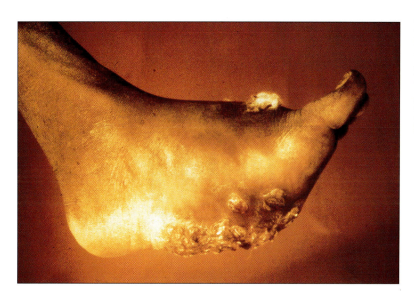

Figure 12-1. "Madura foot." Mycetoma is a chronic, painless, granulomatous infection of the skin, subcutaneous tissues, and underlying bone caused by true fungi (eumycetoma or maduromycetoma) or filamentous aerobic bacteria (actinomycetoma). A well-developed mycetoma is characterized by a painless swelling with multiple sinuses discharging pus and colored grains. Because the foot is the commonest site, some doctors still use the long-standing term "Madura foot."

Common causative organisms of mycetoma		
Color of grain	**Size, *mm***	**Probable organisms**
Black	1–2	*Madurella mycetomatis, Madurella grisea, Leptosphaeria* spp.
White	1–2	*Pseudallescheria boydii, Cephalosporium* spp., *Aspergillus nidulans*
Yellow	0.5–2	*Streptomyces somaliensis*
White	1.5–2	*Actinomadura madurae*
Red	0.2–0.5	*Actinomadura pelletieri*
Beige or orange	0.5–1	*Nocardia* spp.

Figure 12-2. Common causative organisms of mycetoma. Initial identification of mycetoma may be made by examining the characteristics of the grains discharged through the sinuses.

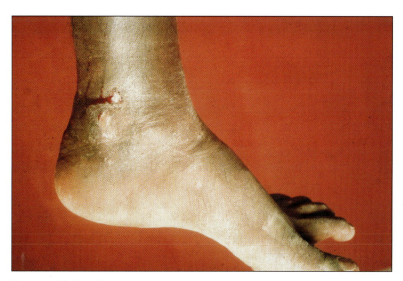

Figure 12-3. The lesion starts as a small, peanut-sized swelling and gradually progresses in size. Grains may be absent, and bloody discharge only may extrude on pressure.

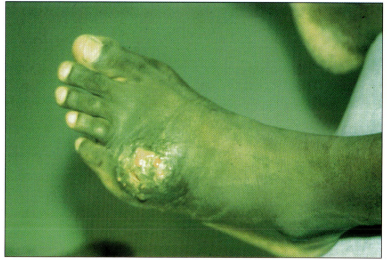

Figure 12-4. Eumycetoma of the dorsum of the foot. Eumycetoma is usually a slow, progressive infection, and the lesion is well demarcated. Note this long-standing mycetoma, which is relatively limited to a small area.

Fungal Infections

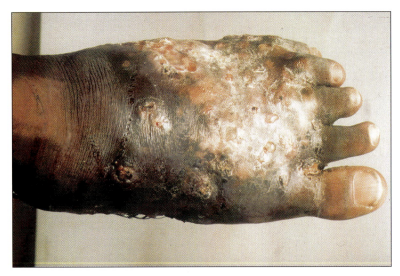

FIGURE 12-5. Actinomycetoma of the dorsum of the foot. In contrast to the infection shown in Fig. 12-4, this infection is an extensive actinomycetoma of the dorsum of the foot caused by *Streptomyces somaliensis*. The lesion has ill-defined margins in the surrounding tissue.

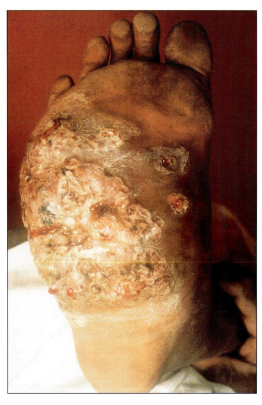

FIGURE 12-6. Actinomycetoma of the sole of the foot. This extensive actinomycetoma caused by *Streptomyces somaliensis* has infected the sole of the patient's right foot. Note the extensive swelling and multiple sinuses.

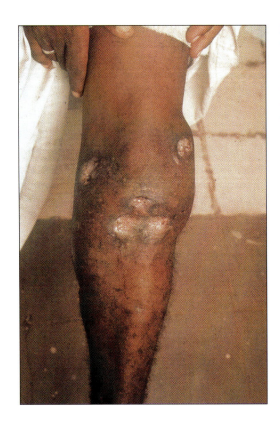

FIGURE 12-7. Mycetoma of the knee. The lower limbs (not necessarily the foot) are affected in about 70% of cases of mycetoma.

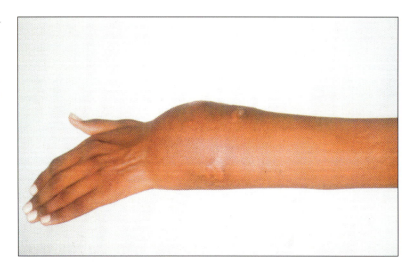

FIGURE 12-8. Mycetoma of the hand. The hand is affected in about 12% of cases of mycetoma.

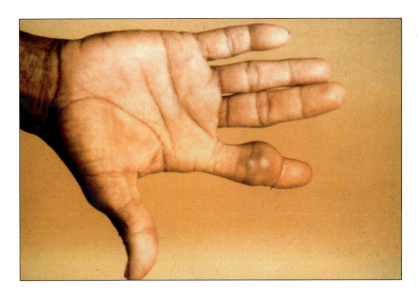

FIGURE 12-9. Mycetoma of the finger. The lesion may be limited to a small site, such as part of a finger, as shown in this figure.

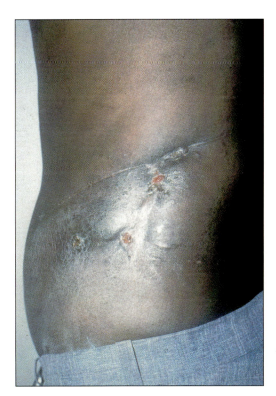

FIGURE 12-10. Mycetoma of the back. In some countries, the back is a common site of mycetoma. The patient previously underwent an operation to remove the lesions, which is indicated by the scar on the patient's back. The infection has since recurred.

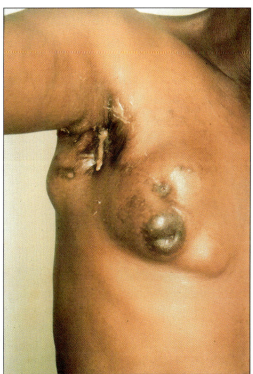

FIGURE 12-11. Mycetoma of the chest wall caused by *Madurella mycetomatis*. Mycetoma usually spreads directly to neighboring tissue, but about 2% of patients may develop a new infection site as a result of lymphatic spread. The figure shows a mycetoma of the chest wall caused by *M. mycetomatis*, which has spread through the axillary lymph nodes to the arm pit.

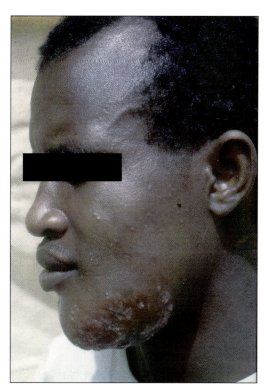

FIGURE 12-12. Mycetoma of the chin caused by *Streptomyces somaliensis*. The head and neck sometimes are afflicted with mycetoma. In fact, mycetoma of the head and neck is more difficult to treat than mycetoma on other parts of the body, due to the blood-brain barrier.

Radiographic Appearance

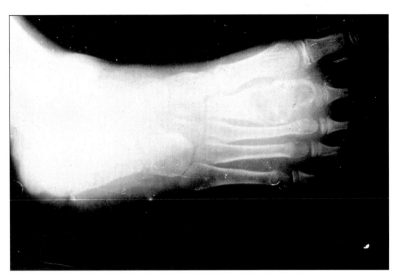

FIGURE 12-13. Radiograph showing a large cavity in the second tarsal bone in the foot of a patient with mycetoma. The presence of a cavity in a bone shown on radiograph is the diagnostic radiologic criterion of mycetoma.

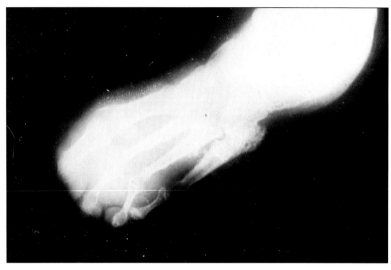

FIGURE 12-14. Radiograph showing periosteal erosion and a start at new bone formation in the foot of a patient with mycetoma. Note this phenomenon in the third and fourth toes.

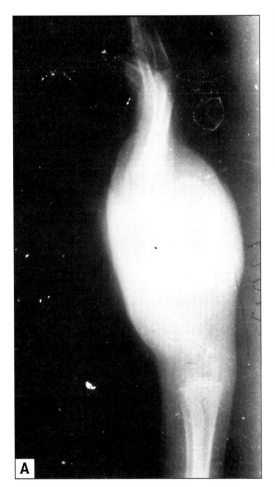
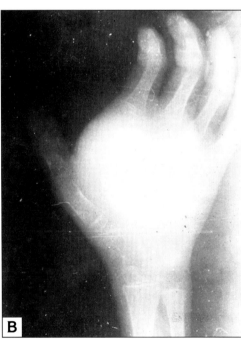

FIGURE 12-15. A and **B**, Radiographs showing osteoporosis (*panel A*) and new bone deposition (*panel B*) in the foot of a patient with mycetoma. The underlying bone may look denser than expected because of the presence of dense granulomata of subcutaneous tissue.

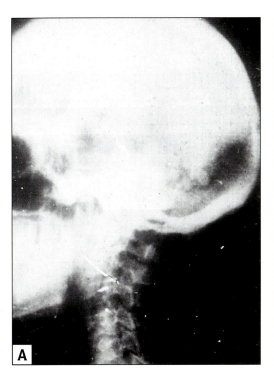
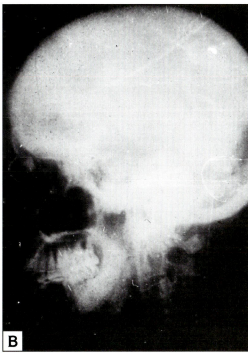

FIGURE 12-16. **A** and **B**, Radiographs of the skull from a patient with mycetoma showing dense amorphous and diffuse bone thickening. When the skull is affected, dense amorphous and diffuse bone thickening is noted rather than cavity formation.

BIOPSY SPECIMENS

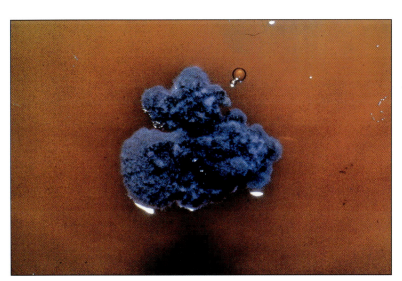

FIGURE 12-17. Biopsy specimen containing grains from a patient with mycetoma. For a successful culture of the organism, a deep-seated biopsy specimen containing grains should be obtained rather than culturing only grains extruded through the sinuses, because the grains are usually dead and contaminated with bacteria. Grains are rinsed quickly in alcohol, washed in normal saline, and cultured on the appropriate media. Actinomycetoma grains are cultured primarily on Löwenstein-Jensen medium (which also is used for culture of *Mycobacterium tuberculosis*) and diagnostic sensitivity test agar. Eumycetoma grains are cultured on ordinary horse or sheep blood agar. No antibacterial or antifungal antibiotics are used. All cultures are incubated at 37°C. Subcultures for all organisms are done on 2% glucose peptone agar (Sabouraud dextrose agar). The culture colonies tend to keep the color of their original grains, but, in addition, some organisms secrete a diagnostic diffusable pigment in the medium. Note the brown pigment in the agar of this black-gray moldlike colony of *Madurella mycetomatis*.

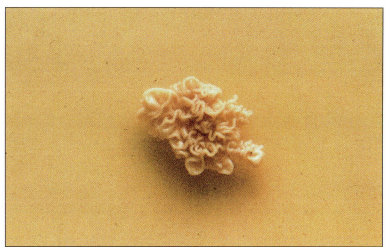

FIGURE 12-18. Culture showing the whitish membranous bacterial colony of *Actinomadura madurae*. No pigment is excreted in the agar.

Histopathology

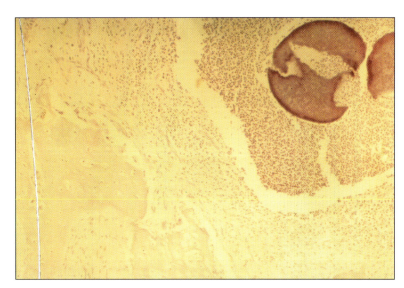

Figure 12-19. Histopathology of mycetoma shown on hematoxylin-eosin stain. No special stain is needed for histopathologic diagnosis of mycetoma. The usual hematoxylin-eosin suffices. The tissue reaction is caused by polymorphonuclear leukocytes, which, together with multinuclear giant cells, are plentiful in actinomycetoma. Diagnosis is only specific when the causative grains are seen. Note the pear-shaped, strongly basophilic, deep-blue grains of *Actinomadura pelletierii*.

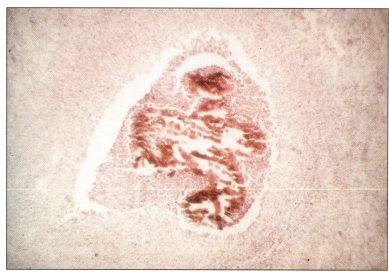

Figure 12-20. Fungal grain of *Madurella mycetomatis*. The fungal grain is shown in the middle of an abscess, which is composed mainly of polymorphonuclear leukocytes. Note the brown color of the large grain.

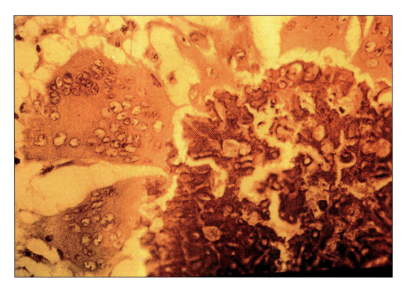

Figure 12-21. Higher magnification of the fungal grain of *Madurella mycetomatis* shown in Fig. 12-20. Note the presence of hyphae and chlamydospores and the grain's brown color. Several multinucleated giant cells surround the grain in an attempt to engulf it.

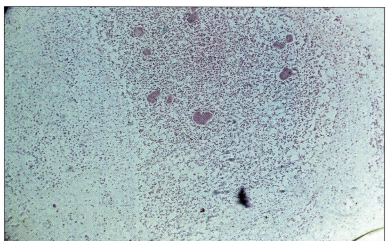

Figure 12-22. Small eosinophilic grains of *Nocardia* species in the middle of an abscess of polymorphonuclear leukocytes and an enclosing band of fibrous tissue.

Diagnostic Tests and Treatment

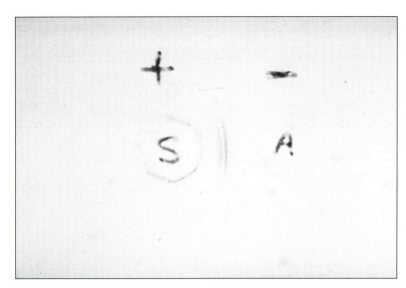

Figure 12-23. Counterimmunoelectrophoresis. Counterimmuno electrophoresis is the serologic test of choice at present for both diagnosis and follow-up of mycetoma. Cytoplasmic extracts of the causative fungus or filamentous bacteria are refined, dried, and reconstituted as antigens. Results are expected in 2 hours. Slide mounts are then dried and stained with naphthalene black for permanent preservation. A—antigen; S—serum.

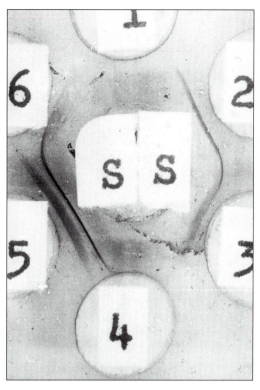

Figure 12-24. Immunodiffusion test. The immunodiffusion test in agar gel also can be used for diagnosis and follow-up of mycetoma, but it is slower than counter-immunoelectrophoresis (results take at least 48 hours). In the figure, the antigen of *Streptomyces somaliensis* (SS) is in the middle surrounded by sera from six patients (1–6). Note the different numbers and intensities of the precipitation lines.

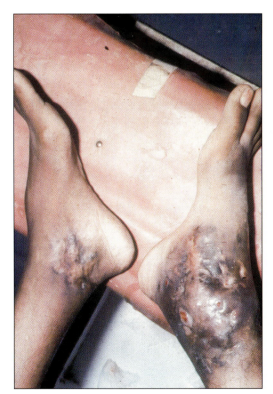

Figure 12-25. Patient with mycetoma of both feet. Some patients are more susceptible to mycetoma than others. Such patients have a deficient cell-mediated immune mechanism. The woman in the figure has mycetoma in both feet with no interconnecting evidence of lymphatic spread. Her lymphocytes were sluggish in transforming into lymphoblasts when challenged with phytohemagglutinin, and the results from her tuberculin skin test were negative.

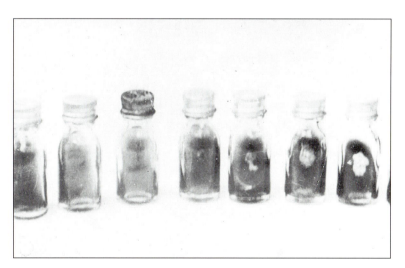

Figure 12-26. Varying dilutions of antibacterial or antifungal agents in a sensitivity test for mycetoma. If the laboratory is well equipped, it is always advisable to do an in vitro sensitivity test for the causative organism before starting treatment. The antibacterial or antifungal agent is incorporated in the agar in varying dilutions, and the lowest titration that inhibits growth is noted.

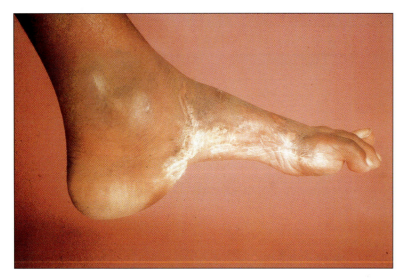

Figure 12-27. Recurrence of mycetoma in a foot after surgical excision. Surgical excision, even if sometimes radical, is accompanied by a high degree of recurrence, which may reach 80%. Note the recurrence of mycetoma in the half foot remaining after this drastic operation. However, bulk-reduction surgery together with medical treatment is recommended.

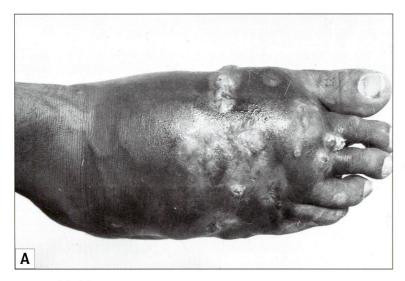
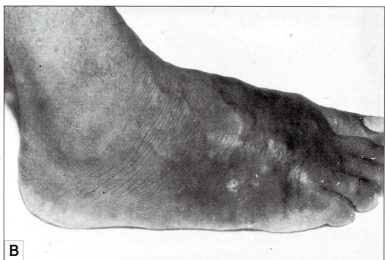

Figure 12-28. **A** and **B**, Before (*panel A*) and after (*panel B*) treatment of an actinomycetoma due to *Streptomyces somaliensis*. The medical regimen for treating actinomycetoma is combination therapy of streptomycin sulfate and trimethoprim sulfamethoxazole. If there is no clinical response, an alternate treatment is streptomycin and dapsone (diaminodiphenylsulfone). In some cases caused by infection with *Nocardia* species, treatment with amikacin and sulfonamides was successful. For eumycetoma due to *Madurella mycetomatis*, ketoconazole 200 mg twice daily is given. The usual treatment continues for 6 to 10 months.

SELECTED BIBLIOGRAPHY

Hay RJ, Mahgoub ES, Leon G, al-Sogair S, Welsh O: Mycetoma. *J Med Vet Mycol>* 1992, 30:41–49.

Mahgoub ES, Gumaa SA: Ketoconazole in the treatment of eumycetoma due to *Madurella mycetomii*. *Trans R Soc Trop Med Hyg* 1984, 78:376–379.

Chapter 13

Dermatophytoses and Other Superficial Mycoses

Roderick J. Hay

The superficial mycoses, which include dermatophytosis or ringworm, superficial candidosis, and *Malassezia* infections, are the commonest of the human fungal infections [1]. The dermatophyte or ringworm fungi invade the stratum corneum of the epidermis and keratinized tissues such as hair or nail derived from it. The dermatophytes affecting humans belong to three genera: *Trichophyton*, *Microsporum*, or *Epidermophyton*. They can be divided into those infections that are spread from human to human (anthropophilic), animal to human (zoophilic), or soil to human (geophilic). The commonest of these organisms is *Trichophyton rubrum*, followed by *Trichophyton violaceum*, *Trichophyton tonsurans*, *Trichophyton interdigitale/mentagrophytes*, *Microsporum canis*, and *Microsporum audouinii*. The initial infection probably follows contact with an infected desquamated scale or hair. The process of skin invasion is initiated by the germination of spores, or arthroconidia, adherent to the stratum corneum [2]. Dermatophyte infections are normally called tinea, followed by the appropriate part of the body involved, in Latin. Other forms include tinea pedis, tinea corporis, tinea cruris, tinea capitis, and tinea facei. Nail infections, or tinea unguium, also are called onychomycosis owing to dermatophytes.

Scytalidium dimidiatum, a plant pathogen found in the tropics and subtropics, and *Scytalidium hyalinum*, which has only been isolated from humans, cause infections of the skin that mimic infections caused by the dermatophyte *T. rubrum*. The *Malassezia* (lipophilic) yeasts are skin-surface commensals, which also have been associated with certain human diseases, the commonest of which are pityriasis versicolor *Malassezia* folliculitis and seborrhoic dermatitis and dandruff. In addition, these organisms rarely cause systemic infections and are usually in neonatal infants receiving intravenous lipid infusions.

White piedra is a chronic infection of the hair shaft caused by the yeast *Trichosporon beigelii*. It is generally sporadic and rare, and the infection mainly is seen in genital hair. It also may affect the axilla and scalp. The lesions are soft yellowish nodules around the hair shafts. Black piedra caused by *Piedraia hortae* is a rare infection confined to the tropics. Scalp hairs are surrounded by a dense black concretion to produce a small nodule.

Tinea nigra is an infection of palmar or plantar skin caused the black yeast *Hortaea* (*Phaeoannelomyces*) *werneckii*. It is seen mainly in the tropics but can present in Europe and the United States. The main differential diagnosis is an acral melanoma because it presents as a flat pigmented mark on the hands or feet. If the lesion is scraped with a glass slide or scalpel, it can be shown to be scaly. Lesions are usually solitary.

Alternaria species cause a rare form of skin granuloma often presenting with ulceration in normal or immunocompromised patients. The lesions most often are located over exposed sites, such as the dorsum of the hands.

Scopulariopsis brevicaulis causes a form of onychomycosis and occasionally may be isolated from toe web spaces. The onychomycosis generally is confined to the great toe nail, which develops a light-tan discoloration. Other fungi also may be isolated from dystrophic nails, including *Fusarium*, *Aspergillus*, and *Pyrenochaeta* species. Generally, they are secondary invaders of already dystrophic nails; however, if they are isolated from this source repeatedly, treatment or nail removal is appropriate.

The superficial mycoses are diagnosed by direct microscopy of scrapings or clippings of skin, hair, and nail [3]. The appearance of the organisms is typical using potassium hydroxide clearance of nail material. With the exception of *Malassezia* species, which requires special conditions, all the superficial pathogenic fungi grow well on Sabouraud's medium.

Generally, most superficial fungal infections are treated topically, whenever practical, using azole or imidazole antifungals. Systemic therapy is more appropriate for extensive infections and those affecting the scalp or nails. Oral terbinafine, itraconazole, fluconazole, or griseofulvin are used in the management of these infections.

Dermatophyte Infections

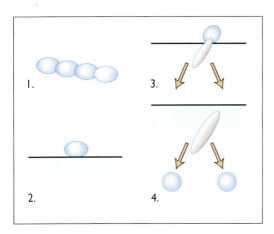

FIGURE 13-1. Pathogenesis of dermatophytosis. The process of skin invasion by a dermatophyte involves a number of stages: survival of transfer from host to host through the production of arthrospores (*1*); adhesion to keratinocytes, which takes 1 to 2 hours (*2*); germination and production of proteases, including keratinases (*3*); and the elicitation of an inflammatory response (*4*).

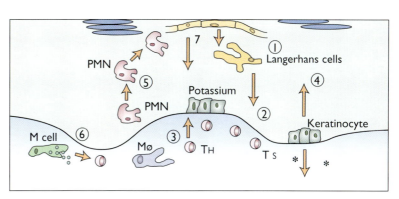

FIGURE 13-2. Summary of immunologic events in dermatophytosis. Immunity against dermatophytes involves the production of inflammatory antigens, which are taken up by Langerhans cells (*1*) and present antigen to T lymphocytes (*2*). Activated T cells (*3*) in turn activate epidermal cells through cytokines such as interferon-γ, which produce other cytokines (*4*) and adhesion molecules such as intracellular adhesion molecules. Neutrophils are attracted to the site of infection and destroy fungal cells through both oxidative and nonoxidative pathways (*5*). In some dermatophyte infections, a TH2 response develops with reduced interferon-γ production (*6*) or inhibitory substances suppress T lymphocyte activation (*7*). *Asterisks* indicate diffusing molecules of cytokines. PMN—polymorphonuclear cells.

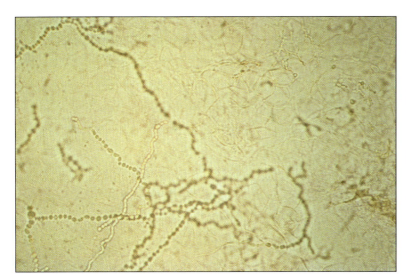

FIGURE 13-3. Direct microscopy of dermatophyte fungi. The diagnosis of dermatophyte infection is confirmed by the techniques of direct microscopy and culture. The direct microscopy of dermatophyte fungi in tissue shows irregular branching and septate hyphae that cross cell boundaries. This preparation used the conventional method with 20% potassium hydroxide and was scanned after 5 minutes.

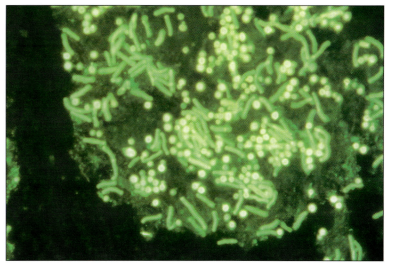

FIGURE 13-4. Direct microscopy of pityriasis versicolor. The yeast and short stubby hyphal forms can be seen. Direct microscopy with fluorescent whitening agents such as calcofluor provides a more distinct preparation, which better highlights the hyphae in tissue. It probably provides a more accurate method of screening nail material, although it has the disadvantage of the need for a fluorescent microscope.

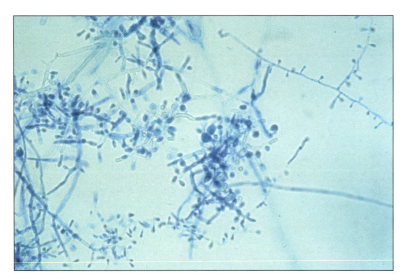

Figure 13-5. *Trichophyton tonsurans.* Cultures from dermatophytes provide the best method of recognition of individual species. The diagnosis is still largely dependent on the gross morphologic appearance and the microscopy of the mounts taken from the culture. Biochemical differences between different organisms can be used but are less helpful. The microscopy of *T. tonsurans* is shown on lactophenol blue stain.

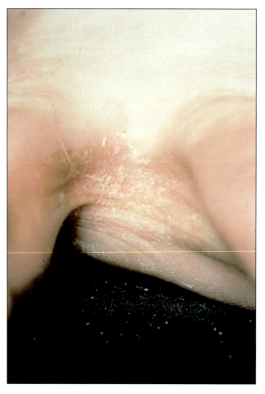

Figure 13-6. Tinea pedis ("athlete's foot"). Tinea pedis is the commonest infection caused by dermatophytes. The figure shows the interdigital type of tinea pedis, which is most commonly caused by infection with *Trichophyton rubrum* and less commonly caused by other organisms such as *Trichophyton interdigitale* (*Trichophyton mentagrophytes*) or *Epidermophyton floccosum*. The infection may spread onto the sole or dorsum of the foot. Treatment with topical azole antifungals or terbinafine is rapidly effective.

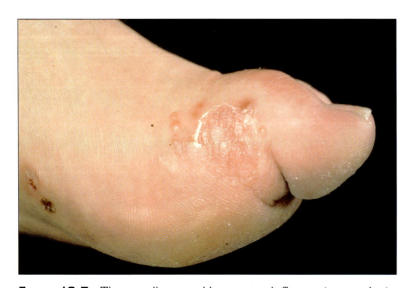

Figure 13-7. Tinea pedis caused by a more inflammatory variant. The figure shows a pronounced vesicular or bullous reaction, in this case on the lateral border of the foot. This reaction generally is caused by *Trichophyton mentagrophytes*, and it often recurs unless treated. The infection often is recurrent and may precipitate an id reaction. Such patients generally have a positive intradermal trichophytin test response.

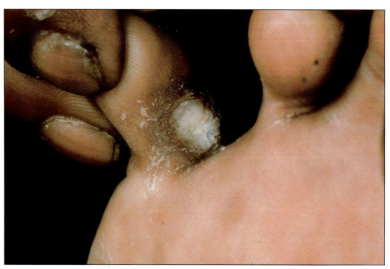

Figure 13-8. Interdigital dermatophyte infection. This infection shows a common complication of long-standing infections, the development of a thickened hyperkeratotic plug, or painful soft corn. It should be removed surgically.

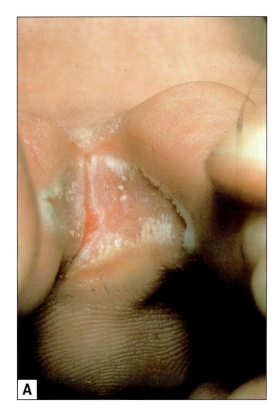
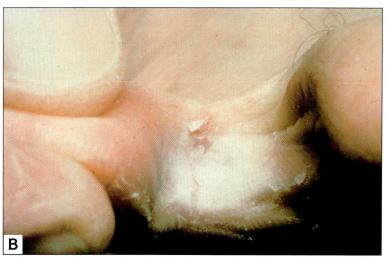

FIGURE 13-9. Interdigital scaling. Interdigital scaling is not always caused by dermatophyte infections, because other organisms such as *Candida albicans* can cause a similar appearance. **A,** Interdigital lesion owing to *Pseudomonas* species is shown. The infection is common in wet or tropical environments and in industrial workers. The lesions are often painful rather than itchy but may be preceded by more typical interdigital fungal infections caused by dermatophytes, dermatophytosis complex. **B,** By contrast, this lesion, which presents with interdigital maceration without significant itching, is caused by *Corynebacterium minutissimum*, erythrasma. It will fluoresce pink with filtered ultraviolet light. Interdigital lesions caused by *Candida* species are similar in appearance.

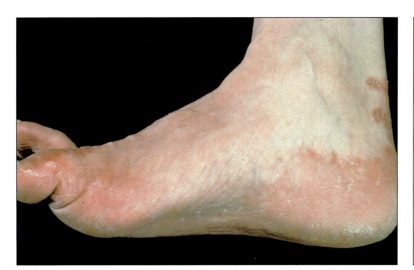

FIGURE 13-10. Dry or moccasin-type tinea pedis. Dry or moccasin-type tinea pedis usually is caused by *Trichophyton rubrum*. It is often asymptomatic and difficult to see where it is confined to the sole of the foot. Itching occurs where the infection spreads onto the lateral borders of the foot. Such infections may run in families. Secondary onychomycosis is common. Oral therapy with terbinafine or itraconazole usually is necessary.

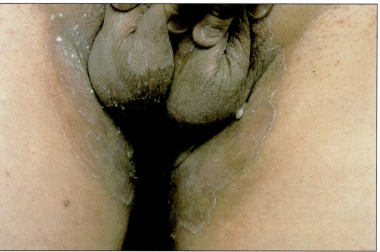

FIGURE 13-11. A man with groin lesions caused by tinea cruris. Tinea cruris is most common in hot environments and the tropics and particularly affects members of the armed forces. The sharply demarcated scaling edge of the groin lesion is typical, and the absence of "satellite" pustules beyond the margin of the rash is useful in distinguishing this rash from *Candida intertrigo*. The main causes are *Trichophyton rubrum* and *Epidermophyton floccosum*. The infection responds to topical antifungal therapy unless it is very extensive or accompanied by lesions elsewhere on the body, such as the feet.

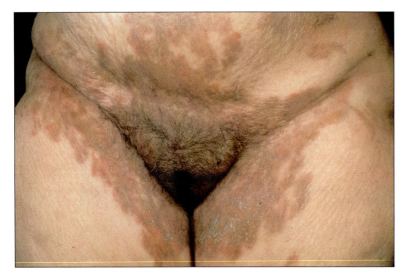

FIGURE 13-12. A woman infected with tinea cruris. Tinea cruris is uncommon in women. When it does occur in women it is usually caused by *Trichophyton rubrum*. It also may spread around the waist region, and sometimes further, to produce tinea corporis.

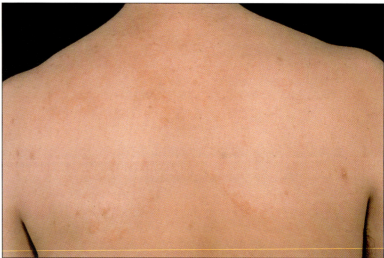

FIGURE 13-13. Tinea corporis caused by *Trichophyton rubrum*. Tinea corporis is a sporadic infection, which affects the trunk of proximal parts of the limbs. If the lesions are well localized, topical therapy is effective; otherwise, oral antifungals are given. Tinea corporis caused by anthropophilic fungi such as *T. rubrum* may be very extensive and often is barely symptomatic. Lesions rarely have an easily discernible raised margin or pustules, although on careful inspection a raised edge usually can be seen at some point on the circumference of the lesion.

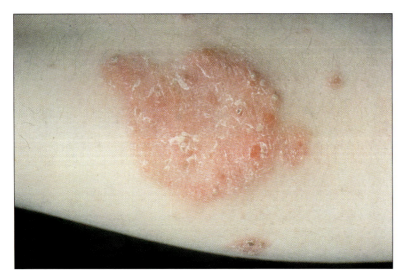

FIGURE 13-14. Tinea corporis caused by *Trichophyton verrucosum*. Tinea corporis caused by zoophilic fungi such as *Microsporum canis* or, in this case, *T. verrucosum* is usually more inflammatory. Lesions are less scattered, and pustules may be present. Itching is common. It is important to screen such patients for infection elsewhere on the body, such as on the scalp, or for infections in other members of the household.

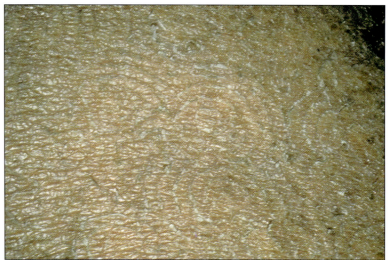

FIGURE 13-15. Tinea corporis caused by *Trichophyton concentricum*. Tinea imbricata is an unusual form of tinea corporis owing to *T. concentricum*. Tinea imbricata is a tropical infection endemic in remote communities in the West Pacific, the Far East, and scattered sites in Mexico, Central America, and Brazil. The typical lesions show multiple concentric rings of scales or confluent large scales. Chronic infections from an early age are common. Lesions are usually hypopigmented.

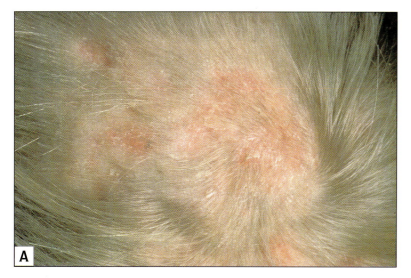
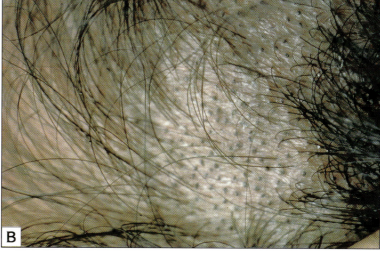
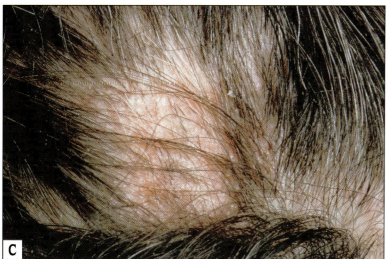

FIGURE 13-16. Tinea capitis. Scalp ringworm is a childhood infection, which is increasingly common in urban areas in the United States and Europe. It also is endemic in parts of the tropics, particularly in Africa. The patterns of infection depend in part on the site where the invading fungus produces Arthroconidia: ectothrix (on the outside of the hair shaft), endothrix (within the hair shaft), or favic (within the hair, but hyphae die leaving air spaces). Oral therapy with griseofulvin is necessary. **A,** Ectothrix scalp infection owing to *Microsporum canis* is shown. The scalp shows a circumscribed patch of alopecia with scaling and inflammation. Hairs have broken 5 mm or more above the scalp surface. **B,** Endothrix infection owing to *Trichophyton tonsurans* is shown. The hairs have broken at scalp level, and minimal scaling is present. Sometimes the scalp shows a scaling response similar to seborrheic dermatitis. The pattern of swollen hair stubs seen at scalp level is known as black dot ringworm. Some *black dots* can be seen in this figure. **C,** Favic pattern of scalp invasion owing to *Trichophyton schoenleinii* is shown. This example is an early infection. Note that hairs are often retained. Later, crusts or scutula (keratin and masses of mycelium) accumulate around the scalp hairs. Scarring alopecia is unusual in tinea capitis but can occur with favus.

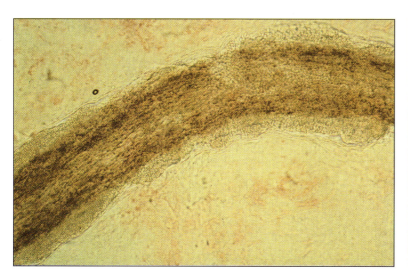

FIGURE 13-17. Direct microscopic appearance of an ectothrix hair with accumulation of arthroconidia outside the shaft. The conidia in this figure are small, and the infection is likely caused by a *Microsporum* species such as *Microsporum canis*.

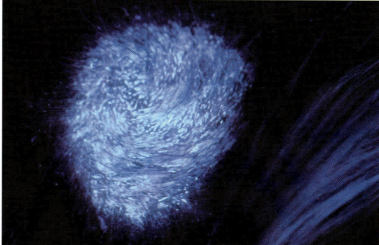

FIGURE 13-18. Lesions of tinea capitis owing to *Microsporum* species. The lesions, after being exposed to filtered ultraviolet light (Wood's light), fluoresce with a greenish light. The technique is useful for screening infected children and also for selecting infected hairs for microscopy and culture. Fluorescent hairs easily are removed by gentle pulling.

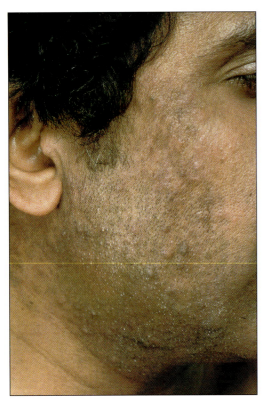

Figure 13-19. Tinea facei. Tinea facei often is difficult to diagnose because lesions may not have a well-demarcated border. They often are mistakenly treated with topical steroids, which further suppresses inflammation and confuses the diagnosis. This reaction is called tinea incognito. Some lesions appear to flare on sun exposure and may be misdiagnosed as photosensitivity. Facial dermatophytosis may be caused by dermatophytes of either human or animal origin. This case is caused by *Trichophyton rubrum* infection.

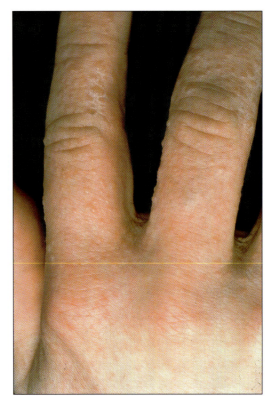

Figure 13-20. The id reaction (dermatophytid) is an immunologically mediated secondary rash (eczema, vasculitis) caused by a secondary inflammatory response to dermatophytosis. It often is precipitated by treatment with antifungal medications. There are a number of different patterns of the id reaction. Pompholyx is shown in this figure. Acute vesicular eczema on the hands or feet may be a feature of an id reaction. In this case, the eruption is asymmetric with pronounced interdigital scaling and blister formation on the side of the initial infection. The infection was on the patient's feet; the hand lesions do not contain fungal elements. A number of different id reactions have been described with tinea corporis or tinea capitis due to zoophilic dermatophytes, once again often precipitated by treatment. These reactions have included multiple papules, small vasculitic lesions, or erythema nodosum following tinea capitis owing to *Microsporum canis*.

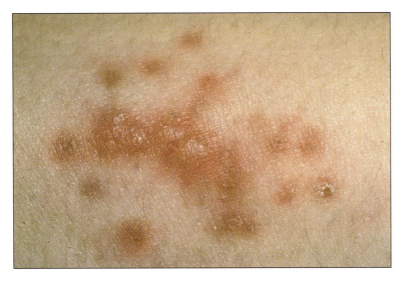

Figure 13-21. Majocchi granuloma. After apparent resolution of highly inflamed dermatophyte lesions of hair-bearing skin, a residual granuloma is sometimes seen, called a Majocchi granuloma. This granuloma does not contain viable fungi. Histologically, the lesion is a well-organized granuloma with a lymphoplasmacytic infiltrate and multinucleate giant cells. The lesion in the figure illustrates the late stage of an infection due to *Trichophyton mentagrophytes* of animal origin (from a pet mouse).

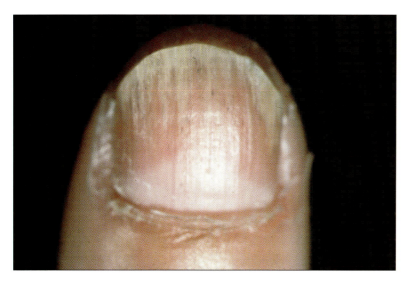

FIGURE 13-22. Onychomycosis. Onychomycosis owing to dermatophyte infections usually affects the distal and lateral margins of the nail plate. Invasion is subungual and from adjacent skin. With time, the nail plate becomes discolored and hyperkeratotic. Gross destruction occurs with well-established lesions. Onychomycosis is very common, affecting more than 3% of the population, and is more common with increasing age. The main cause is *Trichophyton rubrum*, although *Trichophyton mentagrophytes* and *Trichophyton tonsurans* and others also may cause nail infections. An early invasive infection of the nail is shown. There is little thickening, and onycholysis appears around the distal and lateral borders, a pattern known as distal and lateral subungual onychomycosis. The infection is caused by *T. rubrum*. Treatment with oral terbinafine, itraconazole, or fluconazole is indicated.

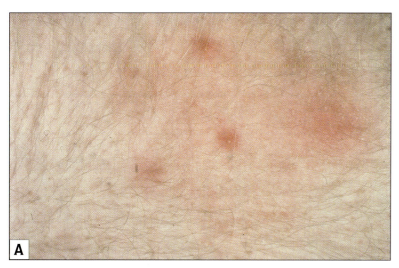
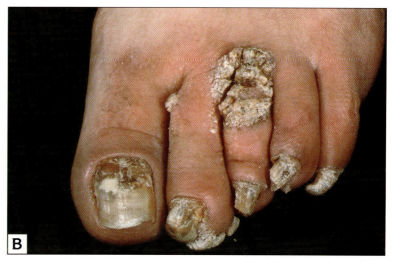

FIGURE 13-23. Dermatophyte infections in immunocompromised patients. Dermatophyte infections in immunocompromised patients are not necessarily more common, but they may appear different clinically. **A,** A patient with an ill-defined oval lesion containing follicular prominences without pustule formation is shown. He is a liver transplant recipient, and the infection is an atypical infection owing to *T. rubrum*. The absence of scaling and follicular invasion is seen often in patients on therapeutic immunosuppressive regimens. **B,** The patient shown has the rare immunodeficiency state of chronic mucocutaneous candidiasis (CMC). In CMC, chronic superficial fungal infections due to *Candida* species or dermatophytes (in this case, *Trichophyton mentagrophytes*) cause a marked hyperkeratotic response. CMC caused by *Candida* infection once was given the misnomer of *Candida* granuloma; however, histologically, the main abnormality is massive hyperkeratosis rather than dermal inflammation such as granuloma formation. This patient also has onychomycosis, and the great toe shows an unusual pattern of toe nail infection where fungal invasion affects the superficial aspect of the nail plate, superficial white onychomycosis. It presents with a powdery infection of the nail plate and is best recognized with *T. mentagrophytes* and some mold fungi such as *Fusarium* species.

Fungal Infections

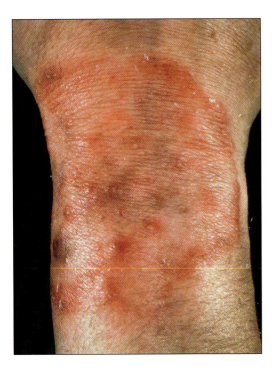

FIGURE 13-24. The application of topical corticosteroids may cause a reduction of inflammation, or tinea incognito. In the patient shown in the figure, the lesion shows reduced scaling but increased erythema and pustule formation. Follicular invasion is a prominent feature. Scrapings from such lesions usually contain large amounts of mycelium.

SCYTALIDIUM INFECTIONS

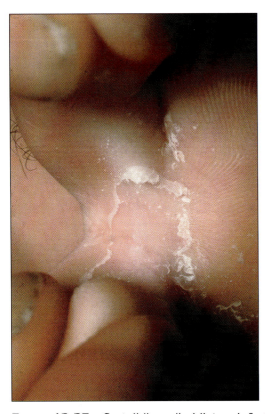

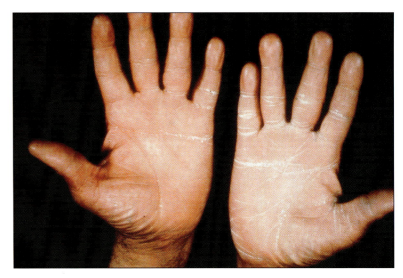

FIGURE 13-26. *Scytalidium hyalinum* infection. A 50-year-old Jamaican patient aged 50 years who has lived in the United Kingdom for 15 years presented with unilateral scaling of the palms of the hand. Although these appearances are typical of *Trichophyton rubrum*, the infection was caused by *S. hyalinum*. Such infections seldom itch.

FIGURE 13-25. *Scytalidium dimidiatum* infection. The patient has what appears to be simple interdigital tinea pedis. However, the organism causing this infection is *S. dimidiatum*. The organism, which is a plant pathogen in the tropics and subtropics, together with a related fungus, *Scytalidium hyalinum*, causes infections that mimic those caused by *Trichophyton rubrum*. Both *Scytalidium* species fail to grow on agar-containing cycloheximide (actidione).

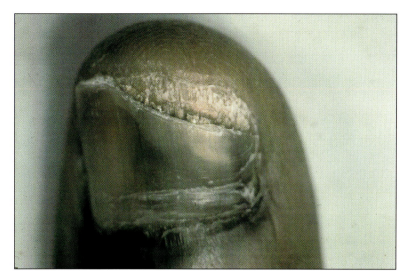

Figure 13-27. An early thumb nail infection caused by *Scytalidium dimidiatum*. The patient also had interdigital scaling and scaling on the soles of the feet. The prominent lateral onycholysis without significant hyperkeratosis is typical. Sometimes nail fold thickening is present, which is suggestive of chronic paronychia.

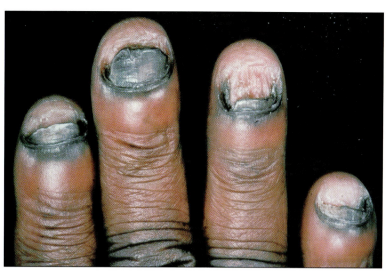

Figure 13-28. A more advanced infection due to *Scytalidium dimidiatum*. The patient's nails are severely undermined without gross hyperkeratosis. *Scytalidium* infections do not respond to the main antifungal agents terbinafine, itraconazole, fluconazole, or griseofulvin. Nail fold swelling is seen in this patient.

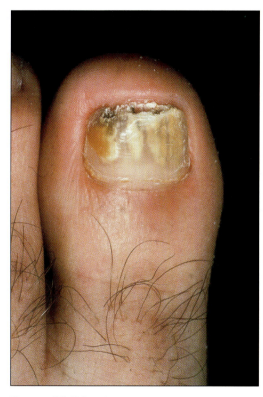

Figure 13-29. *Scopulariopsis brevicaulis* infection. *S. brevicaulis* may cause toe nail infections, usually of the great toe nail. The infection affects the nail plate, which shows a subungual discolored patch with irregular borders. The color is the result of spores of the fungus in the nail plate. Treatment usually involves excision of the nail plate. In some instances, a co-existent dermatophyte infection is present.

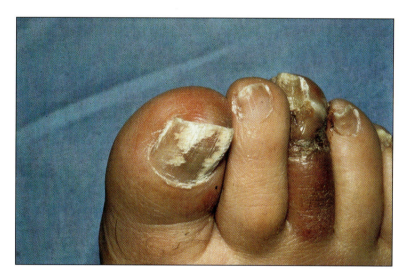

Figure 13-30. *Fusarium* infection. *Fusarium* species may infect the nail plate, causing a white powdery dystrophy on the surface of the nail plate, known as superficial white onychomycosis. In patients with neutropenia, such infections may spread and often are accompanied by a cellulitis of the digit, as seen in the figure. This patient with onychomycosis due to this organism had a disseminated *Fusarium* infection affecting internal organs and skin. The digital cellulitis is clearly seen.

MALASSEZIA YEAST INFECTIONS

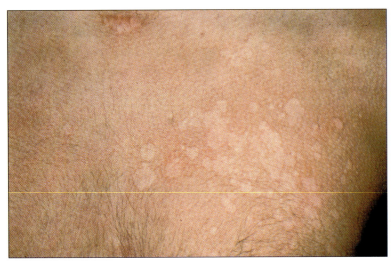

FIGURE 13-31. *Malassezia* infection. *Malassezia* infections are caused by a number of different *Malassezia* species: *Malassezia globosa*, *Malassezia sympodialis*, *Malassezia furfur*, *Malassezia sloofei*, and *Malassezia restricta*. The commonest infection is pityriasis (tinea) versicolor, which usually is a result of *M. globosa* or *M. furfur*. The infection presents with hypo- or hyperpigmented scales on the trunk and upper limbs. The neck and groin areas may be affected. Scaly patches can be highlighted by Wood's light, and they fluoresce with a yellow color. A patient with typical hypopigmented lesions on the trunk is shown in this figure. Sometimes lesions are hyperpigmented and can resemble dermatophyte infections.

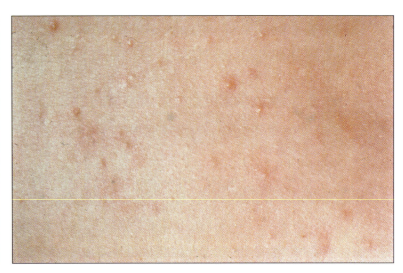

FIGURE 13-32. *Malassezia* folliculitis. *Malassezia* folliculitis usually presents with clusters of itchy papules and pustules on the upper trunk. It is seen in severely ill patients hospitalized for other diseases, but it is also common in young adults who have been exposed to the sun. Itchiness is a charcteristic feature of the condition.

RARER SUPERFICIAL INFECTIONS

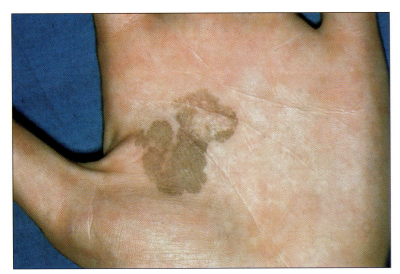

FIGURE 13-33. Tinea nigra. Tinea nigra is a superficial infection of stratum corneum caused by *Hortaea* (*Phaeoanellomyces*) *werneckii*. The hyphae are pigmented in vivo, which provides the clinical appearances of individual lesions. The lesions are diagnosed by scraping, which shows characteristic pigmented hyphae on direct microscopy. The infection usually is acquired in the tropics. Lesions may have to be distinguished from those of acral lentigines.

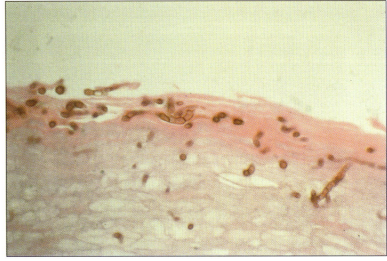

FIGURE 13-34. Biopsy specimen of tinea nigra seen on hematoxylin-eosin stain. The biopsy appearances are typical, and the pigmented hyphae are easily visible with hematoxylin-eosin–stained material (×200).

References

1. Kibbler CC, MacKenzie DWR, Odds FC: *Principles and Practice of Clinical Mycology*. Chichester: John Wiley and Sons; 1996.

2. Hay RJ: Fungal Infections. In *Skin Immune System (SIS)*. Edited by Jan D. Bos. Boca Raton, FL; 1997:593–604.

3. Hay RJ, Moore M: Mycology. In *Textbook of Dermatology, edn. 6*. Edited by Champion RH, Burton JL, Burns DA, Breathnach SM. Oxford: Blackwell Science; 1998:1277–1376.

Selected Bibliography

Friedman-Kien AE: Cutaneous manifestations. In *Atlas of Infectious Diseases*, edn 2. Edited by Mandell GL, Mildvan D. Philadelphia: Current Medicine; 1997:5.2–5.18.

Elgart ML: Cutaneous mycology. *Dematol Clin* 1996, 113–124.

CHAPTER 14

Pneumocystis carinii Infection

Peter D. Walzer

Pneumocystis carinii is an important cause of pneumonia in patients with HIV and in other immunocompromised hosts. The lack of a continuous in vitro culture system has limited knowledge of taxonomy and other features of the basic biology of *P. carinii*. However, molecular studies conducted over the past decade have firmly placed *P. carinii* among the fungi [1], a finding that is reflected by the inclusion of the organism in this chapter.

APPEARANCE AND LIFE CYCLE

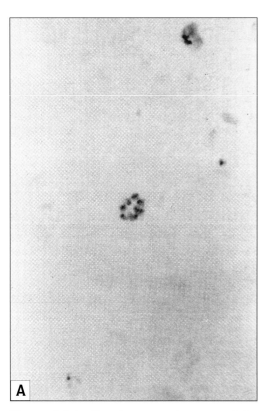
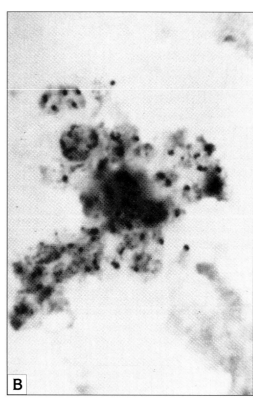
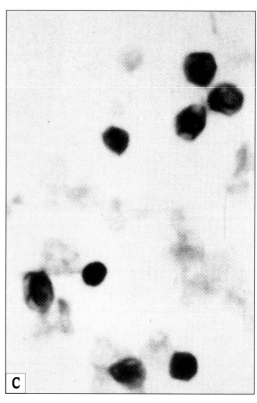

FIGURE 14-1. Developmental stages of *Pneumocystis carinii*. These stages have been identified as the 5- to 8-m cyst (also termed *spore case*), which has a thick cell wall and contains up to eight intracystic bodies ("spores"); the small (1 to 4 m), pleomorphic trophic form, which is the most numerous stage; and the precyst ("sporocyte"), an intermediate stage, which is hard to distinguish from the cyst at the light microscopic level. **A,** Intracystic bodies are shown in a single cyst. The cyst wall is not stained. (Diff Quik stain, x1350.) **B,** Clusters of trophic forms and intracystic bodies are shown in a preparation of rat lung homogenates. (Diff Quik stain, x1700.) **C,** Cysts are stained with the selective cell wall stain cresyl echt violet. The wrinkled appearance is typical. (x1700.) (*From* Walzer *et al.* [2]; with permission.)

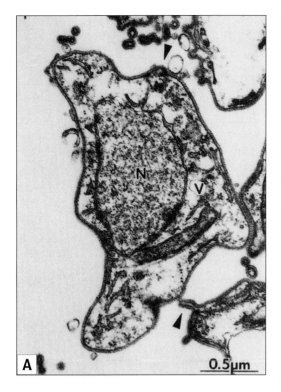
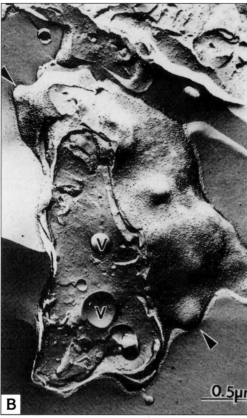

Figure 14-2. Trophic *Pneumocystis carinii*. **A**, Thin-section photograph of a trophic *P. carinii* is shown. Note the irregular shape, a central nucleus (N) and mitochondria, and a few vacuoles (V). Filopodia (*arrowheads*) are seen stretching from the cell body. (Uranyl acetate and lead citrate stain, x28,000.) **B**, Freeze-fracture image shows a trophic *P. carinii*. Note two layers of the pellicle. Filopodia (*arrowheads*) can be seen as bulges of cytoplasm. The smoothness of the vacuolar wall (V) is evident. (x28,000.) (*From* Yoneda *et al.* [3]; with permission.)

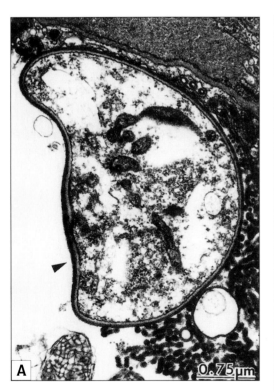
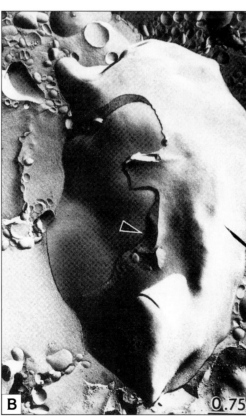

Figure 14-3. *Pneumocystis carinii* precyst. **A**, Thin-section photograph of a *P. carinii* precyst is shown. Note the tightly packed outer layer of the cell wall (*arrowhead*). (x19,000.) **B**, Freeze-fracture image shows a *P. carinii* precyst. Note the smoothness of the surface and thickness of the wall (*arrowhead*). (x19,000.) (*From* Yoneda *et al.* [3]; with permission.)

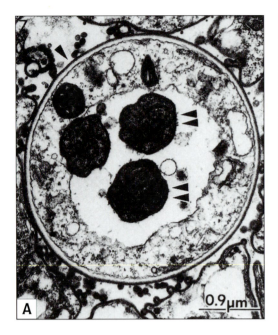
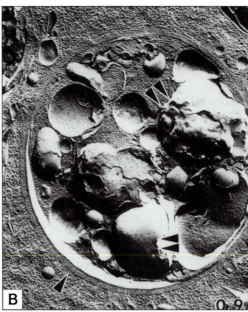

FIGURE 14-4. *Pneumocystis carinii* cyst. **A**, Thin-section photograph of a *P. carinii* cyst is shown. Note the tightly packed wall and intracystic bodies (*double arrowheads*). (Uranyl acetate and lead citrate strain, x16,000.) **B**, Freeze-fracture image shows a *P. carinii* cyst. The fracture plane crossed the center of the cyst. Notice the tightly packed wall (*arrowhead*) and intracystic bodies (*double arrowheads*). (x16,000.) (*From* Yoneda *et al.* [3]; with permission.)

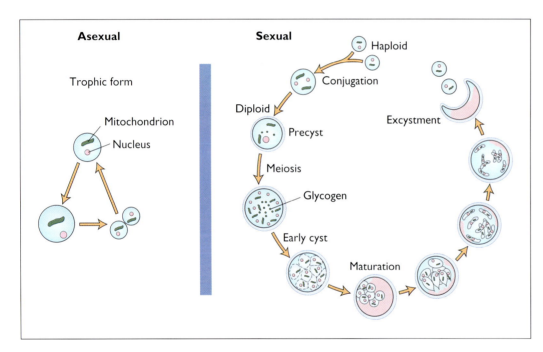

FIGURE 14-5. Proposed life cycle of *Pneumocystis carinii*. Information about the life cycle mainly has come from light and electron microscopic studies of *P. carinii* in the lungs of animals and short-term culture. Photographs depict living tropic and cyst forms by Nomarski interference contrast microscopy. In the asexual phase, the trophic forms replicate by mitosis and cell division. In the sexual phase, the haploid trophic forms (mating types) conjugate to form a diploid zygote (early phase), which undergoes meiosis and subsequent mitosis to form eight haploid nuclei (late-phase sporocyte). The spores or intracystic bodies are formed by compartmentalization of nuclei and cytoplasmic organelles (*eg*, mitochondria). The spores exhibit different shapes, including spherical and elongated forms. It is postulated that the elongation of the spores preceeds release from the spore case or cyst. Release is believed to occur through a rent in the cell wall. After evacuation, the empty ascus usually collapses but retains some residual cytoplasm. (*Adapted from* Cushion [4].)

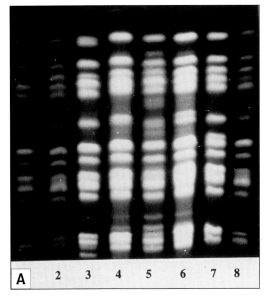
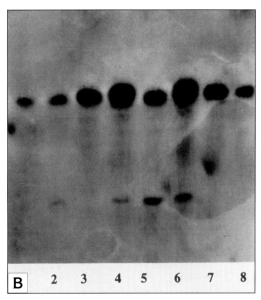

FIGURE 14-6. Pulsed field gel electrophoresis (PFGE) analysis of rat *Pneumocystis carinii*. This technique, which involves the separation of chromosomes, has been very helpful in studying the genetic diversity of *P. carinii*. Studies of *P. carinii* in rat colonies conducted by academic institutions and commercial breeders have revealed species or differences in the organism that have contributed to the development of new nomenclature [6–8]. The two principal forms of *P. carinii* in rats have been termed *prototype* (*P. carinii* sp.f. *rattus*) and *variant* (*P. carinii* sp.f. *carinii*). Chromosome patterns of PFGE can distinguish prototype, variant, or mixtures of the two forms of *P. carinii*. **A**, Ethidium bromide–stained clamped homogeneous electrical field (CHEF) gel (a type of PFGE) of prototype and variant *P. carinii* populations form the lungs of individual rats in a Charles River Wistar rat colony. *Lane 1*: rat 1083, prototype; *lane 2*: rat 1085, mixed prototype-variant; *lane 3*: rat 1086, prototype; *lane 4*: rat 1089, prototype with small amount of variant; *lane 5*: rat 1090, mixed prototype and variant; *lane 6*: rat 1091, mixed; *lane 7*: rat 1092, prototype; *lane 8*: rat 1097, prototype. Sizes of the chromosomes are based on labda concatamers. **B**, Southern blotted CHEF gel of specimen from *panel A* was probed with a *P. carinii*–enolase gene probe to identify prototype and variant populations. *Lanes* correspond with those in *panel A*. The enolase gene is found on a 527 kb chromosome of prototype populations and a 400 kb chromosome of variant populations. (*Courtesy of* Dr. Melanie Cushion.)

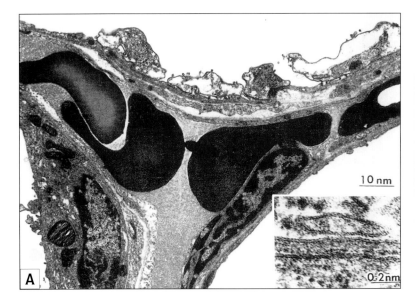
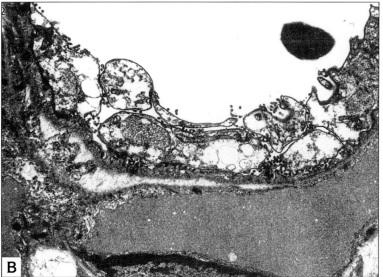

FIGURE 14-7. Sequential changes in the interaction of *Pneumocystis carinii* with alveolar type I cell in immunosuppressed rat. **A**, Pulmonary alveoli are shown at 4 weeks of corticosteroid therapy. Note the attachment of trophic forms on the type I pneumocyte. Alveolar epithelial and capillary endothelial cells are intact. (Lead citrate and uranyl acetate, x7650.) *Inset*: High magnification of the site of attachment. The trophic form cytoplasm is above, and the type I pneumocyte is below. (Lead citrate and uranyl acetate, x163,800.) **B**, Pulmonary alveolus is shown at 7 weeks of treatment. Note extensive attachment of the organisms, completely covering one surface. (Lead citrate and uranyl acetate, x7650.) (*From* Yoneda and Walzer [5]; with permission.)

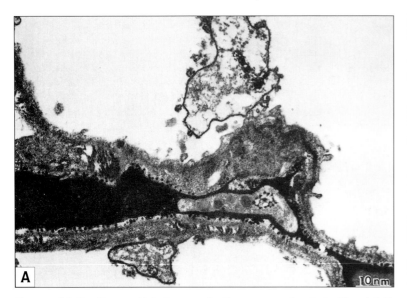 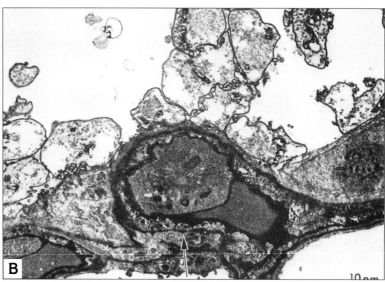

FIGURE 14-8. Sequential changes in the same animals in Fig. 14-7 using horseradish peroxidase (HRP) as an ultrastructural marker. **A**, HRP is confined in the vascular space at 4 weeks, suggesting an intact alveolar–capillary membrane. (×7650.) **B**, By week 7, HRP has leaked into the intercellular space of the endothelium and the basement membrane. The changes suggest increased alveolar–capillary permeability. (×7650.) (*From* Yoneda and Walzer [5]; with permission.)

CLINICAL PRESENTATION

Clinical features of *Pneumocystis carinii* pneumonia

Feature	Patients with HIV	Patients without HIV
Occurrence	Common	Sporadic
Presentation	Subacute illness	Acute illness
Symptoms	Fever, dyspnea, nonproductive cough	Fever, dyspnea, nonproductive cough
Signs	Few	Few
Blood gasses	Hypoxemia with respiratory alkalosis	Hypoxemia with respiratory alkalosis
Organism burden	High	Moderate
Diagnostic yield	Excellent	Good
Prognosis	Good/excellent	Fair/good
Recurrence	Common	Variable
Adverse drug reaction	Common	Variable

FIGURE 14-9. Clinical features of *Pneumocystis carinii* pneumonia. Pneumocystosis in patients with HIV has been characterized by frequent occurrence, relatively mild presentation, and propensity to recur. Prognosis has been improved by the advances in diagnosis and treatment; however, patients with HIV frequently experience adverse effects to antimicrobial drugs. Pneumocystosis occurs less commonly in other immunocompromised hosts, has a more dramatic presentation, and still has a high mortality rate.

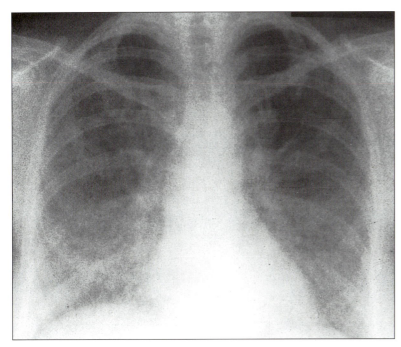

Figure 14-10. Chest radiograph demonstrating the typical bilateral infiltrates of *Pneumocystis carinii* in a patient with HIV [13]. (*From* Rosen [6].)

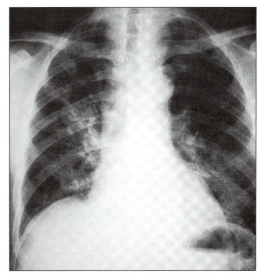

Figure 14-11. Chest radiograph of a patient who developed pneumocystosis during the first 2 weeks of symptomatic, primary HIV infection. The development of *Pneumocystis carinii* pneumonia in this individual and another patients with HIV described in the report was associated with profound CD4 lymphopenia [15]. CD4 counts and percentages in these patients returned to normal within 4 months, and remained normal for 24 to 48 months of follow-up. During this time, there were no other symptoms of progression of HIV to AIDS. (*From* Dore and Cooper [7].)

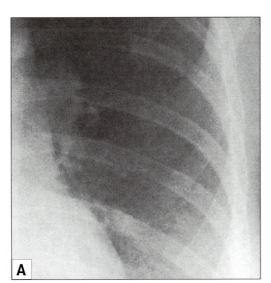
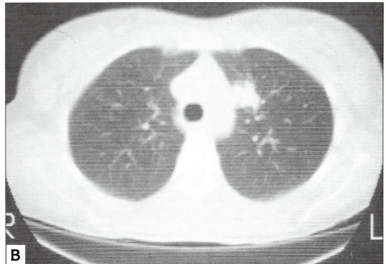
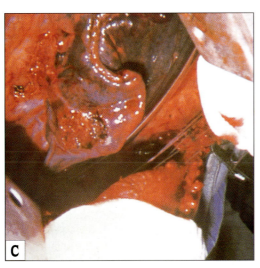

Figure 14-12. Atypical presentation of *Pneumocystis carinii* pneumonia. **A,** Detail of a chest radiograph shows a mass in the para-aortic area. **B,** Computed tomogram of the chest confirms this nodule. **C,** A nodule as seen during surgery. On histologic section, this nodule contained granulomas and *P. carinii* organisms. (*From* Rosen [6].)

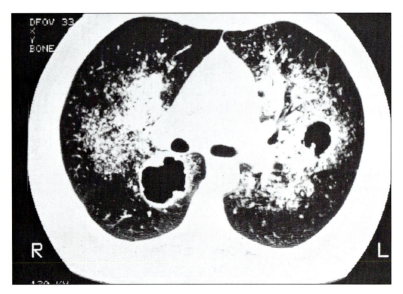

FIGURE 14-13. Computed tomogram showing cystic *Pneumocystis carinii* pneumonia. Cysts and pneumatoceles may complicate this infection. Rupture leads to pneumothorax and sometimes bronchopleural fistula. Pleural effusion and mediastinal adenopathy rarely occur in pneumocystosis and suggest other pathology. (*From* Froude [8].)

DIAGNOSIS

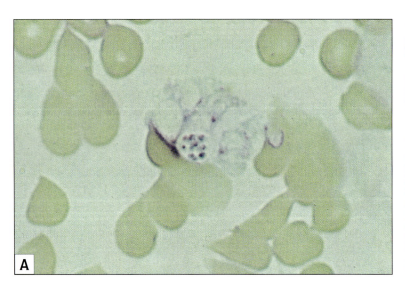

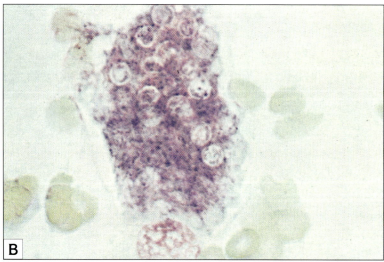

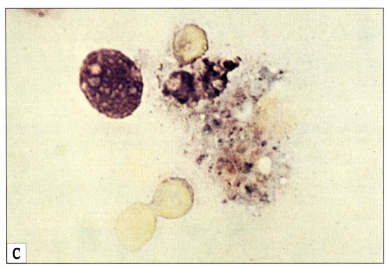

FIGURE 14-14. Diagnosis of *Pneumocystis carinii*. Diagnosis of pneumocystosis is made by histologic demonstration of the organism. Stains such as methenamine silver, cresyl echt violet, and toluidine blue O selectively stain *P. carinii* cysts. Stains such as Giemsa stain the nuclei of all *P. carinii* developmental stages. Immunofluorescence and immunoperoxidase techniques also have been used. Induced sputum has been used to obtain specimens for analysis, but its success rate is highly variable. Bronchoalveolar lavage (BAL) has been the widely used diagnostic procedure, with a success rate of more than 90%. If BAL is unsuccessful, more invasive procedures (*eg*, transbronchial biopsy, open lung biopsy) can be used. **A,** A touch imprint of an open lung biopsy specimen shows an oval cyst of *P. carinii* containing eight intracystic bodies. The cyst wall is unstained, and cytoplasm of intracystic bodies stain blue with excentric nuclei staining reddish purple. (Giemsa stain, x1000.) **B,** A BAL specimen shows a cluster of *P. carinii* cysts in varying stages of maturity, admixed with innumerable free trophic forms. The lavender-staining, honeycombed matrix enveloping the organisms may be readily discerned by low power (*eg*, x100) microscopy. (Giemsa stain, x1000.) **C,** A smear of BAL lavage fluid shows a cyst of *P. carinii* and numerous free trophic forms. The cyst is distinguished by the clear halo surrounding it, whereas trophic stages are crescent-shaped and contain a reddish-purple nucleus. The presence of numerous trophic forms and a sparsity of cysts often characterize the microscopic presentation of acute *P. carinii* pneumonia. (Giemsa stain, x1000.)

(continued on next page)

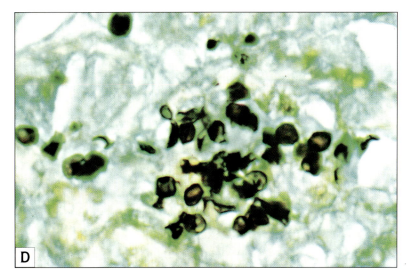

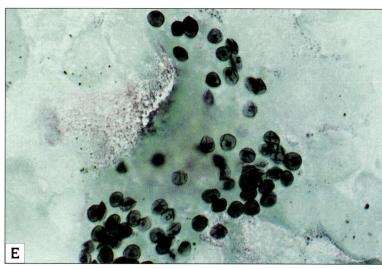

FIGURE 14-14. *(continued)* **D**, A touch print from an open lung biopsy specimen shows clusters of black-to-brown–staining cysts of *P. carinii*. Cysts are located within a "foamy exudate" in the alveoli and may display a variety of shapes, including collapsed sickle-shaped cysts. Thickening or indentation of the cyst wall also may occur. Intracystic bodies, unlike the cyst wall, are not stained with this stain. Budding, as in yeastlike organisms (*eg*, *Histoplasma* or *Candida* species), is never observed with *P. carinii*. (Gomori methenamine silver stain, x1000.) **E**, Methenamine silver stain of BAL fluid shows cysts of *P. carinii*, which often are characterized by the presence of parenthesis- or comma-shaped collapsed cell wall material. (x1000.) (*From* Bottone [9].)

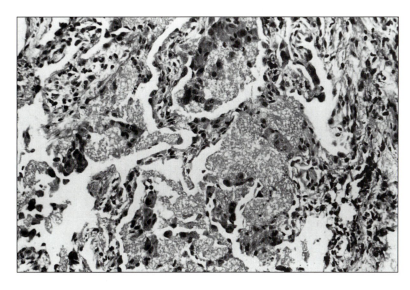

FIGURE 14-15. Typical features of human *Pneumocystis carinii* pneumonia. Alveolar lumens are filled with frothy honeycombed material. A small number of pulmonary macrophages are intermixed. Alveolar septa reveal features of interstitial pneumonia with hyperplasia and hypertrophy of type II pneumocytes, edema, mononuclear cell infiltrates, and mild fibrosis. (Hematoxylin-eosin stain, x250.) (*From* Walzer *et al.* [2]; with permission.)

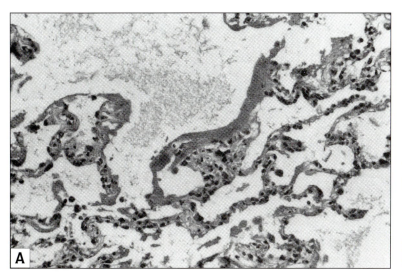

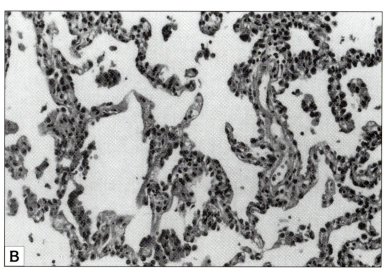

FIGURE 14-16. Atypical histologic features of human *Pneumocystis carinii* pneumonia. **A**, Prominent hyaline membranes are shown along the alveolar septa. Clusters of cysts usually are found by Grocott's methenamine silver stain. (Hematoxylin-eosin stain, x140.) **B**, Lack of alveolar honeycombed material. The alveolar septa reveal interstitial inflammation identical to usual interstitial pneumonia. Organisms rarely are found in this histologic picture. (Hematoxylin-eosin stain, x140.)

(continued on next page)

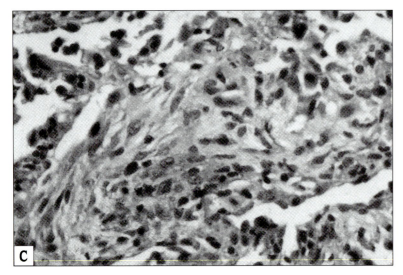
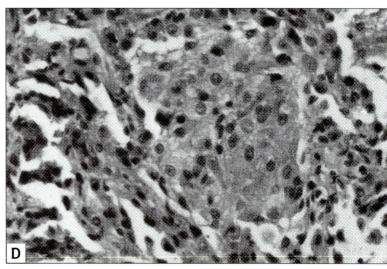

FIGURE 14-16. *(continued)* **C**, Organizing exudate obliterate the alveolar lumen, resulting in features of organizing pneumonia. (Hematoxylin-eosin stain, x250.) **D**, Changes resembling noncaseating epithelioid granuloma are shown. (Hematoxylin-eosin stain, x250.) (*From* Walzer *et al.* [2]; with permission.)

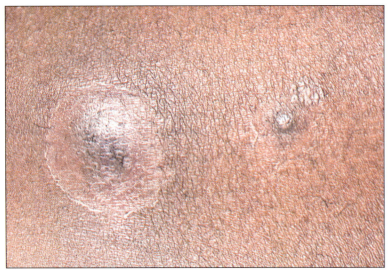

FIGURE 14-17. Cutaneous pneumocystosis. Dissemination of a pulmonary infection with *Pneumocystis carinii* rarely causes skin lesions in the immunocompromised host. Cutaneous papular lesions owing to *P. carinii* have been seen in patients with HIV receiving aerosolized pentamidine prophylaxis. The 2- to 6-mm papular skin lesions are flesh-colored to deep red and can resemble the lesions of molluscum contagiosum. (*From* Friedman-Kien [10].)

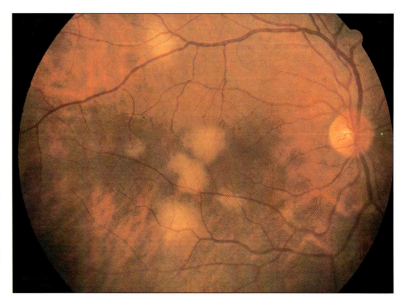

FIGURE 14-18. *Pneumocystis carinii* choroiditis. A man aged 41 years recovered from *P. carinii* pneumonia 3 months earlier and was being maintained on monthly aerosol pentamidine. Despite the posterior location of the lesions, his vision was 20/15. He was hospitalized at the same time with *P. carinii* pneumonia. Treatment of *P. carinii* with systemic prophylactic agents rather than inhalational pentamidine may reduce the risk of disseminated disease, including choroiditis [11,12]. (*From* Davis and Palestine [13].)

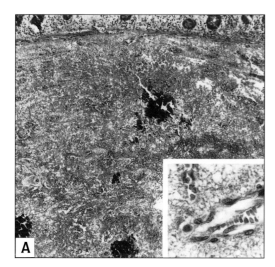 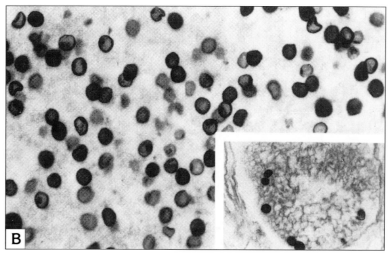

FIGURE 14-19. Disseminated pneumocystosis in a patient with HIV who presented with an acute abdomen. A plaquelike tumor of the small intestine was resected and found to consist of masses of *Pneumocystis carinii* organisms, which also exhibited a perivascular and intravascular distribution. Identical changes were found in regional lymph nodes. **A**, Histologic examination of the intestinal lesion shows confluent lakes of eosinophilic, foamy, focally calcified material abutting muscularis mucosae. (Hematoxylin-eosin stain, x65.) *Inset*: Perivascular foamy material. (Hematoxylin-eosin stain, x37.) **B**, Cysts of *P. carinii* are shown on methenamine silver stain. (x790.) *Inset*: Foamy material and cysts within thin-walled vessel. (Methenamine silver stain, x375.) (*From* Carter *et al.* [14]; with permission.)

TREATMENT AND PREVENTION

Treatment of pneumocystis

Indication	Drug of choice	Alternative drugs
Mild disease	TMP/SMX	Trimethoprim and dapsone
		Clindamycin and primaquine
		Atovaquone
Moderate to severe disease	TMP/SMX	Pentamidine
		Trimetrexate
		Clindamycin and primaquine

TMP/SMX—trimethoprim and sulfamethoxazole.

FIGURE 14-20. Treatment of pneumocystosis. The severity (and prognosis) of *Pneumocystis carinii* pneumonia can be classified on the degree of hypoxemia in mild disease, the arterial oxygen pressure is greater than 70 mm Hg and the alveolar–arterial oxygen gradient on room air is less than 35 mm Hg. In moderate to severe disease, these corresponding values are 70 mm Hg or greater and 35 mm Hg or greater, respectively. Trimethoprim-sulfamethoxazole is the drug of choice in all forms of pneumocystosis, but it causes a high frequency of adverse reactions in patients with HIV. The treatment recommendations for patients without HIV are similar to those for patients with HIV except that the role of corticosteroids as adjunctive therapy has not been established.

Prevention of pneumocystosis	
Intervention	Comments
Antimicrobial drugs	Highly effective and widely practical. TMP/SMX is agent of choice; dapsone ± pyrimethamine, aerosol pentamidine are alternatives
Patient isolation	Not officially recommended by CDC; however, many authorities place patients with *Pneumocystis carinii* in private rooms
Removal of predisposing conditions	Cure of the underlying condition and/or restoration of normal immune function should remove the risk of *P. carinii*

CDC—Centers for Disease Control and Prevention; TMP/SMX—trimethoprim and sulfamethoxazole.

FIGURE 14-21. Prevention of pneumocystosis. Chemoprophylaxis can be directed toward first episode (primary) or recurrent episodes (secondary) of *Pneumocystis carinii* pneumonia. Specific indications (*eg*, CD4 count less than 200, thrush) for primary chemoprophylaxis in patients with HIV have been developed. Patients with HIV who recover from pneumocystosis have a high risk of developing recurrent episodes; therefore, chemoprophylactic drugs are administered indefinitely. Recent studies showing that about half of these recurrent episodes are caused by different strains of *P. carinii* have increased interest in isolating patients with *P. carinii* from other immunocompromised hosts [1]. The introduction of protease inhibitors and other powerful anti-HIV drugs has raised the possibility that patients who restore their immune function may not need chemoprophylaxis of opportunistic infections. The general preventive measures for patients without HIV are similar to those for patients with HIV except that the specific guidelines are less well defined. This is because the incidence of pneumocystosis is lower in patients without HIV and the underlying conditions are more heterogeneous.

REFERENCES

1. Stringer JR, Walzer PD: New biologic insights. In *Pneumocystis carinii*. Edited by Sattler F, Walzer PD. London: Baillere Tindall LTD; 1995:415–430.

2. Walzer PD, Kim CK, Cushion MT: *Pneumocystis carinii*. In *Parasitic Infections in the Compromised Host*. Edited by Walzer PD, Genta RM. New York: Marcel Dekker; 1989:463–526.

3. Yoneda K, Walzer PD, Richey CS, *et al.*: *Pneumocystis carinii*: freeze-fracture study of various stages of the organism. *Exp Parasitol* 1982, 53:68–76.

4. Cushion M: *Pneumocystis carinii*. In *Topley and Wilson's Microbiology and Microbial Infections*. Edited by Balows A, Sussman M. New York: Oxford University Press; 1998:645–683.

5. Yoneda K, Walzer PD. Mechanism of alveolar injury in experimental *Pneumocystis carinii* pneumonia in the rat. *Br J Exp Pathol* 1981, 62:339–346.

6. Rosen MJ: Pulmonary complications. In *Atlas of Infectious Diseases*, vol 1, 2nd ed. Edited by Mandell GL, Mildvan D. Philadelphia: Current Medicine; 1997:8.1–8.10.

7. Dore GL, Cooper DA: Classification and spectrum. In *Atlas of Infectious Diseases*, vol 1, 2nd ed. Edited by Mandell GL, Mildvan D. Philadelphia: Current Medicine; 1997:4.1–4.11.

8. Froude J: Protozoan and helminthic infections of the lungs. In *Atlas of Infectious Diseases*, vol 6. Edited by Mandell GL, Simberkoff MS. Philadelphia: Current Medicine; 1996:8.1–8.30.

9. Bottone EJ: Microbiology of opportunistic infections. In *Atlas of Infectious Diseases*, vol 1, 2nd ed. Edited by Mandell GL, Mildvan D. Philadelphia: Current Medicine; 1997:13.1–13.16.

10. Friedman-Kien AE: Cutaneous manifestations. In *Atlas of Infectious Diseases*, vol 1, 2nd ed. Edited by Mandell GL, Mildvan D. Philadelphia: Current Medicine; 1997:5.1–5.18.

11. Rao NA, Zimmerman PL, Boyer D, *et al.*: A clinical, histopathologic, and electron microscopic study of *Pneumocystis carinii* choroiditis. *Am J Ophthalmol* 1989, 107:218–228.

12. Dugel PU, Rao NA, Forster DJ, *et al.*: *Pneumocystis carinii* choroiditis after long-term aerosolized pentamidine therapy. *Am J Ophthalmol* 1990, 110:113–117.

13. Davis JL, Palestine AG: Ophthalmic manifestations. In *Atlas of Infectious Diseases*, vol 1, 2nd ed. Edited by Mandell GL, Mildvan D. Philadelphia: Current Medicine; 1997:6.1–6.15.

14. Carter TR, Cooper PH, Petri WA, *et al.*: *Pneumocystis carinii* infection of the small intestine in a patient with the acquired immunodeficiency syndrome. *Am J Clin Pathol* 1988, 89:679–683.

Chapter 15

Phaeohyphomycosis and Hyalohyphomycosis

Patrícia P.C. Pacheco
Deanna A. Sutton
Michael G. Rinaldi

Phaeohyphomycosis and hyalohyphomycosis are artificial categories created to avoid the proliferation of new disease names each time a filamentous septate fungus is implicated in human disease. Phaeohyphomycosis (*phaeo*, black in Greek; *hypho*, hyphae) comprises mycotic diseases caused by moulds that form septate hyphae with darkly pigmented cell walls in tissue or culture. Hyalohyphomycosis comprises mycotic diseases caused by moulds whose basic tissue/culture form is in septate hyphae with colorless walls and distinctive hyphal shapes.

With this designation system, based on the presence or absence of melanin, when a specific organism is identified as the cause of a disease, the phrase "caused by" may be added (*eg*, cerebral phaeohyphomycosis caused by *Exophiala dermatitidis*). This approach is intended to simplify matters; however, it is purely artificial, and completely unrelated organisms fall in the same category. Another nuance is that chromoblastomycosis and mycetoma are excluded from this classification (because they have distinctive clinical and histologic patterns), even if they can be caused by moulds also implicated in phaeohyphomycosis. In the same way, the genus *Aspergillus* and more recently the species *Penicillium marneffei*, nevertheless being filamentous hyaline moulds, are no longer considered agents of hyalohyphomycosis, because their frequency justifies assignment to separate clinic categories (aspergillosis and penicilliosis).

Despite the ubiquitous nature of these fungi and their worldwide distribution with unavoidable exposure, human disease usually does not occur unless some impairment of host defense mechanisms (either decreased immune function or a loss of normal epithelial barriers) is present. The improvement of medical technology is a major reason for the escalating number of cases of hyalohyphomycosis and phaeohyphomycosis in recent years, which are now considered truly emerging opportunistic infections, some among the most aggressive and refractory ever reported.

This chapter provides an overview of these diseases, including general characteristics of the fungi, major risk factors, clinical manifestations, and diagnostic procedures. Some selected fungi are reviewed as related to the more severe or frequent diseases that they promote, including some illustrative clinical cases. The reader must be aware that this revision is not inclusive, and all these moulds can cause varied clinical manifestations depending on the immune state of the host, route of infection, and degree of exposure.

Treatment is covered briefly. In localized infections, surgical excision seems essential, whereas in invasive infections, which frequently are severe and life threatening, no standard treatment is available, and antifungal susceptibility tests may prove useful to guide the optimal therapeutic approach.

General Characteristics

General characteristics of agents of phaeohyphomycosis and hyalohyphomycosis

	Phaeohyphomycosis	Hyalohyphomycosis
Phylogenetic relations	Heterogenous group (Ascomycetes, Hyphomycetes, Coelomycetes)	Homogenous group (Hyphomycetes)
Morphologic characteristics	Septate hyphae	Septate hyphae
	Hyphae/conidia with darkly pigmented wall and distinctive moniliform appearance	Hyphae/conidia with colorless wall and distinctive moniliform appearance
Habitat	Nature (many are plant pathogens)	Nature (many are plant pathogens)
	Worldwide distribution	Worldwide distribution
Route of infection	Inhalation	Inhalation
	Inoculation	Inoculation
Human disease	Opportunistic infection	Opportunistic infection
	Some can be pathogenic for immunocompetent hosts	
	Localized	Localized
	Disseminated	Disseminated
Genera most frequently involved	*Alternaria*	*Acremonium*
	Bipolaris	*Fusarium*
	Curvularia	*Paecilomyces*
	Cladophialophora	*Penicillium*
	Cladosporium	*Scopulariopsis*
	Exophiala	
	Exserohilum	
	Fonsecaea	
	Exophiala	
	Ochroconis	
	Scedosporium*	

*Although *Scedosporium* spp grow as dematiaceous moulds in the laboratory, they resemble agents of hyalohyphomycosis in tissue; therefore, these species are sometimes referred to as agents of hyalohyphomycosis.

FIGURE 15-1. General characteristics of phaeohyphomycosis and hyalohyphomycosis agents.

Major Risk Factors

Major risk factors for development of phaeohyphomycosis and hyalohyphomycosis

Disruption of skin barrier
  Trauma
  Surgery
  Intrabody devices (IV or peritoneal catheters/prosthetic devices)
  IV drug abuse
  Wounds
  Chronic injured skin/mucosa
Depressed cellular immune response
  Hematologic malignancies (neutropenia)
  Organ transplant recipients
  Immunosuppressive therapy (corticosteroids/immunosuppressors)
  Chronic granulomatous disease
Increased environmental exposure (?)

FIGURE 15-2. Major risk factors for development of phaeohyphomycosis and hyalohyphomycosis. The majority of infections are opportunistic because they occur in patients with local or general impairment of host defense. However, neurotropic dematiaceous agents occasionally infect normal individuals, and in those cases, the exposure to an environmental source of the organism may be significant [1]. Due to the possible pathogenic role [2] and respiratory route of infection, all laboratory studies with those moulds should be accomplished within a biologic safety hood. HIV infection does not appear to constitute a risk factor (with the exception of *Penicillium marneffei* infection) because the immunodeficiency chiefly affects the T-cell population and granulocytes are preserved until late-stage infection.

Clinical Manifestations

Clinical spectrum of phaeohyphomycosis and hyalohyphomycosis*

	Phaeohyphomycosis	Hyalohyphomycosis

Localized infections	Skin and keratinized structures
	  Mycotic keratitis
	    Curvularia spp
	    Exophiala spp
	  Onychomycosis
	    Nattrassia mangiferae
	    Scedosporium spp
	  Dermatomycosis
	    Alternaria spp
	Subcutaneous tissue
	  Subcutaneous cyst
	    Bipolaris spp
	    Exophiala spp
	    Exophiala dermatitidis
	  Cellulitis
	    Scedosporium apiospermum
	Sinus
	  Alternaria spp
	  Curvularia spp
	  Bipolaris spp
	Central nervous system
	  Bipolaris hawaiiensis
	  Cladophialophora bantiana
	  Exophiala dermatitidis
	  Ochroconis gallopavum
	  Ramichloridium obovoideum
	Osteoarticular structures
	  Scedosporium spp
	Other deep organ infection possible but more rarely described
		Skin and keratinized structures
		  Mycotic keratitis
		    Fusarium spp
		  Onychomycosis
		    Fusarium spp
		Subcutaneous tissue
		  Cellulitis
		    Fusarium spp
		Peritoneum (continuous ambulatory peritoneal dialysis)
		  Paecilomyces spp
		  Penicillium spp
		  Fusarium spp
		Eye
		  Endophthalmitis
		    Fusarium spp
		    Paecilomyces spp
		Heart (prosthetic valves)
		  Paecilomyces spp
		Other deep organ infection possible but more rarely described

Disseminated infections	Rare *Scedosporium* spp are the most frequently involved	Increasingly described in patients with neutropenia *Fusarium* spp are the most frequently involved

*Includes the most frequent etiologic agents.

Figure 15-3. Clinical spectrum of phaeohyphomycosis and hyalohyphomycosis. Classically, the clinical manifestations are categorized in four types by the region of the body in which the infection occurs: superficial, cutaneous, subcutaneous, and systemic [3]. However, this classification excludes frequent clinical forms of presentation such as sinus or deep-organ infection. Therefore, the authors suggest the use of a more practical clinical division: localized infections versus disseminated infections (defined as infection occurring in two or more noncontiguous organs). In immunocompetent patients, the disease tends to remain localized at the site of traumatic inoculation or within the sinus after inhalation. Disseminated infection characteristically occurs in immunocompromised patients and may be severe and life threatening. In general, cases of phaeohyphomycosis are reported more frequently as localized infections, and cases of hyalohyphomycosis reported as disseminated infections.

Diagnostic Procedures

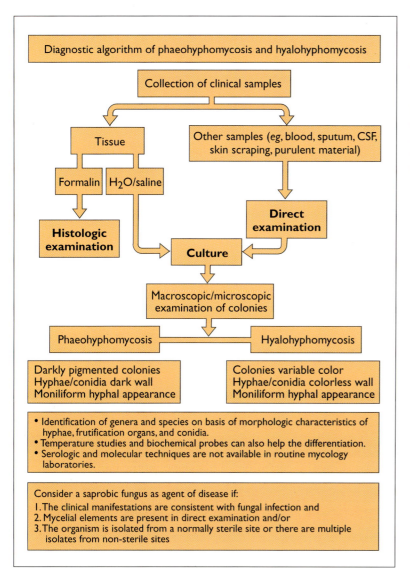

FIGURE 15-4. Diagnostic algorithm of phaeohyphomycosis and hyalohyphomycosis. Identification of genus and species is made on the basis of morphologic characteristics of hyphae, frutification organs, and conidia. Temperature studies and biochemical probes also can help the differentiation. Serologic and molecular techniques are not available in routine mycology laboratories. A saprobic fungus should be considered as the agent of disease if the clinical manifestations are consistent with fungal infection, and mycelial elements are present in direct examination, and/or the organism is isolated from a normally sterile site or there are multiple isolates from nonsterile sites.

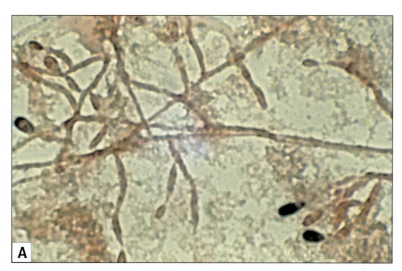
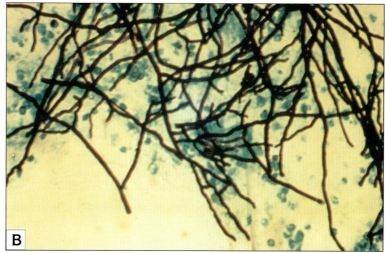

FIGURE 15-5. Direct examination of clinical specimens. The direct examination of clinical specimens can provide rapid and essential information because the presence of hyphae are diagnostic of fungal disease. **A**, Gram stain of *Scedosporium prolificans* in blood in a disseminated infection is shown (×920). **B**, Gomori-methenamine silver stain of hyphae of *Fusarium semitectum* in vitreous fluid in a case of endophthalmitis is shown (×460).

Moulds such as *Acremonium*, *Fusarium*, *Paecilomyces*, and *Scedosporium* species more frequently are found in blood in disseminated infections, possibly as a result of the production and dispersion of a large number of conidia. However, direct observation of fungi in blood is rare, and commercial blood culture systems should be used to improve the rate of detection of fungi.

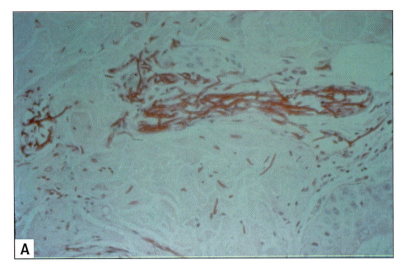
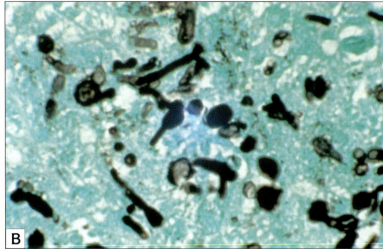
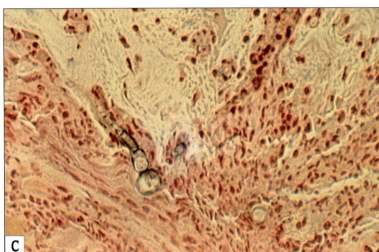

FIGURE 15-6. Histologic examination of clinical specimens. **A,** Hematoxylin-eosin stain of hyphae of *Fusarium* species in tissue is shown (×230). **B,** Gomori-methenamine silver stain of moniliform hyphal elements of *Ramichloridium obovoideum* in brain tissue is shown (×920). **C,** Positive Masson-Fontana stain of a dematiaceous mould in tissue is shown (×920). Histologic stains such as hematoxylin-eosin and Gomori-methenamine silver are appropriate for fungal recognition. However, the accurate identification of dematiaceous organisms in tissue often requires the use of a melanin-specific stain such as Masson-Fontana [4]. The fungus agents of phaeohyphomycosis and hyalohyphomycosis can assume various morphologic forms in tissue including yeastlike cells, pseudohyphae-like elements, septate hyphae, or combinations of these forms. The differentiation between genera frequently is difficult or impossible in histologic examination, for example, *Aspergillus* and *Fusarium* species easily can be confused in tissue; therefore, a microbiologic diagnosis based on culture should always be performed. Depending on the immune state of the patient and localization of the infection, a variable inflammatory reaction can be present: epithelioid granulomas, giant cells, abscess formation, and eosinophilic/lymphocytic infiltration.

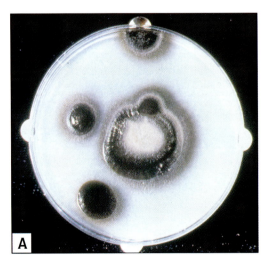
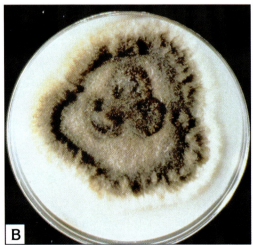
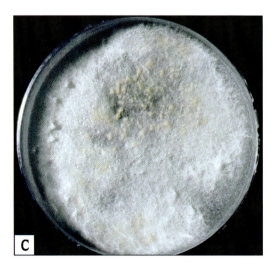

FIGURE 15-7. Macroscopic characteristics of cultures. **A,** *Exophiala castellanii* with a yeastlike appearance colony is shown on potato flakes agar (PFA) after 10 days. Some dematiaceous moulds, such as *Exophiala* species, appear initially as "black yeasts" with a shining, mucoid appearance, which becomes filamentous at maturity. **B,** *Bipolaris spicifera* filamentous colony is shown on PFA after 2 weeks. Genera such as *Alternaria*, *Bipolaris*, *Curvularia*, and *Exserohilum* present rapidly growing filamentous colonies. **C,** *Fusarium solani* colony shown on PFA after 5 days. Hyaline fungi such as *Fusarium* species can produce light or colored colonies, but the reverse side of the culture is always nonpigmented. The use of a plant-based medium such as PFA for culture is highly recommended. Although Sabouraud dextrose agar supports the growth of these fungi, it often fails to promote characteristic pigmentation as well as adequate conidiation and diagnostic structures for identification. The incubation period is 4 to 6 weeks at 25° to 30°C. Among these agents are rapid and slow growers, but most produce visible colonies within 2 weeks. (*From* Sutton *et al.* [5]; with permission.)

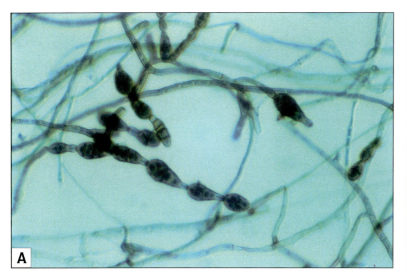
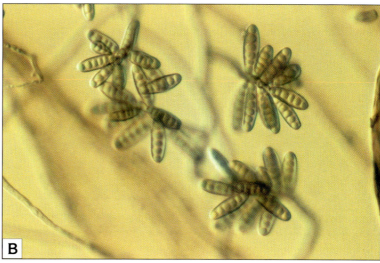

FIGURE 15-8. A, *Alternaria alternata* (×230). **B,** *Bipolaris hawaiiensis* (×460). The genera *Alternaria*, *Bipolaris*, *Curvularia*, and *Exserohilum* produce large, air-borne conidia. When inhaled by humans, they usually remain in the sinus due to their large conidial dimensions and, therefore, commonly are implicated in sinusoidal fungal infection, both in competent and immunosuppressed individuals. Two major clinical forms of fungal sinusitis usually are reported. The first is allergic fungal sinusitis (AFS), a noninvasive pansinusitis resulting from allergic mechanisms that occurs in immunocompetent individuals with a strong history of atopy. AFS is characterized by the presence of abundant green-brown material constituted of mucin and fungal hyphae. The second is an invasive form, with granuloma formation and tissue invasion. Erosion of bone structures can occur in both forms; however, in AFS it probably results from reabsorption due to pressure mechanisms. Whether the invasive form results from the progression of AFS or is a distinct clinicopathologic entity is still not clear. Both infections are insidious in normal patients, but can be rapidly progressive in immunocompromised hosts. In chronic injured sinus mucosa there is a potential risk of central nervous system invasion, usually after destruction of the cribriform plate, resulting in brain abscess or cerebritis. The treatment of AFS is usually surgical (debridement and sinus aeration). The invasive form also requires antifungal therapy. (Panel B *from* Sutton *et al.* [5]; with permission.)

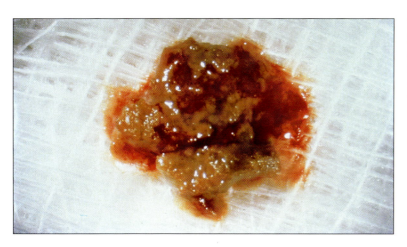

FIGURE 15-9. Allergic fungal sinusitis. An 11-year-old boy with a history of bronchial asthma presented with a 6-month history of nasal obstruction and discharge. On examination, a right periorbital swelling and proptosis was present, and the computed tomogram revealed a soft-tissue mass with involvement of the right nasal cavity, maxillary, ethmoid, and sphenoid sinuses. Surgical resection of the soft-tissue mass was performed. The resected material was constituted of mucin and hyphal elements. The mould was later identified as a species of *Exserohilum* [6].

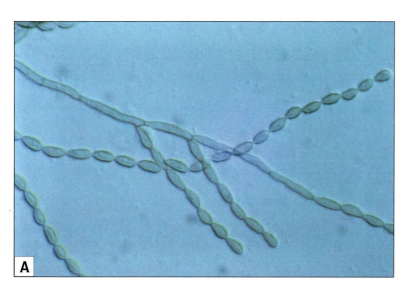

FIGURE 15-10. Dematiaceous fungi. **A–C,** The dematiaceous fungi, *Cladophialophora bantiana* (panel A, ×460), *Ramichloridium obovoideum* (panel B, ×920), and *Exophiala dermatitidis* (panel C, ×920), show a remarkable predilection for the brain (neurotropism). The clinical expression of cerebral involvement can be either abscess lesions in the parenchyma or chronic meningitis/meningoencephalitis. *C. bantiana* is the agent most frequently implicated. Cerebral involvement is by far more frequent in immunosuppressed patients, but it also occurs in immunocompetent hosts, which has lead some authors to postulate a possible pathogenic adaptation of the fungus [2].

(continued on next page)

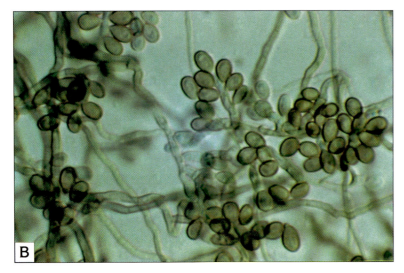
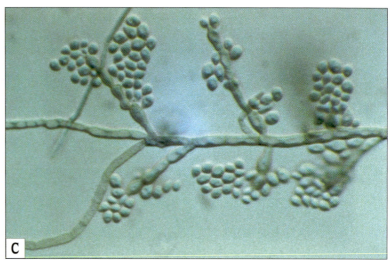

Figure 15-10. *(continued)* The infection follows inhalation or inoculation, and in immunocompetent hosts, it is typically a community-acquired disease, often with a significant occupational history (*eg*, farmers, miners, laborers) [1]. *R. obovoideum* (*R. mackenziei*) appears to be endemic in the Middle East, where it is among the most frequent agents of brain infection. The cerebrospinal fluid usually reveals nonspecific inflammatory parameters, and the detection of the organism from cerebrospinal fluid cultures is rare. Histopathologic examination and culture of tissue can provide the diagnosis. Cerebral phaeohyphomycosis has high morbidity and mortality, requiring early and aggressive therapy (surgical excision plus amphotericin B). Surgical resection appears to be the most important factor for cure and survival.

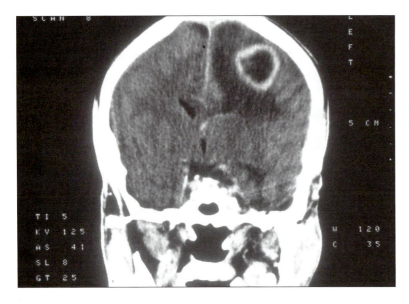

Figure 15-11. Cerebral phaeohyphomycosis caused by *Ramichloridium obovoideum*. An immunocompetent 36-year-old man residing in the Middle East had a several-month history of fatigue, weight loss, and decreased memory with a more recent history of right arm paresis. The computed tomogram revealed a ring-enhancing hypodense lesion in the left parietal subcortical region with surrounding edema. On histopathologic examination, the characteristic hyphae of agents of phaeohyphomycosis were apparent, and *R. obovoideum* was identified in culture. Treatment consisted of surgical excision of the lesion and oral itraconazole. Despite an initial clinical improvement, the patient's condition deteriorated, and he died while still receiving itraconazole therapy. (*From* Sutton *et al.* [7]; with permission.)

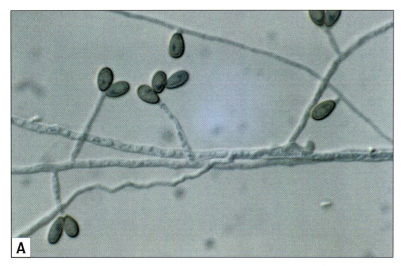 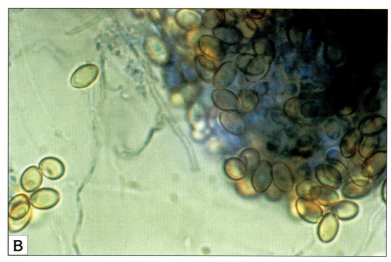

FIGURE 15-12. *Scedosporium* species. Classically, the genus *Scedosporium* has been associated with eumycotic mycetoma; however, in recent years it has become clear that it can incite a much broader spectrum of disease, ranging from cutaneous to disseminated infections. **A** and **B**, Two species of clinical significance have been identified: 1) *Scedosporium apiospermum* (panel A, ×920), which is the anamorphic stage of *Pseudallesheria boydii* (panel B, ×920) and 2) *Scedosporium prolificans*. The importance of species differentiation (note the swollen, flask-shaped, conidiogenous cells of *S. prolificans* shown in Fig. 15-13) assumes great significance in this genus. In addition to subcutaneous infections, *S. apiospermum/P. boydii* is a frequent agent of disease in cases of near-drowning in contaminated or stagnant water, causing pneumonia, meningitis, or brain abscesses [8]. *S. prolificans* has emerged as an important agent of osteoarticular infection both in immunocompromised and competent hosts, usually following traumatic inoculation. Rapidly fatal disseminated infections in patients with neutropenia due to this multiresistant fungal pathogen also have been reported [9]. Because both species present innate amphotericin B resistance, other therapeutic options must be considered. Itraconazole has been successfully used to treat infections caused by *P. boydii*. *S. prolificans* infections are usually more difficult to control due to their significant antifungal resistance. Antifungal susceptibility tests may be performed to optimize therapy because some isolates can express susceptibility to itraconazole or miconazole [10]. For focalized infections, surgical resection or debridement seems to be essential. (*From* Sutton *et al*. [5]; with permission.)

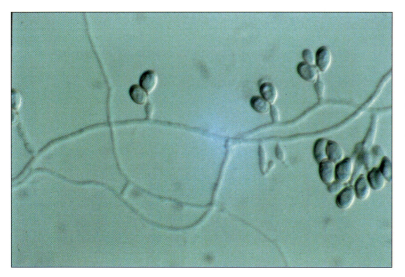

FIGURE 15-13. Articular hyalohyphomycosis due to *Scedosporium prolificans*. A previously healthy 11-year-old boy put his foot through a glass aquarium containing dried marine soil and sustained deep lacerations to his right ankle. Five weeks later he presented with septic arthritis. Surgical drainage revealed purulent joint fluid and an embedded piece of glass. *S. prolificans* was isolated in pure culture from the fluid and the glass particle. Treatment with amphotericin B was ineffective, and the clinical cure was achieved with drainage and oral itraconazole [11].

Fungal Infections

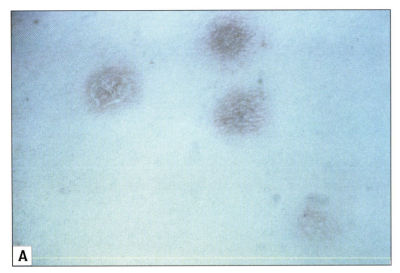
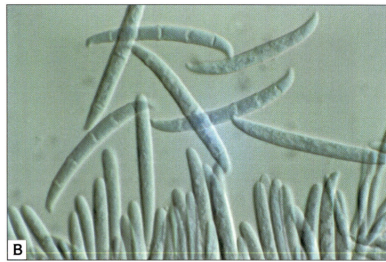
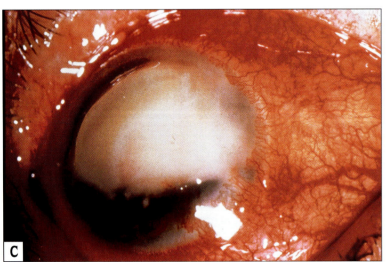

FIGURE 15-14. *Fusarium* species. The more aggressive cytostatic regimens used for patients with hematologic malignancies have favored the emergence of *Fusarium* infections. This genus, well known as a plant pathogen, recently has become a major agent of disseminated infection in patients with neutropenia. **A**, Fever unresponsive to broad-spectrum antibiotics, multiorgan dysfunction, and disseminated skin lesions (shown) are the usual clinical manifestations. Skin biopsy and blood cultures can establish the diagnosis (60% to 75% of patients with *Fusarium* disseminated infection have documented fungemia). The prognosis is closely related to neutrophil count recovery, and colony-stimulating factors are an essential part of the treatment. Resistance to amphotericin B and azoles is frequent, contributing to the high mortality (60%, irrespective of the antifungal used) [12]. *Fusarium solani*, *Fusarium moniliforme*, and *Fusarium oxysporum* are the species most frequently involved. **B**, *F. solani* macroconidia are shown on potato flakes agar ($\times 920$). Because dissemination can follow minor localized infection (*eg*, onychomycosis), adequate vigilance and treatment of all potential foci of infection must be performed in hematooncologic patients. In immunocompetent hosts, the infection usually is confined to keratinized tissues and occurs following traumatic inoculation with contaminated material. **C**, *Fusarium* species are among the most frequent causes of mycotic keratitis worldwide. (Panel B *from* Sutton *et al.* [5]; with permission.)

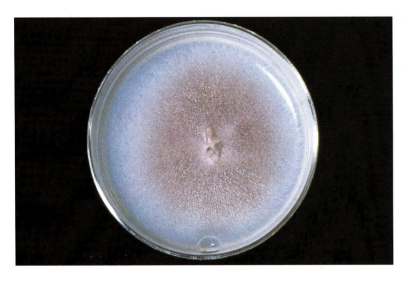

FIGURE 15-15. Disseminated hyalohyphomycosis due to *Fusarium moniliforme*. A 69-year-old man with acute myelogenous leukemia developed fever and bilateral pulmonary infiltrates during a neutropenic phase after the second cycle of chemotherapy. Despite treatment with broad-spectrum antibiotics and amphotericin B, his condition did not improve. The patient began to complain of myalgia, and he developed multiple small cutaneous lesions. *F. moniliforme* was identified in sputum and blood cultures. The patient died within the first week of treatment despite continued amphotericin B therapy [13]. (*From* Sutton *et al.* [5]; with permission.)

Phaeohyphomycosis and Hyalohyphomycosis

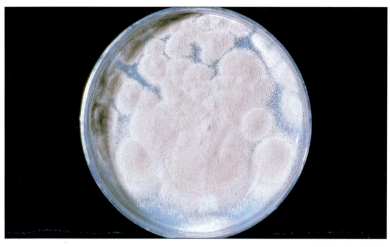

FIGURE 15-16. Macroscopic morphology of *Paecilomyces lilacinus* shown on potato flakes agar at 2 weeks. The most common species of *Paecilomyces* involved in human hyalohyphomycosis are *P. variotii* and *Paecilomyces lilacinus*. Because these organisms are common saprobes in the hospital environment and are resistant to most sterilizing techniques, the risk of a patient contracting a nosocomial infection is increased. Contaminated medical devices have been at the origin of most cases reported in the literature, many in an outbreak form (*eg*, endophthalmitis following lens implantation, fungal peritonitis in patients receiving continuous peritoneal dialysis, endocarditis in prosthetic heart valves). Disseminated infection in immunodepressed patients following contaminated intravenous catheter placement usually has resulted in a rapid and fatal outcome. Treatment requires removal of the contaminated material and antifungal therapy. *Paecilomyces* species tend to be resistant to many antifungal agents; therefore, antifungal susceptibility tests may guide treatment options.

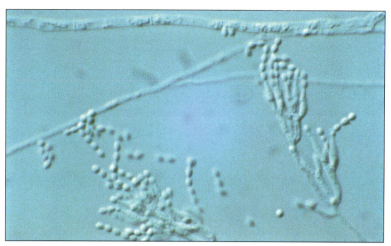

FIGURE 15-17. Nosocomial outbreak of *Paecilomyces lilacinus*. An outbreak of invasive mycosis due to *P. lilacinus* occurred in 1993 in a hematooncology unit of the University Hospital in Basel, Switzerland. During a period of 2 months, 12 patients were found to be infected or colonized with *P. lilacinus*. Nine patients developed invasive infections with skin eruptions. Multidrug resistance was found, and two patients died. The origin of the contamination was a commercially available skin lotion used in the unit. The outbreak ended after the skin lotion was recalled [14].

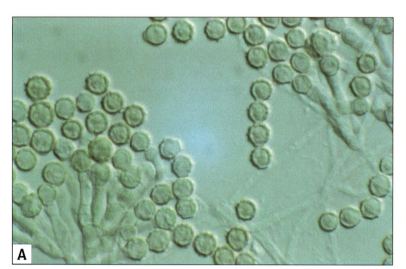

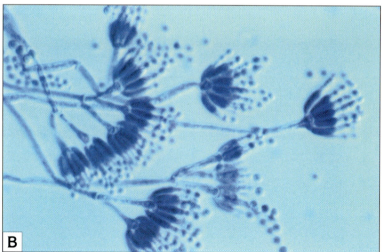

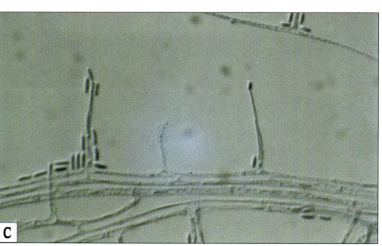

FIGURE 15-18. **A**, *Scopulariopsis brevicaulis* (×920). **B**, *Penicillium* species (×460). **C**, *Acremonium strictum* (×460). These genera are less commonly involved in human hyalohyphomycosis. Localized infections occasionally are described, but invasive and disseminated infections usually are limited to severely immunocompromised patients, particularly those who are neutropenic. As with other hyalohyphomycotic agents, antifungal resistance is common and the overall prognosis is poor, depending essentially on recovery of neutrophil count.

Documented infection with *Penicillium* species is relatively rare, except in Southeast Asia, where *Penicillium marneffei* has emerged as a frequent opportunistic agent in patients with AIDS. This disease currently is named penicilliosis and is reviewed in Chapter 11. (Panel A *from* Sutton *et al.* [5]; with permission.)

SPECIES

Currently documented agents of phaeohyphomycosis*

Acrophialophora fusispora	*Cladosporium* spp	*E. salmonis*	*Phialemonium* spp
Alternaria spp	*C. cladosporioides*	*E. spinifera*	*P. curvatum*
A. alternata	*C. elatum*	*Exserohilum* spp	*P. obovatum*
A. chartarum	*C. herbarum*	*E. longirostratum*	*Phialophora* spp
A. chlamydosporum	*C. oxysporum*	*E. mcginnisii*	*P. bubakii*
A. dianthicola	*C. sphaerospermum*	*E. rostratum*	*P. repens*
A. infectoria	*Colletotrichum* spp	*Fonsecaea pedrosoi*	*P. richardsiae*
A. stemphyloides	*C. coccodes*	*Hormonema dematioides*	*P. verrucosa*
A. tenuissima	*C. dematium*	*Hortae werneckii*	*Phoma* spp
Anthopsis deltoidea	*C. gloeosporioides*	*Lecythophora* spp	*P. cava*
Arthrinium phaeospermum	*Coniothyrium fuckelii*	*L. hoffmannii*	*P. cruris-hominis*
Aureobasidium pullulans	*Corynespora cassiicola*	*L. mutabilis*	*P. eupyrena*
Bipolaris spp	*Curvularia* spp	*Microascus* spp	*P. herbarum*
B. australiensis	*C. brachyspora*	*M. cinereus*	*P. hibernica*
B. hawaiiensis	*C. clavata*	*M. cirrosus*	*P. minutella*
B. spicifera	*C. geniculata*	*Moniliella suaveolens*	*P. oculo-hominis*
Botryodiplodia theobromae	*C. lunata*	*Myceliophthora thermophila*	*Phomopsis* spp
Botryomyces caespitosus	*C. pallescens*	*Mycocentrospora acerina*	*Phyllostictina* spp
Chaetomium spp	*C. senegalensis*	*Nattrassia mangiferae*	*Pleurophoma pleurospora*
C. atrobrunneum	*C. verruculosa*	*Nigrospora sphaerica*	*Pseudomicrodochium suttonii*
C. funicolum	*Dichotomorhthora portulacae*	*Ochroconis gallopavum*	*Pyrenochaeta unguis-hominis*
C. globosum	*Dichotomophoropsis*	*Oidiodendron cerealis*	*Ramichloridium obovoideum*
C. purpulchrum	*nympheaurm*	*Peyronellaea glomerata*	*Rhinocladiella schulzeri*
C. strumarium	*Dissitimurus exedrus*	*Phaeoacremonium* spp	*Sarcinomyces phaeomuriformis*
Cladorrhinum bulbillosum	*Exophiala* spp	*P. inflatipes*	*Sarcinosporon inkin*
Cladophialophora spp	*E. castellanii*	*P. parasiticum*	*Stenella araguata*
C. arxii	*E. dermatitidis*	*P. rubrigenum*	*Tetraploa aristata*
C. bantiana	*E. jeanselmei*	*Phaeoannellomyces elegans*	*Thermomyces lanuginosa*
C. boppii	*E. lecanii-corni*	*Phaeosclera dematioides*	*Trichomaris invadens*
C. carrionii	*E. moniliae*	*Phaeotrichonis crotalariae*	*Ulocladium chartarum*
C. devriesii	*E. pisciphila*		*Veronaea botryosa*

*List is not inclusive.

FIGURE 15-19. Currently documented agents of phaeohyphomycosis [15,16].

Currently documented agents of hyalohyphomycosis*			
Acremonium spp	*Chrysosporium* spp	*F. pallidoroseum*	*Penicillium* spp
A. alabamensis	*C. pannicola*	*F. solani*	*P. chrysogenum*
A. falciforme	*C. zonatum*	*F. subglutinans*	*P. citrinum*
A. kiliense	*Coprinus delicatulus*	*F. verticillioides*	*P. commune*
A. potroni	*Cylindrocarpon* spp	*Gymnascella* spp	*P. decumbens*
A. recifei	*C. destructans*	*G. dankaliensis*	*P. expansum*
A. roseo-griseum	*C. lichenicola*	*G. hyalinospora*	*P. marneffei*[†]
A. strictum	*C. vaginae*	*Myriodontium keratinophilum*	*Schizophyllum commune*
Aphanoascus fulvescens	*Emmonsia parva*	*Onychocola canadensis*	*Scopulariopsis* spp
Arthrographis kalrae	*Engyodontium album*	*Paecilomyces* spp	*S. acremonium*
Beauveria spp	*Fusarium* spp	*P. javanicus*	*S. brevicaulis*
B. alba	*F. aqueductuum*	*P. lilacinus*	*Scytalidium hyalinum*
B. bassiana	*F. chlamydosporum*	*P. marquandii*	*Trichoderma* spp
Cephaliophora irregularis	*F. coeruleum*	*P. variotii*	*T. viride*
Chrysonilia sitophila	*F. dimerum*	*P. viridi*	*T. longibrachiatum*
	F. moniliforme		*Tritirachium oryzae*
	F. napiforme		*Tubercularia vulgaris*
	F. nivale		*Verticillium serrae*
	F. oxysporum		*Volutella cinerescens*

*List is not inclusive.
[†]Most authorities refer to disease incited by this species as penicillosis.

FIGURE 15-20. Currently documented agents of hyalohyphomycosis [15–19].

Synonyms/obsolete names of phaeohyphomycotic and hyalohyphomycotic agents	
Agent	**Synonym/obsolete name**
Acremonium spp	*Cephalosporium* spp
Alternaria spp	*Macrosporium* spp
Alternaria alternata	*Alternaria tenuis*
Bipolaris hawaiiensis	*Drechslera hawaiiensis*
Cladophialophora bantiana	*Xylohypha bantiana*
	Xylohypha emmonsii
	Cladosporium trichoides
	Cladosporium bantianum
	Cladosporium trichoides var. *chlamydosporum*
Cladosporium spp	*Hormondendrum* spp
Exophiala jeanselmei	*Phialophora jeanselmei*
	Phaeoannellomyces elegans (in part)
Hortae werneckii	*Exophiala werneckii*
	Phaeoannellomyces werneckii
Ochroconis gallopavum	*Dactylaria gallopava*
	Dactylaria constricta var. *gallopava*
Pseudallescheria boydii	*Allescheria boydii*
Scedosporium apiospermum	*Monosporium apiospermum*
Scedosporium prolificans	*Scedosporium inflatum*
Ochroconis spp	*Dactylaria* spp
Ramichloridium obovoideum	*Ramichloridium mackenziei*
Exophiala dermatitidis	*Wangiella dermatitidis*
	Phialophora dermatitidis
	Fonsecaea dermatitidis
	Hormiscium dermatitidis
	Hormodendrum dermatitidis

FIGURE 15-21. Synonyms and obsolete names of agents of phaeohyphomycosis and hyalohyphomycosis.

References

1. Dixon DM, Walsh TJ, Merz WG, McGinnis MR: Infections due to *Xylohypha bantiana* (*Cladosporium trichoides*). *Rev Infect Dis* 1989, 11:515–525.

2. de Hoog GS: Significance of fungal evolution for the understanding of their pathogenicity, illustrated with agents of phaeohyphomycosis. *Mycoses* 1997, 40(suppl 2):5–8.

3. Fader RC, McGinnis MR: Infections caused by dematiaceous fungi: chromoblastomycosis and phaeohyphomycosis. *Infect Dis Clin North Am* 1988, 2:925–938.

4. Rinaldi MG: Phaeohyphomycosis. *Dermatol Clin* 1996, 14:147–153.

5. Sutton DA, Fothergill AW, Rinaldi MG: *Guide to Clinically Significant Fungi*. Philadelphia: Lippincott Williams & Wilkins; 1998.

6. Torres C, Ro JY, El-Naggar AK, *et al.*: Allergic fungal sinusitis: a clinicopathologic study of 16 cases. *Hum Pathol* 1996, 27:793–799.

7. Sutton DA, Slifkin M, Yakulis R, Rinaldi MG: US case report of cerebral phaeohyphomycosis caused by *Ramichloridium obovoideum* (*R. mackenziei*): criteria for identification, therapy and review of other known dematiaceous neurotropic taxa. *J Clin Microbiol* 1998, 36:708–715.

8. Ender PT, Dolan MJ: Pneumonia associated with near-drowning. *Clin Infect Dis* 1997, 25:896–907.

9. Berenguer J, Rodriguez-Tudela JL, Richard C, *et al.*: Deep infections caused by *Scedosporium prolificans*: a report of 16 cases in Spain and a review of the literature. *Medicine* 1997, 76:256–265.

10. Salkin IF, McGinnis MR, Dykstra MJ, Rinaldi MG: *Scedosporium inflatum*, an emerging pathogen. *J Clin Microbiol* 1988, 26:498–503.

11. Wood GM, McCormack JG, Muir DB, *et al.*: Clinical features of human infection with *Scedosporium inflatum*. *Clin Infect Dis* 1992, 14:1027–1033.

12. Bodey GP: New fungal pathogens. *Curr Clin Topics Infect Dis* 1997, 17:205–235.

13. Freidak H: Hyalohyphomycosis due to *Fusarium* spp.: two case reports and review of literature. *Mycoses* 1995, 38:69–74.

14. Orth B, Frei R, Itin PH, *et al.*: Outbreak of invasive mycoses caused by *Paecilomyces lilacinus* from a contaminated skin lotion. *Ann Intern Med* 1996, 125:799–806.

15. de Hoog GS, Guarro J: *Atlas of Clinical Fungi*. Baarn, The Netherlands: Centraalbureau voor Schimmelcultures; 1995.

16. Matsumoto T, Ajello L, Matsuda T, *et al.*: Developments in hyalohyphomycosis and phaeohyphomycosis. *J Med Veterinary Mycol* 1994, 32(supp 1):329–349.

17. Rogers AL, Kennedy MJ: Opportunistic hyaline hyphomycetes. In *Manual of Clinical Microbiology*, 5th ed. Edited by Balows A, Hausler WJ Jr, Herrmann KL, *et al*. Washington, DC: American Society for Microbiology; 1991:659–673.

18. Kennedy MJ, Sigler L: *Aspergillus*, *Fusarium*, and other opportunistic moniliaceous fungi. In *Manual of Clinical Microbiology*, 6th ed. Edited by Murray PR, Baron EJ, Pfaller MA, *et al*. Washington, DC: American Society for Microbiology; 1995:765–790.

19. Roilides E, Sigler L, Bibashi E, *et al.*: Disseminated infection due to *Chrysosporium zonatum* in a patient with chronic granulomatous disease and review of non-Aspergillus fungal infections in patients with this disease. *J Clin Microbiol* 1999, 37:18–25.

INDEX

Abscesses, in *Candida* myocarditis, 107
  in coccidioidomycosis, 31, 32
  hepatic, in hepatosplenic candidiasis, 102
Acquired immunodeficiency syndrome (AIDS). *See* AIDS (acquired immunodeficiency syndrome)
Actinomadura madurae, biopsy specimen showing, 187
Addison's disease, associated with histoplasmosis, 11
Adrenal lesions, in histoplasmosis, 11
  in paracoccidioidomycosis, 61
AFS (allergic fungal sinusitis), 223
AIDS (acquired immunodeficiency syndrome). *See also* HIV infection
  aspergillosis with, 143
  cryptococcosis with, 83
  histoplasmosis with. *See* Histoplasmosis, with AIDS
  oropharyngeal candidiasis with, pathogenesis of, 127
  Penicillium marneffei infections with. *See Penicillium marneffei* infections
Alcian blue stain, In cryptococcosis, 89
Allergic aspergillosis, bronchopulmonary, 140
  treatment of, 141
Allergic fungal sinusitis (AFS), 223
Alternaria alternata, 223
Alveolitis, allergic, in aspergillosis, 140
Amphotericin B, for aspergillosis, 156, 157
  for blastomycosis, 51
  for candidiasis, esophageal, 129
    oropharyngeal, 128
    systemic, 115
  for cryptococcosis, 85
  for histoplasmosis, 19, 20
  for mucormycosis, 167
  for *Penicillium marneffei* infection, 180
  for sporotrichosis, 76
Angioinvasion, in mucormycosis, 164
  in pulmonary invasive aspergillosis, 149
Antifungal drugs. *See also* specific drugs
  for histoplasmosis, 19, 20
  resistance to, with *Cryptococcus neoformans*, 85
Antigen assay, for histoplasmosis diagnosis, 17–18
Aspergillomata, pulmonary, 141
Aspergillosis, 135–159. *See also Aspergillus* species
  allergic, bronchopulmonary, 140
    treatment of, 141
  disease manifestations of, 139
  invasive, 142–159
    in AIDS, 143
    of central nervous system, 155
    classification of, 142
    cutaneous, 154
    endocarditis due to, 155
    epidemiology of, 142–143
    experimental pathogenesis and clinical risk factors for, 143–147
    in immunocompromised hosts, 142
    mastoiditis due to, 154
    otomycosis due to, 154
    pulmonary, 147–153
    risk factors for, 147
    sinusitis due to, 153–154
    treatment of, 156–159
    of vomer, 154
  noninvasive, 140–141
    pulmonary aspergillomata in, 141
    saprophytic, treatment of, 141
Aspergillus species, clearance of inhaled conida from lung tissue and, 145
  colonial morphology of, 137
  host defenses against, 143
  microscopic morphology of, 138–139, 149
  portals of entry for, 139
  recovery from respiratory tract, 150
Athlete's foot, 194–196
Azole-resistant candidiasis, 132–133

Back, mycetoma of, 185
BAL (bronchoalveolar lavage), in invasive pulmonary aspergillosis, 150–151
Balanoposthitis, *Candida*, 122
Bamboo rat, *Penicillium marneffei* infection and, 179
Blastomycosis, 39–51
  of central nervous system, 48
  clinical classification of, 40
  clinical manifestations of, 41
  cutaneous, 44–46
  differential diagnosis of, 46
  histopathologic features of, 44
  lesions in, 44–46
    diagnosis of, 41
    disseminated, in immunocompromised patient, 49
    endemic areas for, 40
    histopathology of, 41
  ocular, 48
  osteoarticular, 47
  pulmonary, 42–43
    in immunocompromised patient, 50
  treatment of, 51
Bone, blastomycosis of, 47
Brain. *See* Central nervous system
Brain parenchymal involvement, in cryptococcosis, 90
Bronchoalveolar lavage (BAL), in invasive pulmonary aspergillosis, 150–151
Bronchopulmonary aspergillosis, allergic, 140
Bursal swelling, in sporotrichosis, 74
Butoconazole, for vulvovaginal candidiasis, 125

Candida albicans. *See also* Systemic candidiasis
  colony appearance of, 98
  culture of, 87
  Gram stain of, 98
  identification of, 99–100
Candida species. *See also* Cutaneous candidiasis; Esophagitis, *Candida*; Mucocutaneous candidiasis; Oropharyngeal candidiasis; Systemic candidiasis; Vulvovaginal candidiasis
  differentiation of, 99
  distribution in hematogenously disseminated candidiasis, 97
  in human disease, 97
  microabscess due to, 100
Central nervous system, aspergillosis of, 155
  blastomycosis of, 48
  candidiasis of. *See* Systemic candidiasis, of central nervous system

Central nervous system, aspergillosis of, *continued*
   coccidioidomycosis of, 33
   cryptococcosis of, 92
   paracoccidioidomycosis of, 61
   sporotrichosis of, 75
Cerebral phaeohyphomycosis, *Ramichloridium obovoideum*, 224
Chest wall, mycetoma of, 185
Choroiditis, *Pneumocystis carinii*, 214
Clotrimazole, for oropharyngeal candidiasis, 128
   for vulvovaginal candidiasis, 125
Coccidioides immitis. *See also* Coccidioidomycosis
   histologic appearance of, 35–36
   life cycle of, 27
   outcomes after infection with, 27
Coccidioidomycosis, 23–36. *See also Coccidioides immitis*
   areas of skin-test positivity for, 25
   cutaneous manifestations of, 29–30
   diagnosis of, 33–36
   disseminated, 30–33
     cutaneous manifestations of, 30
     infectious manifestations of, 31, 32
     musculoskeletal manifestations of, 31–32
     neurologic manifestations of, 33
     ocular manifestations of, 33
   dust storms associated with outbreaks of, 26
   endemic areas for, 24, 25, 26
   epidemiology of, 24–27
   gross pathologic appearance of, 35
   with HIV infection, pneumonia in, 29
   incidence over past decade, 27
   Lower Sonoran Life Zone and, 25
   pulmonary manifestations of, 28–29
   treatment of, 36
Colonic lesions, in histoplasmosis, with AIDS, 15
Complement fixation antibody response, in coccidioidomycosis, 34
Conidiobolus infection, 169
Corticosteroids, suppressive effects on antifungal activity of neutrophils against *Aspergillus* hyphae, 144
   tinea incognito and, 200
Cotrimoxazole, for paracoccidioidomycosis, 62
Counterimmunoelectrophoresis, in mycetoma, 189
Cryptococcosis, 79–92. *See also Cryptococcus neoformans*
   clinical manifestations of, 84–85, 90–92
   culture and histopathology of, 87–89
   disseminated, 90
   with HIV infection, 92
   molecular epidemiologic studies for, 88
   pulmonary, 92
   risk groups for, 83
   species contracting, 81
   treatment of, 85–86
   with and without AIDS, 83
Cryptococcus neoformans. *See also* Cryptococcosis
   antifungal drug resistance with, 85
   comparison of varieties of, 82
   culture and histopathology of, 87–89
   life cycle of, 81
   molecular biology of, 82
   virulence phenotypes for, 82
Cutaneous aspergillosis, 153–154
Cutaneous blastomycosis, 44–46
Cutaneous candidiasis, 130–131. *See also* Mucocutaneous candidiasis
   classification of, 130
   diaper, 131
   granuloma in, 130
   intertriginous, 130
   periungual, 131
Cutaneous lesions, in coccidioidomycosis, 30
   in cryptococcosis, 91
   in hematogenous candidiasis, 132
   in histoplasmosis, 13
   in paracoccidioidomycosis, 60
   in *Penicillium marneffei* infections, 173–175
   in sporotrichosis, 67
   with HIV infection, 75
   in systemic candidiasis, 105
   in vulvovaginal candidiasis, 122
Cutaneous mucormycosis, 168
Cutaneous pneumocystosis, 214

Dematiaceous fungi, 223–224
   Masson-Fontana stain of, 222
Dermatophytoses, 193–200
   cultures in, 194
   direct microscopy of fungi in, 194
   id reaction in, 198
   in immunocompromised patients, 199
   immunologic events in, 193
   interdigital, 195
   Majocchi granuloma in, 199
   onychomycosis, 199
   pathogenesis of, 193
   tinea capitis, 197–198
   tinea corporis, 196–197
   tinea cruris, 196
   tinea facei, 198
   tinea incognito, 200
   tinea pedis, 194–196
Dexamethasone, suppressive effects on macrophages against *Aspergillus* conida, 144
Diaper candidiasis, 131
Dust storms, coccidioidomycosis associated with, 26

Electrocardiogram (ECG), in *Candida* myocarditis, 107
Emphysema, following paracoccidioidomycosis, 59
Endocarditis, *Aspergillus*, 155
   due to systemic candidiasis, 106–107
   postmortem findings in, 107
   risk factors for, 106
Endophthalmitis, in systemic candidiasis. *See* Systemic candidiasis, hematogenous endophthalmitis due to
Entomophthoramycosis, 169
Epiglottis, destruction of, in paracoccidioidomycosis, 59
Erythema, in vulvovaginal candidiasis, 122
Erythema multiforme, in coccidioidomycosis, 29
Erythema nodosum, in coccidioidomycosis, 30
   in histoplasmosis, 8
Esophagitis, *Candida*, 128–129
   differential diagnosis of, 129
   invasive, 128–129
   treatment of, 129
Exophalia castellanii, culture of, 222

Face, mycetoma of, 185
Finger, mycetoma of, 185
Fluconazole, for candidiasis, systemic, 115
   candidiasis resistant to, 133
   for cryptococcosis, 85

for esophageal candidiasis, 129
for oropharyngeal candidiasis, 128
for *Penicillium marneffei* infection, 180
for vulvovaginal candidiasis, 125
Flucytosine, for cryptococcosis, 85
for *Penicillium marneffei* infection, 180
Folliculitis, *Malassezia*, 202
Foot, mycetoma of. See Mycetoma
tinea pedis of, 194–196
Fusarium infection, 201
Fusarium moniliforme, 226
Fusarium species, 226
hematoxylin-eosin stain of, 222

G

Gastric mucosa, hemorrhagic necrosis of, in mucormycosis, 167
G-CSF (granulocyte colony-stimulating factor), enhancement of neutrophil-induced hyphal damage to *Aspergillus* by, 158
reversal of neutrophil-induced damage of *Aspergillus* hyphae by, 158
Genital lesions, in paracoccidioidomycosis, 60
Genitourinary candidiasis, 108–109
Gomori methenamine silver stain, in cryptococcosis, 89
of *Histoplasma capsulatum*, 17
of *Penicillium marneffei*, 175, 177
of *Ramichloridium obovoideum*, 222
Granulocyte colony-stimulating factor (G-CSF), enhancement of neutrophil-induced hyphal damage to *Aspergillus* by, 158
reversal of neutrophil-induced damage of *Aspergillus* hyphae by, 158
Granulocytopenia, incidence of pulmonary aspergillosis and, 146
Granulomas, *Candida*, cutaneous, 130
in histoplasmosis, liver biopsy showing, 17
Majocchi, 199

H

Hand, mycetoma of, 184
Hematogenous candidiasis, 132
Hematoxylin-eosin stain, in cryptococcosis, 89, 90
of *Fusarium* species, 222
in mycetoma, 188
of *Penicillium marneffei*, 177
Hepatosplenic candidiasis. See Systemic candidiasis, hepatosplenic
Histoplasma capsulatum. See also Histoplasmosis
course of infection after exposure to, 5
macrophage engorged with, 4
mold and yeast culture of, 16
mold phase of, 2
lactophenol cotton blue stain of, 17
phagocytosis of, 4
sources of exposure to, 3
Histoplasmosis, 1–20. See also *Histoplasma capsulatum*
acute, clinical manifestations of, 5
course of resolution of, 6
pulmonary, 6–7
symptoms of, 6
adrenal masses in, 11
with AIDS, 14–15
clinical findings in, 14
colonic lesions in, 15
chronic, pulmonary, 9, 11
diffuse, pulmonary, 7
disseminated, with adrenal masses, 11
bone marrow aspirate in, 13
chest radiographic findings in, 13
clinical findings in, 12
head MRI in, 15
laboratory diagnosis of, 17
liver biopsy in, 5

miliary infiltrate in, 12
risk factors for, 12
skin lesions in, 13
treatment of, 19, 20
endemic distribution of, 3
laboratory diagnosis of, 16–18
lymphadenopathy in, 9
mediastinitis with, fibrosing, 10
granulomatous, 8–9
pericarditis due to, 8
pulmonary, treatment response in, 19
rheumatologic manifestations of, 8
self-limited, diagnosis of of milder forms of, 18
treatment of, 19–20
HIV infection. See also AIDS (acquired immunodeficiency syndrome)
aspergillosis in, sinusitis and, 153–154
cryptococcosis with, 92
invasive pulmonary aspergillosis in, 150
Pneumocystis carinii infections in. See *Pneumocystis carinii* infections
sporotrichosis in, 74–75
cutaneous lesions in, 75
disseminated, 74
Hortaea werneckii infection, 202
Human immunodeficiency virus (HIV). See HIV infection
Hyalohyphomycosis, 217–227, 229
clinical manifestations of, 220
diagnosis of, 221–227
general characteristics of, 219
risk factors for, 219
species causing, 229

I

Id reaction, 198
IFN-γ (interferon-γ), enhancement of neutrophil-induced hyphal damage to *Aspergillus* by, 158
reversal of neutrophil-induced damage of *Aspergillus* hyphae by, 158
Immune system, dermatophytoses and, 193
Immunocompromised hosts. See also AIDS; HIV infection
aspergillosis in, 142
blastomycosis in, 49–50
pulmonary, 50
dermatophytoses in, 199
Immunodiffusion test, in mycetoma, 189
Immunosuppression, pathogenesis of pulmonary aspergillosis and, 146
India ink examination, in cryptococcosis, 88
Infection control, for aspergillosis prevention, 159
Interdigital scaling, in tinea pedis, 195
Interferon-gamma (IFN-gamma), enhancement of neutrophil-induced hyphal damage to *Aspergillus* by, 158
reversal of neutrophil-induced damage of *Aspergillus* hyphae by, 158
Intestinal lymphangiectasia, in paracoccidioidomycosis, 57
Itraconazole, for aspergillosis, 156, 157
for blastomycosis, 51
for cryptococcosis, 85
for esophageal candidiasis, 129
for histoplasmosis, 19, 20
for oropharyngeal candidiasis, 128
for paracoccidioidomycosis, 62
for *Penicillium marneffei* infection, 180
for sporotrichosis, 76
for vulvovaginal candidiasis, 125

K

Ketoconazole, for oropharyngeal candidiasis, 128
for paracoccidioidomycosis, 62
for *Penicillium marneffei* infection, 180
for vulvovaginal candidiasis, 125

Knee, mycetoma of, 184
KOH (potassium hydroxide) microscopy, in vulvovaginal candidiasis, 124
KOH (potassium hydroxide) sputum preparation, for coccidioidomycosis diagnosis, 33

Lactophenol cotton blue stain, of *Histoplasma capsulatum*, 17
　of *Rhizopus* species, 163
Laryngeal lesions, in paracoccidioidomycosis, 59
Leptomeningitis, in cryptococcosis, 90
Leukemia, invasive pulmonary aspergillosis in, 149, 154
Liver abscesses, in hepatosplenic candidiasis, 102
Liver biopsy, in disseminated histoplasmosis, 5, 17
Lower Sonoral Life Zone, 25
Lung. *See* Pulmonary entries
Lymphadenopathy, in histoplasmosis, 9
　in paracoccidioidomycosis, 57
Lymphangiectasia, intestinal, in paracoccidioidomycosis, 57
　mediastinal, in paracoccidioidomycosis, 58
Lymphangitis, nodular, from sporotrichosis, 69
Lymphocutaneous sporotrichosis. *See* Sporotrichosis, lymphocutaneous

Madura foot. *See* Mycetoma
Madurella mycetomatis, fungal grain of, 188
Majocchi granuloma, 199
Malassezia infections, 202
Masson-Fontana stain, of dematiaceous mold, 222
Mastoiditis, *Aspergillus*, 153–154
Mediastinitis, in histoplasmosis, 8–9, 10
Meningitis, cryptococcal, treatment failure in, 85
Methenamine silver stain, in candidiasis, 109
Miconazole, for *Penicillium marneffei* infection, 180
　for vulvovaginal candidiasis, 125
Mucicarmine stain, in cryptococcosis, 89
Mucocutaneous candidiasis, 117–133
　chronic, 130
　dermatophytosis in, 199
　　cutaneous. *See* Cutaneous candidiasis
　drug-resistant, 132–133
　esophageal. *See* Esophagitis, *Candida*
　hematogenous, skin lesions in, 132
　onychomycosis due to, 131
　oropharyngeal. *See* Oropharyngeal candidiasis
　vulvovaginal. *See* Vulvovaginal candidiasis
Mucorales. *See also specific organisms*
　classification of, 162
　morphologic features of, 163
Mucormycosis, 161–168
　blood vessel invasion in, 164
　clinical syndromes of, 164
　cutaneous, 168
　disseminated, gastric involvement in, 167
　histopathologic appearance of, 163–164
　predisposing factors for development of, 165
　pulmonary, 166–167
　rhinocerebral, 165–166
　　computed tomography of sinuses in, 166
　　in diabetes, 165
　　residual infection following surgical debridement in, 166
　treatment of, 167
Muscle, abscesses of, in coccidioidomycosis, 32
Mycetoma, 181–190
　of back, 185
　biopsy specimens in, 187
　of chest wall, 185
　clinical appearance of, 183–185
　coccidioidal, 28
　diagnostic tests for, 189
　　treatment of, 189–190
　of face, 185
　of finger, 185
　of hand, 184
　histopathology of, 188
　of knee, 184
　organisms causing, 183
　radiographic appearance of, 186–187
　recurrent of, 190
Myocarditis, *Candida*, 107
　electrocardiogram findings in, 107
　microabscesses in, 107

Neurologic disorders. *See* Central nervous system
Neutropenia, cutaneous aspergillosis in, 153–154
　invasive pulmonary aspergillosis in, 149
Nocardia, eosinophilic grains of, 188
Nodules, cutaneous, in sporotrichosis, 70–71
　in systemic candidiasis, 105
　subcutaneous, in blastomycosis, 44

Ocular blastomycosis, 48
Ocular coccidioidomycosis, 33
Ocular pneumocystosis, 214
Onychomycosis, 199
　Candida, 131
Optic neuropathy, in cryptococcosis, 91
Oral lesions, in histoplasmosis, with AIDS, 14
　in *Penicillium marneffei* infections, 174
Oropharyngeal candidiasis, 126–128
　in AIDS, pathogenesis of, 127
　atrophic, 128
　chronic hyperplastic, 127
　microbiology of, 127
　pharyngeal, 128
　pseudomembranous, 127
　risk factors for, 126
　treatment of, 128
Osteoarticular blastomycosis, 47
Osteomyelitis, *Candida*, 111–112
　coccidioidal, 31–32
　in sporotrichosis, 73
Osteoporosis, in mycetoma, 186
Otomycosis, *Aspergillus*, 153–154

Paecilomyces lilacinus, 227
Paecilomyces variotii, 227
Paracoccidioides brasiliensis, culture of, 62
Paracoccidioidomycosis (PCM), 53–62
　clinical classification of, 56
　clinical manifestations of, 56–61
　differential diagnosis of, 61
　geographic distribution of, 54
　histopathology of, 62
　laboratory diagnosis of, 62
　mycology of, 55
　natural history of, 56
　pathophysiology of, 56
　pulmonary, 58–59
　risk groups for, 55
　treatment of, 62

Paronychia, *Candida*, 131
PCM. *See* Paracoccidioidomycosis (PCM)
Penicillium marneffei infections, 171–180
  bamboo rats and, 179
  culture of, 177–178
  cutaneous lesions in, 173–175
  distribution of, 172
  endemic areas for, 172
  incidence of, 172
  microscopic appearance of, 175–177
  route of infection and, 180
  signs and symptoms of, 173
  treatment of, 180
Pericarditis, in histoplasmosis, 8
Periodic acid-Schiff stain, of *Penicillium marneffei*, 177
  in systemic candidiasis, 105
Periungual candidiasis, 131
Phaeohyphomycosis, 217–228, 229
  cerebral, *Ramichloridium obovoideum*, 224
  clinical manifestations of, 220
  diagnosis of, 221–227
  general characteristics of, 219
  risk factors for, 219
  species causing, 228, 229
Phase contrast microscopy, in vulvovaginal candidiasis, 124
Pityriasis versicolor, direct microscopy of, 194
Plaquelike lesions, in blastomycosis, 46
  in paracoccidioidomycosis, 60
Pleural effusions, coccidioidal, 28
Pneumocystis carinii, cyst of, 208
  development stages of, 206
  interaction with alveolar type I cell, 209–210
  life cycle of, 208
  precyst of, 207
  pulsed field gel electrophoresis of, 209
  trophic, 207
Pneumocystis carinii infections, 205–216
  atypical presentation of, 211
  CD4 lymphopenia and, 211
  clinical features of, 210
  cutaneous, 214
  diagnosis of, 212–215
  imaging in, 211, 212
  infiltrates in, 211
  intestinal, 215
  ocular, 214
  prevention of, 216
  treatment of, 215
Pneumonia, *Candida*, 113
  coccidioidal, 28–29
  Pneumocystis carinii. *See Pneumocystis carinii* infections
Pneumonitis, in cryptococcosis, 92
Potassium hydroxide (KOH) microscopy, in vulvovaginal candidiasis, 124
Potassium hydroxide (KOH) sputum preparation, for coccidioidomycosis diagnosis, 33
Pruritus, in vulvovaginal candidiasis, 122
Pseudomembranous candidiasis, 127
Pulmonary aspergillosis, allergic, 140
  aspergillomata in, 141
  invasive, 147–153
    anatomic relation of airways and major vessels in lung and, 148
    angioinvasion in, 149
    bronchoalveolar lavage in, 150–151
    differential diagnosis of, 151
    granulocytopenia and incidence of, 146
    with HIV infection, 150
    imaging in, 151, 152–153
    in leukemia, 149, 154
    management of, 153
    microscopic morphology of *Aspergillus* in, 149
    necrotizing tracheitis caused by, 148
    nodular lesions in, 148–149
    organ involvement in, 147
    pathogenesis of, in immunosuppressed hosts, 146
    patterns of lung involvement in, 147
    recovery of *Aspergillus* species from respiratory tract in, 150
Pulmonary blastomycosis, 42–43
  in immunocompromised patient, 50
Pulmonary cryptococcosis, 92
Pulmonary histoplasmosis, chest radiographs in, 6, 7, 11
  pulmonary infiltrates in, 9
Pulmonary mucormycosis, 166–167
Pulmonary paracoccidioidomycosis, 58–59
Pulmonary sporotrichosis, 72
  differential diagnosis of, 72
  risk factors, pathogenesis, and clinical features of, 72
Pyopneumothorax, coccidioidal, 28

Ramichloridium obovoideum, cerebral phaeohyphomycosis caused by, 224
  Gomori methenamine silver stain of, 222
Renal tubular casts, in genitourinary candidiasis, 108
Rhinocerebral mucormycosis. *See* Mucormycosis, rhinocerebral
Rhizopus species, lactophenol cotton blue stain of, 163
Ringworm, of scalp, 197–198

Saline microscopy, in vulvovaginal candidiasis, 123
Saprophytic aspergillosis, treatment of, 141
Scalp, tinea capitis of, 197–198
Scedosporium prolificans, 225
Scedosporium species, 225
Scopulariopsis brevicaulis, 227
Scopulariopsis brevicaulis infection, 201
Scytalidium dimidiatum infection, 200, 201
Scytalidium hyalinum infection, 200
Sensitivity tests, for mycetoma, 189
Serologic tests, for coccidioidomycosis diagnosis, 34
Sinusitis, allergic, 223
  Aspergillus, with HIV infection, 153–154
Skin. *See also* Cutaneous lesions
  local innoculation of, coccidioidomycosis acquired by, 30
Skull, in mycetoma, 187
Spinal osteomyelitis, *Candida*, 111–112
  imaging in, 111, 112
  microscopic findings in, 112
Spondylitis, coccidioidal, 32
Sporothrix schenckii. *See also* Sporotrichosis
  characteristics of, 65
  growth at various temperatures, 67
  primary lesions of infection with, 69
Sporotrichosis, 65–76. *See also Sporothrix schenckii*
  diagnosis of, 76
  epidemiology of, 66
  in HIV infection, 74–75
    brain MRI in, 75
    cutaneous lesions in, 75
    disseminated, 74
    lymphocutaneous, 68–71

Sporotrichosis, *continued*
   clinical manifestations of, 68
   differential diagnosis of, 68
   fixed cutaneous sporotrichosis, 69
   lymphangitic spread of, 69
   multiple lesions in, 70–71
   multiple primary lesions in, 69
   nodular lesions in, 70–71
   nodular lymphangitis and, 69
   primary lesion at site of inoculation and, 69
   tissue response patterns in, 71
   ulcerated lesions in, 70, 71
  manifestations of, 68
  osteoarticular, 73–74
  pulmonary, 72
   differential diagnosis of, 72
   risk factors, pathogenesis, and clinical features of, 72
   treatment of, 76
Stomach, hemorrhagic necrosis of gastric mucosa and, in mucormycosis, 167
Stomatitis, "mulberry-like," in paracoccidioidomycosis, 59
Subcutaneous abscesses, in coccidioidomycosis, 31
Sweet's syndrome, in coccidioidomycosis, 30
Synovitis, coccidioidal, 31–32
Systemic candidiasis, 95–115. *See also Candida albicans; Candida* species
  Candida species implicated in, 97
  of central nervous system, 110–111
   computed tomography in, 110
   microabscesses in, 110
   postmortem findings in, 110
  cutaneous lesions in, 105
  endocarditis due to, 106–107
   postmortem findings in, 107
   risk factors for, 106
  genitourinary, 108–109
  hematogenous endophthalmitis due to, 102–104
   complications and variations of, 104
   eyeball in, 102
   fundoscopic findings in, 102–104
   lesions of, 104
   predisposing factors for, 103
  hematogenously disseminated, distribution of *Candida* species in, 97
   risk factors for, 97
  hepatosplenic, 101–102
   imaging in, 101
   liver abscess in, 102
   postmortem findings in, 101
  management of, 114–115
   algorithm for, 114
   fluconazole versus amphotericin B for, 115
  myocarditis due to, 107
   electrocardiogram findings in, 107
   microabscesses in, 107
  osteomyelitis due to, 111–112
   imaging in, 111, 112
   microscopic findings in, 112
  pneumonia due to, 113

Terconazole, for vulvovaginal candidiasis, 125
Thrush, 127
Tinea capitis, 197–198
Tinea corporis, 196–197
Tinea cruris, 196
Tinea facei, 198
Tinea incognito, 200
Tinea nigra, 202
Tinea pedis, 194–196
Tioconazole, for vulvovaginal candidiasis, 125
Trichophyton concentricum, tinea corporis due to, 197
Trichophyton rubrum, tinea corporis due to, 196
  tinea pedis due to, 196
Trichophyton tonsurans, culture of, 194
Trichophyton verrucosum, tinea corporis due to, 197

Ulcers, colonic, in histoplasmosis, 15
  cutaneous, in blastomycosis, 44
  in cryptococcosis, 91
  in sporotrichosis, 70–71
  oral, in histoplasmosis, with AIDS, 14

Vaginal candidiasis. *See Candida albicans; Candida* species; Vulvovaginal candidiasis
Vaginal discharge, in vulvovaginal candidiasis, 122
Vena cava, compression of, by paracoccidioidomycosis, 57
Verrucous lesions, in blastomycosis, 45
Vomer, aspergillosis of, 153–154
Vulvovaginal candidiasis, 118–126. *See also Candida albicans; Candida* species
  Candida virulence factors and, 118–119
  classification of, 119
  clinical manifestations of, 122
  diagnostic procedures for, 123–124
  differential diagnosis of, 123
  epidemiology of, 119
  etiology of, 120
  in HIV infection, CD4 cell count and, 121
  microbiology of, 120
  natural anti-*Candida* defense mechanisms of vagina and, 120
  pathogenesis of, 121
  risk factors for, 121
  symptoms of, 122
  treatment of, 124–125

Wright's stain, of *Penicillium marneffei*, 175, 176